Suicidal Behaviour

T0229621

Suicidal Behaviour: Underlying dynamics is a wide ranging collection of articles that builds upon an earlier volume by the same editor, *Suicidal Behaviour: Assessment of people-at-risk*, 2010, and delves deeper into the dynamics of suicide by synthesizing significant psychological and interdisciplinary perspectives. The volume brings together varied conceptualizations by scholars across disciplines from around the globe, adding to available theoretical understanding as well as providing research-based inputs for practitioners in the field of suicidal behaviour.

The book has sixteen chapters divided into two broad sections, opening with a discussion of the theoretical underpinnings of suicidal behaviour in the first half, conceptualizing the phenomenon from different vantage points of genetics, personality theory, cognitive and affective processes, stress and assessment theories. The second half brings in varied research evidences and assessment perspectives from different populations and groups, building on theoretical foundations and discussing the nuances of dealing with suicidal behaviours among sexual minority populations, alcoholics, military personnel, and specific socio-cultural groups. It closes with a focus on a significant issue encountered often in clinical practice – assessment of suicide risk and ways of resolving the cultural, ethical and legal dilemmas.

Updesh Kumar is a Scientist 'F' and Head, Mental Health Division, Defence Institute of Psychological Research, the Defence Research and Development Organization (DRDO), New Delhi, India.

Suicidal Behaviour

Underlying dynamics

**Edited by
Updesh Kumar**

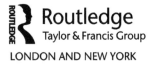
Routledge
Taylor & Francis Group

LONDON AND NEW YORK

First published 2015 by Routledge

2 Park Square, Milton Park, Abingdon, Oxfordshire OX14 4RN
711 Third Avenue, New York, NY 10017

Routledge is an imprint of the Taylor & Francis Group, an informa business

First issued in paperback 2018

British Library Cataloguing in Publication Data
A catalogue record for this book is available from the British Library

Library of Congress Cataloging in Publication Data
    pages cm
    1. Suicidal behavior—Risk factors.   I. Kumar, Updesh.
    RC569.S8954 2015
    616.85′844505—dc23
                                        2014019822

ISBN: 978-1-138-79381-1 (hbk)
ISBN: 978-1-138-58021-3 (pbk)

Typeset in Galliard
by RefineCatch Limited, Bungay, Suffolk

To His Holiness Sri Sri Ravi Shankar Ji
Founder, Art of Living

Contents

Contributors

The Editor

Updesh Kumar, PhD, is Scientist 'F' and chair of the Mental Health Division at the Defence Institute of Psychological Research (DIPR), R&D Organization, Ministry of Defence, Delhi. He obtained his doctorate degree in the area of suicidal behaviour from Punjab University, Chandigarh and has 23 years of experience as a scientist in R&D organizations. He specializes in low intensity conflict, suicidal behaviour and terrorism research. He edited six volumes: *Recent Developments of Psychology, Counseling: A practical approach, Suicidal Behaviour: Assessment of People-at-Risk* (Sage Publications, 2010), *Countering Terrorism: Psychosocial Strategies* (Sage Publications, 2012), *Understanding Suicide Terrorism: Psychosocial Dynamics* (Sage Publications, 2014), and recently *Positive Psychology: Applications in Work, Health and Well-being* (in press, Pearson Education). He has written the manuals *Suicide and Fratricide: Dynamics and management* for defence personnel, *Managing Emotions in Daily Life and in Work Place* for general publication, *Overcoming Obsolescence and Becoming Creative in the R&D Environment* for R&D organizations and *Self-Help Techniques in Military Settings*. He has written more than 50 other academic publications in the form of research papers, journal articles and book chapters and represented his institute at national and international level. Dr Kumar has been a psychological assessor (psychologist) in various services selection boards for eight years for the selection of officers in the Indian armed forces. He is certified by The British Psychological Society with level A and level B Certificate of Competence in Occupational Testing. He has to his credit many important research projects relating to the armed forces. He was conferred with the DRDO's Best Popular Science Communication Award, 2009 by the Honourable Defence Minister of India. He has also been the recipient of the DRDO Technology Group Award in 2001 and 2009, Professor Manju Thakur Memorial Award, 2009 and 2012 by the Indian Academy of Applied Psychology (IAAP) and Professor N. N. Sen Best Paper Award for the year 2010 by the Indian Association of Clinical Psychologists (IACP). The Indian government recently conferred the Laboratory Scientist of the Year Award, 2012–2013 and the prestigious DRDO's Scientist of the Year Award, 2013.

Contributors

Michael D. Anestis, PhD, is Assistant Professor and Director of Suicide and Emotion Dysregulation Laboratory, Department of Psychology, University of Southern Mississippi, USA. His work focuses primarily on risk factors for suicidal behaviour and efforts to empirically test widely held assumptions about suicide. He has published numerous journal articles in the field of suicidal behaviour in *Suicide and Life-Threatening Behaviour, Journal of Psychiatric Research, Journal of Affective Disorders, Archives of Suicide Research, Personality, Behaviour Research, Clinical Psychology Review* and *Therapy and Mental Health*. He is the author of several book chapters in the area of suicidal behaviour published by the Oxford University Press and Guilford Press. He has been the reviewer of various international journals of suicidal behaviour and clinical psychology. He is affiliated to various professional societies like the American Association of Suicidology (AAS) and Military Suicide Research Consortium (MSRC) and is the recipient of Resident Outstanding Contribution to the Consortium Award 2011 and Leonard Krasner Student Dissertation Award 2009.

Alan Apter, MD, is Professor of Psychiatry at the Sackler School of Medicine at the University of Tel Aviv, where he served as Chair of the department. He is also the director of the Feinberg Child Study Center at Schneider Children's Medical Center of Israel, a member of numerous professional societies and organizations and has published more than 300 articles and chapters as well as two books. He is a member of the Israel government inter-ministerial committee on suicide prevention and is also an adviser on suicide prevention to the Israel Defense Force and a recipient of the American Foundation for Suicide Prevention's Distinguished Investigator Award.

Ella Arensman is Professor and Director of Research with the National Suicide Research Foundation (NSRF) and Adjunct Professor with the Department of Epidemiology and Public Health, University College Cork, Ireland. She has been involved in research and prevention into suicide and self-harm over the last 25 years, with a particular emphasis on risk and protective factors associated with suicide and self-harm, cross-cultural differences, clustering and contagion of suicidal behaviour, and effectiveness of suicide prevention and self-harm intervention programmes. In Ireland, she played a key role in developing Reach Out, the National Strategy for Action on Suicide Prevention (2005–2014). She has been involved in many international research consortia, such as the European Alliance against Depression (EAAD) and Optimising Suicide Prevention Programmes and their Implementation in Europe (OSPI-Europe).

Bruce Bongar, PhD, ABPP, FAPM, is the Calvin Professor of Psychology at Palo Alto University, California and Consulting Professor of Psychiatry and the Behavioral Sciences at Stanford University School of Medicine. He is a past president of the Section on Clinical Crises and Emergencies of the Division of

Clinical Psychology of the American Psychological Association, a diplomat of the American Board of Professional Psychology, and a distinguished fellow of numerous psychological organizations. He has won the Edwin Shneidman Award for outstanding early career contributions to suicide research, the Louis I. Dublin award for lifetime achievement in suicidology research, and the Florence Halpern award for distinguished contributions to the practice of clinical psychology. His research and published work reflect his interest in the wide-ranging complexities of therapeutic interventions with difficult patients in general, and in suicide and life-threatening behaviours in particular.

Craig J. Bryan, PsyD, ABPP, is a board-certified clinical psychologist in cognitive behavioural psychology, and is currently the Associate Professor/Director of the National Center for Veterans' Studies (NCVS) at The University of Utah, USA. He is on the Board of Directors of the American Association for Suicidology and is considered a leading national expert on military suicide. He is a consultant to the Department of Defense for psychological health promotion initiatives and suicide prevention and has briefed Congressional leaders on these topics. He regularly provides training to clinicians and medical professionals about managing suicidal patients and has authored over 60 scientific publications and book chapters, including the book *Managing Suicide Risk in Primary Care*. For his contributions to military suicide prevention, posttraumatic stress disorder, and traumatic brain injury, he was recognized in 2009 by the Society for Military Psychology with the Arthur W. Melton Award for Early Career Achievement and in 2013 by Psychologists in Public Service with the Peter J. N. Linnerooth National Service Award.

Qijin Cheng, PhD, is a postdoctoral fellow at HKJC Centre for Suicide Research and Prevention, the University of Hong Kong and Adjunct Senior Instructor in the Department of Psychiatry, University of Rochester Medical Center, USA. Her research focuses on suicide, media and social context. She has published in the *Lancet, BMJ, Journal of Clinical Psychiatry, Journal of Affective Disorders* and *BMC Public Health*. She was a journalist before pursuing her PhD and is devoted to promoting better cooperation between suicide prevention professionals and media professionals.

Joyce Chu, PhD, is Assistant Professor at Palo Alto University, USA. She earned her BA and MA in psychology at Stanford University, her PhD in clinical psychology from the University of Michigan, and did a postdoctoral fellowship at the University of California, San Francisco. Her specialties include geriatrics, ethnic minority populations and diversity. Her research is focused around understanding and improving mental health services for ethnic minority individuals with depression, suicide, particularly among older adults and Asian Americans.

Tracy A. Clemans, PhD, is a research psychologist with the National Center for Veterans' Studies (NCVS), University of Utah. She works collaboratively with the Associate Director of NCVS, on military and veteran-related research projects, publications and national presentations. From 2010 to 2012, she completed a postdoctoral fellowship at the University of Texas Health Science Center, where she worked as a research therapist with STRONG STAR, a PTSD Research Consortium funded by the Department of Defense. She serves as a consultant on the VISN 19 MIRECC Suicide Consultation Service, providing suicide and psychological assessment to veterans considered to be at risk for suicide. In addition, she provides individual psychotherapy with veterans with PTSD, substance abuse/dependence and suicidality.

Philippe Courtet, PhD, is Professor of Psychiatry at the University of Montpellier, and Head of the Department of Emergencic Psychiatry at the Academic Hospital, Montpellier, France. His areas of interest and expertise involve vulnerability to suicidal behaviour, genetics and brain imaging of suicidal behaviours, bipolar disorders and eating disorders. He is president of the French Association of Biological Psychiatry and Neuropsychopharmacology, chairman of the suicide network of the European College of Neuropsychopharmacology (ECNP), chairman of the task force 'suicide' of the World Federation of Societies of Biological Psychiatry (WFSBP), and he was the President of the Local Organizing Committee of the 2013 Congress of the European Psychiatric Association (EPA). He has published about 100 articles in the field of suicidal behaviour in peer-reviewed journals, including *Archives of General Psychiatry*, *American Journal of Psychiatry*, *Molecular Psychiatry* and *Biological Psychiatry*. He is author of several book chapters and editor of two books on suicidal behaviour in France.

Peter Dome, PhD, received his medical diploma in 2000 at the Semmelweis University, Budapest, Hungary. Until 2007 he worked as a psychiatric resident and – after 2006 – as a psychiatrist at the National Institute for Psychiatry and Neurology, Budapest. Since 2007 he has been a psychiatrist and a researcher at the Department of Clinical and Theoretical Mental Health, Semmelweis University, Faculty of Medicine, Budapest. In 2011, he defended his PhD dissertation entitled 'Treatises on psychiatric disorders as risk factors of somatic disorders and risk factors of suicide'. His research interest includes the background mechanisms of mood-disorders-associated high risk of cardiovascular disorders, suicide risk factors and various aspects of smoking in patients with psychiatric disorders. He received the Research Prize of the Association of European Psychiatrists twice in 2008 and 2011.

David Giannini is currently pursuing a doctoral research program in clinical psychology at Palo Alto University, California. His research interests include the experience of trauma, military psychology, suicide and substance abuse. He is currently researching bravery and the links between military service and suicidality.

Peter Goldblum, PhD, MPH, is a Professor of Psychology, Director of the Center for LGBTQ Evidence-Based Applied Research (CLEAR), Director of the LGBTQ Area of Emphasis, Co-Director of the Multicultural Suicide

Research Center, and Director of the Transgender Research Consortium at Palo Alto University, California. He was a founder and original deputy director of the UCSF AIDS Health Project and a visiting scholar and director of the HIV Bereavement and Caregiver Study at Stanford. He is a pioneer in the development of community-based mental health programmes for LGBTQ clients, and has contributed to the professional literature related to gay men's health, AIDS-related suicide, end of life issues, HIV and work and AIDS bereavement. He has co-authored two highly acclaimed books: *Strategies for Survival: A gay men's health manual for the age of AIDS* and *Working with AIDS Bereavement*. In 2013, he received two awards from the American Psychological Association for his work on LGBTQ issues in psychology.

Xenia Gonda, PhD, is a clinical psychologist and pharmacist currently working as Assistant Professor at the Department of Clinical and Theoretical Mental Health at Semmelweis University, Budapest. She is also affiliated with the Department of Pharmacodynamics at Semmelweis University, with the Neuropsychopharmacology and Neurochemistry Research Group of the Hungarian National Academy of Sciences and Semmelweis University, and the Laboratory for Suicide Research and Prevention of the National Institute of Psychiatry and Addictions. She is the recipient of the Bolyai Janos Research Fellowship of The Hungarian Academy of Sciences. She is engaged in full clinical work in addition to teaching at various universities and research. Her main research fields include the genetic background of personality and psychiatric illnesses, pharmacotherapy of bipolar disorders and biopsychosocial approach to suicidal behaviour. She is the author of more than 100 scientific publications, primarily on the biopsychosocial and genetic aspects of personality, mood disorders, and suicide.

Yari Gvion, PhD, is a supervising clinical psychologist who has worked for many years in a psychiatric hospital and in private clinic and has 20 years' experience with patients who engaged in suicide attempts. She teaches in the Clinical Division of the Psychology Departments at Bar-Ilan University and Tel Aviv-Yaffo College. Her thesis examined the multi-dimensional effects of risk factors for suicide attempts. Specifically she studies trait and state impulsivity and aggression variables as distinguishing between different levels of attempts severity.

Lori Holleran is currently a doctoral researcher in clinical psychology at Palo Alto University, California. Her research interests include examining elements influencing suicide and risk, implications of experiencing trauma, and dynamics affecting criminal offending, as well as potential relationships between these factors. Currently she is involved in research examining factors related to predicting an individuals likelihood of experiencing chronic post traumatic stress disorder (PTSD) at the National Center for PTSD. In the future she is interested in integrating technology and treatment to offer more comprehensive, accessible care to a broader group of individuals.

Kasie Hummel is a doctoral researcher in clinical psychology at Palo Alto University, California. She earned her MA in clinical psychology from Minnesota State University in Mankato, MN, where her thesis focused on geriatric psychology. Furthermore, she conducted research for a global health disparities study focusing on sudden infant death syndrome (SIDS), stillbirth and fetal alcohol syndrome (FAS). Currently, she is a member of the Clinical Emergencies and Crises research group at Palo Alto University led by Bruce Bongar. Her main research interests include military psychology, trauma and correctional psychology.

Miriam Iosue is Lecturer of Psychology and Psychiatric Rehabilitation at the University of Molise. She participated as investigator in studies assessing impulsive and self-harm behaviours among inmates, as well as evaluating genetic and neurobiological correlates of depression and suicide. She conducted screening campaigns and programs aimed at raising adolescents' awareness of suicide and mental health within several European Union funded projects. She is involved in the study of mental health problems and suicidal behaviour among patients with obesity, diabetes and dermatological diseases. She is member of the Section of Suicidology and Suicide Prevention of the European Psychiatric Association and member of the International Association for Suicide Prevention.

Hardeep Lal Joshi, PhD, is Assistant Professor, Department of Psychology, Kurukshetra University, Kurukshetra. He has more than 15 years' teaching as well as research experience. He completed his specialized degree in Clinical Psychology from the Institute of Human Behaviour and Allied Sciences (IHBAS) which is affiliated to the University of Delhi. His specialization is in the areas of clinical psychology, psychological testing, and mental health. He has published twenty-five research papers in journals of national and international repute.

Uri Kugel, MS, is a doctoral researcher in clinical psychology at Palo Alto University, California. Uri earned his MS in clinical psychology from the Leiden University in the Netherlands. He is a member of Clinical Emergencies and Crises research group at Palo Alto University led by Bruce Bongar. His main research interests include clinical emergencies and in particular suicide in the US Military, within the US veteran population and suicide terrorism. Additionally he conducts research in the field of evidence-based internet assessment and clinical oriented artificial intelligence.

Carmel McAuliffe, PhD, currently divides her assignments between suicide research with the National Suicide Research Foundation (NSRF) in Cork, Ireland and as a cognitive-behavioural psychotherapist with St Patricks University Hospital at the Dean Clinic in Cork. She previously worked as a senior researcher with the National Suicide Research Foundation. In 2010 she was awarded the Andrej Marusic prize for young suicide researchers. Prior to this, she worked most of the time at the National Suicide Research Foundation and with the HSE Southern area in Cork. She has been involved in research into suicide and deliberate self-harm over the last 17 years, with a special interest in patients who engage in deliberate self-harm and the efficacy of psychotherapy in preventing repeated suicidal behaviour as well as in psychological autopsy studies and families bereaved by suicide. Since the mid-1990s she has been involved in various international collaborative studies including the WHO/Euro Multicentre Study on Suicidal Behaviour, the Saving and Empowering Young Lives in Europe (SEYLE) project and the Optimising Suicide Prevention Programs and their Implementation in Europe (OSPI Europe) project. She has published in scientific peer reviewed journals and contributed to international textbooks on suicidal behaviour.

Swati Mukherjee is Scientist 'D' at the Defence Institute of Psychological Research (DIPR), Delhi. She is involved in many major research projects of the Institute including suicide in the armed forces. She has written journal articles and book chapters. She has been the associate editor of a volume on *Recent Developments in Psychology* and has co-authored a manual on *Suicide and Fratricide: Dynamics and management* for armed forces personnel and a manual on *Overcoming Obsolescence and Becoming Creative in the R&D Environment* for R&D organizations. Her areas of interest are social psychology, positive mental health practices and suicidal behaviour. She was a recipient of the Defence Research & Development Organization (DRDO) Best Performance Award in 2008.

Emilie Olié, MD, is a psychiatrist in the Department of Psychiatric Emergencies and Post-emergencies of the University Hospital and member of the INSERM team 'Vulnerability to suicidal behaviour' in Montpellier, France. Her areas of interest are suicidal behaviours, bipolar disorders and psychological pain. She has expertise in functional neuroimaging. She has published scientific articles in peer-reviewed journals and is the author of several book chapters dealing with suicidal behaviours and pain. She coordinates the section for suicidal behaviours study of the French Association of Biological Psychiatry.

Vijay Parkash, PhD, is Scientist 'C' at the Defence Institute of Psychological Research (DIPR), Defence R&D Organization, Delhi. After completing his post-graduate degree, he was awarded the DRDO Research Fellowship, and he completed his doctorate degree in psychology from Kurukshetra University, Kurukshetra. His interest areas are health psychology, personality and psychometrics. He has ten years of research experience. He also served as a psychologist on the Air Force Selection Board, Dehradun for two years. He has been involved in many major research projects related to suicidal behaviour and test constructions for personnel selection in the armed forces and paramilitary forces. He has been an editor of three volumes – *Recent Developments in Psychology, Counseling: A practical approach* and *Positive Psychology: Applications in work, health and well-being*, and he has more than 15 other academic publications in the form of journal articles and book chapters.

Samantha Pflum, MS, is a fourth-year doctoral researcher in clinical psychology at Palo Alto University, California. She is a member of the LGBTQ psychology and child and family areas of emphasis. She is a lead student in Palo Alto University's Transgender Research Consortium, and is currently conducting research related to social support and mental health outcomes in the transgender population. She is a student editor and chapter co-author of a forthcoming Oxford University Press book, *The Challenge of Youth Suicide and Bullying*. Clinically, Samantha conducts individual, group and family therapy in a community mental health clinic and an elementary school. She is passionate about working with underserved populations, particularly sexual and gender minorities. Samantha also serves as a teaching assistant, tutor and adjunct adviser to fellow students. Her areas of professional interest include suicidology research, as well as LGBTQ, child/paediatric and family psychology.

Yury E. Razvodovsky, MD, PhD, is a psychiatrist specializing in social psychiatry. He has worked as an associate professor at the Department of Psychiatry in Grodno State Medical University, Belarus. Currently he is research scientist at the Central Scientific Laboratory in Grodno State Medical University. He has published more than 500 articles in English and Russian peer-reviewed journals and conference papers focusing on epidemiology of suicides and alcohol-related problems in transitional society. He is a founding member of the International Society of Addiction Medicine (ISAM) and an active member of the National Association of Psychiatrists.

Zoltán Rihmer is a professor of psychiatry at Semmelweis University, Budapest, Hungary. His special interest is the clinical and biological/genetic aspects of mood and anxiety disorders, with particular regard to the prediction of treatment response and prediction and prevention of suicide. He has published more than 440 scientific articles and book chapters and five books. He received the Nyírő Gyula Award from the Hungarian Psychiatric Association 1987, the Award of the Medicina Publishing House 1987 and 2012, the Brickell Suicide Research Award of the Department of Child and Adolescent Psychiatry, Columbia University, New York 1999, the Premio Aretaeus of the Associazione per lo Studio della Malatia Maniaco-Depressiva 2010, the 'Szabó György Award' of the Hemingway Foundation 2010, Lifetime Achievement Award of the European Bipolar Forum 2011, the Lifetime Achievement Award of the Hungarian Psychiatric Association 2012, the 'Széchenyi Award' of the Government of Hungary 2012, and the Aristotle Gold Medal of Lifetime Achievement in Mental Health given by the International Society of Neurobiology and Psychopharmacology. He is a member of several Hungarian and international scientific associations and boards.

Vsevolod A. Rozanov, MD, PhD, has an extensive background in the study of suicidal behaviour, starting with educational training at the Karolinska Institute to his current position as Professor and Chair of Clinical Psychology at Odessa Mechnikov University and lecturer in the Suicide Research and Prevention Centre. In 1997 he created a non-government non-profit organization 'Human Ecological Health' that became contractor for several educational, research and implementation projects in suicide prevention supported by different charities. In 1999 he started collaborating with Professor Danuta Wasserman from Karolinska Institute, Stockholm, and in 2000 became director of the Ukrainian part of the Swedish-Ukrainian genetic project on suicidal behaviour. In 2000, he also started collaboration with the European Network on Suicide Attempts Monitoring and Prevention (led by Wurzburg University) and headed the corresponding Collaborating Centre in Odessa. In 2008 he established a collaborative Suicide Research and Prevention Centre under the Odessa National Mechnikov University and Human Ecological Health, developed curricula and established on-going education in suicide prevention and mental health promotion for psychologists, GPs, school teachers, military and other focus groups. He is the author and co-author of more than 300 published articles, reviews, books for students and chapters in international textbooks.

Marco Sarchiapone, psychiatrist and psychoanalyst, is a professor at the University of Molise, Italy. He has been involved in research in the field of suicidology for more than 20 years in an interdisciplinary perspective, ranging from biological aspects to social and psychological correlates. He is Vice President of IASP (the International Association of Suicide Prevention). He is deputy co-ordinator of SEYLE (Saving and Empowering Young Lives in Europe) and WE-STAY (Working in Europe to Stop Truancy Among Youth) – two research projects regarding the prevention of suicidal and other risk behaviours in adolescence, funded under the EU 7th Framework Programme. He is also one of the promoters of SUPREME (Suicide Prevention by Internet and Media Based Mental Health Promotion), funded by the European Agency for Health and Consumers and a site leader in the European project, MONSUE (Monitoring Suicide in Europe). In Italy, he has been responsible for a large research project on psychological and genetic factors associated with violence and self-harm behaviour in prisoners. He was the President of the 13th European Symposium on Suicide and Suicidal Behaviour.

Elvin Sheykhani is a doctoral researcher in clinical psychology at Palo Alto University, California. His main research interests include crisis management and military psychology. He is interested in working with the US veteran population within the domain of suicide prevention within active duty and reservist personnel. He conducts research on suicide prevention within the US military and assessment of special operations personnel.

Joseph Tomlins is a doctoral researcher in clinical psychology at Palo Alto University, California. His graduate work focuses on clinical emergencies such as suicide. His current interests include military suicide risk assessment, intervention, treatment, and post-intervention practices. He has presented on clinical emergencies at national conventions such as the American Psychological Association (APA). Most recently, he presented a presidential symposium on military suicide risk assessment at the 2013 APA convention. He also has two years' experience in clinical work. He has received specialized training in LGBTQ issues at the Sexual and Gender Minorities Clinic in Los Alto, CA.

Kaitlin Venema, is a doctoral researcher in clinical psychology at Palo Alto University, California. Her previous research at the University of Washington includes the study of early biomarkers of autism spectrum disorders and perceived tool use in infancy. At Palo Alto University, she is working under Bruce Bongar examining suicidality in sexual minorities, military populations, and terrorists. She is also involved in research exploring institutional review boards (IRBs) practices surrounding suicide research, as well as bravery during heroic acts. In terms of clinical work, she is interested in working with children, adolescents, LGBTQ youth, families, and individuals with trauma histories. Particularly, she is interested in preventative interventions for high-risk populations in the community and interventions for bullying.

Paul S. F. Yip is the Director of the Centre for Suicide Research and Prevention and a professor in the Department of Social Work and Social Administration, The University of Hong Kong. He has served as a national representative of the IASP since 2002 (Hong Kong Region) and a fellow of the International Association of Suicide Research. He has research interests in population health and suicide prevention areas. He has published papers in bio-medical-socio areas. His recent monograph *Suicide in Asia: Causes and prevention*, published by the Hong Kong University Press, has provided an important contribution in understanding suicide and its prevention in Asia. He has served as an honorary governor on the board of Suicide Prevention Service and a consultant for Beijing and Shenzhen Suicide Prevention Service and for the Hong Kong Government on population health issues. He received a Distinguished Alumni Award from La Trobe University in 2008 for his excellent research and service on population health. He is also a recipient of an Excellent Research Award 'Charcoal Burning Suicide' by the Health and Welfare Bureau of Hong Kong SAR Government, 2007 and a Silver Asian Innovation Award, by Asian Wall Street Journal and Singapore Economic Development Board, 2005.

Foreword

For those involved in suicide prevention and suicide research, every new contribution to this field represents a further step forward in the dissemination of the principles operating in such an area. However, among the hundreds of papers and books that are published each year, not all try to shed a real light on the understanding and prevention of suicidal behaviours. The book edited by Updesh Kumar, the suicidal behaviour researcher and senior military psychology scientist in India, is the kind of contribution that helps the reader gain a new insight into the suicidal phenomenon.

Nowadays, we are witnessing a new era in the research and prevention of suicide. This enigmatic phenomenon has attracted the attention of many different thinkers in centuries of human history, from philosophers to clergy, from doctors to sociologists. Needless to say, that an integrated view of the phenomenon has always been much needed. We have now a rare opportunity to discover the delicate mechanisms that mediate genetics, environment and suicide risk, which were not foreseeable even a few years ago. Furthermore, when dealing with suicide risk, one needs proper assessment, regardless of family history, environment and past trauma. This book guides the readers to reach a detailed understanding of suicidal behaviour which is the key concept in suicide prevention, being assessment and management of suicide features traceable in the same person.

My view as a dedicated suicidologist and psychiatrist is that my model for depicting suicide refers to the two distinct dimensions that often overlap, the one comprising psychiatric disorders and the other referring to suicidality. When substantial overlapping exists, there is major risk of suicide as the patient is 'attacked' in two ways. However, suicide can occur with no psychiatric disorders when profound distress and psychological pain become unbearable and when suicide is seen as the perfect solution. In suicidal individuals, psychological pain affects the very core of their human condition and threatens life, which cannot be accepted in its present condition. It is this aspect that characterizes suicide deaths, and it is absent in the vast majority of psychiatric patients. A psychiatric disorder alone, therefore, is not sufficient to precipitate suicide. There must be the suicidality dimension that carries some variant of negative emotions. I found this book very helpful in providing a detailed analysis of the psychological pain.

Unbearable psychological pain has been labelled by my mentor and dear friend Edwin Shneidman, 'psychache' which can be clearly distinguished from depression or other psychiatric disorders because of the uniqueness of suffering perceived by the subject and because of the fact that the subject cannot stand it. The individual cannot see a way out and believes that ending their life is the solution. I considered psychache to be the main ingredient of suicide and if tormented individuals could somehow stop consciousness and still live, they would opt for that solution. Suicide occurs when the psychache is deemed by that individual to be unbearable. It is an escape from intolerable suffering; and this views suicide not as a movement towards death but rather as a remedy to escape from intolerable emotion, unendurable or unacceptable anguish.

Having said that, there are, however, interventions that must be considered beyond the single individual. These include interventions to change the attitudes of the mass media when reporting suicide, which in turn may influence clusters of suicide. Knowledge of genetics and the biology of suicide is also of paramount importance to accomplish the new target of science, that is personalized medicine; grouping together biological markers and the clinical picture. Moreover, intervention through policies, for example, regulating alcohol consumption, has proved to be very effective as well as other interventions that regulate access to lethal methods, the integration of minority groups and getting to know the medical consequences when dealing with suicide risk.

This book, with an extraordinary panel of contributors, contains a comprehensive synthesis of the underlying dynamics of suicidal behaviour and is no doubt a must read book for anyone involved in suicide prevention and those who want to familiarize themselves with the phenomenon. This will serve as a beacon for contemporary researchers in this field and is also a practical tool for stakeholders and policy-makers.

Maurizio Pompili, MD, PhD
Professor of Suicidology,
Director, Suicide Prevention Centre,
Sapienza University of Rome,
Italy

Preface

Suicidal behaviour has been a matter of growing research interest among social scientists and psychiatrists in the recent past as it is one of the major causes of death across the globe. Suicide accounts for a life approximately every 40 seconds and it is considered to be one of the three leading causes of death among young people. The World Health Organization estimates that more than one million people lose their lives every year by means of suicide and this figure is likely to increase above 1.5 million per annum by 2020. Suicidal behaviour includes a process that occurs in varied forms of varying degree of severity, starting from ideation or thought level to completed suicide. On the one hand, it may be as fatal as an act of killing oneself and, on the other, it can be the non-fatal behaviour of a person just wishing him or herself dead that also constitutes suicidal behaviour. Suicide is widely regarded as a personal act deeply rooted in the subjective will of a person. Suicide is currently among the major public health problems in most countries around the world and the seriousness and scope of this maladaptive behaviour have projected a pressing need for a better understanding of the situation from a multidimensional perspective and forced planning and implementation of effective preventive strategies, as well as health care policies to curb suicidal behaviour.

Although a growing number of social scientists and health care professionals have recently been dedicating their efforts to research on various aspects of suicidal behaviour, a relatively small and constrained body of existing literature on the precipitating factors fundamental to suicidal behaviour reveals the relative paucity of a comprehensive focus on the understanding of the specific origin, roots and channels of occurrence of suicidal behaviours. The associated factors and underlying dynamics behind varying trends of suicide have always remained complex. To tackle suicide crisis from the core it is important to identify and analyse these covert aspects. Addressing these calls, this volume *Suicidal Behaviour: Underlying dynamics* tries to challenge the elements of randomness about suicidal behaviour and describes how suicidal behaviour is modelled, both socially and spatially. It is an attempt to minutely delineate the process in which all the biological, psychological, sociological and even geographical factors contribute significantly to the varying trends of suicide worldwide. The volume presents a multifaceted approach to understanding the epidemiological side of *suicidal behaviour*, to appreciate and comprehensively portray the *underlying dynamics* in a single resource and to open further avenues for researchers and academia to expand and delve into the diversity of suicide research.

In order to systematically uncover the underlying dynamics of suicidal behaviour, the volume bases its matter of discourse on sixteen chapters contributed by internationally acclaimed scholars and experts in the field of suicidal behaviour, and attempts to eliminate the existing gaps in the subject by reflecting upon the phenomenon across different communities and countries. The text has been divided into two parts. Part I is focused on elaborating the theoretical underpinnings and comprises eight chapters on various psycho-sociocultural aspects of suicidal behaviour. It begins with a conceptual arena on the subject matter, which primarily concentrates on thorough understanding of the roots of a suicidal process, ranging from genetics through personality to environment, and it further thoroughly unfolds the relation of suicidality to aggression, emotion dysregulation and psychological stress. Simultaneously, along with the theoretical comprehension of the process, it also focuses on specific risk assessment and various theoretical approaches to prevention and intervention particular to the kind of dynamics that underlie any particular suicidal act. Part I begins with 'Conceptualizing suicidal behaviour', from a broad perspective including various definitions, theories and models to enumerate the entire domain of suicidality from different scientific perspectives. In this crucial introductory chapter Hardeep Lal Joshi, Vijay Parkash and Updesh Kumar have delved into suicide as a multidimensional phenomenon, and put forth a detailed conceptual framework of suicidal behaviour. They have attempted to delineate the wide latitude of suicidality and tried to elaborate the conceptual underpinnings from varied interdisciplinary perspectives explaining the vast domain of suicidal behaviours. Considering it essential to list effective preventive strategies and intervention techniques, they briefly cite some concrete ways that can be utilized to help suicidal people and save their lives.

Suicidal behaviour is a complex and multi-factorial phenomenon and epidemiological genetic studies suggest that the genes of the serotonergic system are linked to suicidal vulnerability. Building on the conceptual framework in Chapter 1 and bringing out the hereditary links, in Chapter 2 of the volume, Sarchiapone and Iosue try to explicate the 'Genetics of suicidal behavior'. The authors demonstrate the familial transmission of suicide and the way in which it is distinct from the familial transmission of psychiatric disorders associated with suicidal behaviour. The authors very well exemplify a specific clinical phenotype of suicidal behaviour related to attempted and completed suicides by elucidating various adoption and twin studies. Citing the role of heredity, they emphasize that vulnerability to suicidal behaviour may involve interactions between genetic factors, acting via the transmission of personality traits and environmental factors. The authors also describe various gene approach studies and suggest the role of different genes coding in suicidal aberration. They indicate that the Genome Wide Association studies and epigenetics have a significant potential to examine large sets of gene polymorphisms and heritable changes and thus improve our understanding of the association between gene expression and suicidal vulnerability.

Ranging from the exploration of genetic factors to understanding of the personality and temperamental make-up of an individual, probably social scientists have delved deep into the roots of suicidal behaviour to understand the pathways leading to its evolution and sustenance. The forthcoming chapters focus on the linkage of various psychological constructs of personality, emotion dysregulation and impulsiveness with various types of suicidal behaviour. Describing in Chapter 3, 'Suicidality and personality: linking pathways', Parkash and Kumar delve into various personality factors linked to different aspects of suicidality. Considering the widely accepted personality descriptive models including the big-three and the big-five, they have attempted to highlight all the important paths that link an individual's personality make-up with various suicidal dimensions, thereby making an individual vulnerable. The genetically determined side of personality – temperament – has also been elaborated to reveal its precipitative effects on suicidality. In the attempt to uncover all personality-related linking pathways to suicidality, they have also tried to concisely explain various related personality aberrations in the form of disorders and the way they form a bridge to suicidal behaviour. The need to focus on very specific narrower personality traits has been highlighted for a deeper understanding of the suicidal dynamics.

Covering the more specific and abstract personality aspects, in Chapter 4, 'Emotion dysregulation and suicidality', Anestis investigates the influence of negative affect on vulnerability to suicidal ideation. The author has defined emotion dysregulation as a multifaceted construct connected with problematic outcomes of anti-social behaviour, non-suicidal self-injury and substance use. Using the Interpersonal-Psychological Theory of suicidal behaviour, the author differentiates between the desire for suicide and the capability for suicide and states that most individuals with a suicidal desire will not have the capability and those with the capability will not have the desire to commit suicide. Theories of Dialectical Behaviour Therapy and Emotion Regulation Group therapy have been regarded as effective psycho-social approaches to enhance an individual's capacity to regulate their emotions and teach distress tolerance skills. Taking the discourse on personality-suicidality link further and deeper is the task of Chapter 5, 'Role of aggression and impulsivity in suicide attempts and in suicide completion'. Gvion and Apter examine the influence of each construct independently as well as in association and elaborate on how these contribute to various aspects of suicidality. The authors amply cite that aggression has been linked to the act of suicide in multiple epidemiologic, clinical, retrospective, prospective, and family studies. They highlight that direct, proximate and indirect causal factors have been studied while evaluating impulsivity within the context of suicidal behaviour. While focusing on patients with disorders, the authors emphasize how impulsive-aggressive personality disorders and alcohol abuse were two independent predictors of suicide in major depression and aggression but impulsivity does not appear to be a factor for patients with bipolar disorder.

Making the evidently perceived underlying dynamics explicit, in Chapter 6 Rozanov comprehensively describes the connections between psycho-social stress and suicidal behaviour. In addition to the individual psychological factors, the author here suggests various macro-, meso- and micro-level factors that mediate the effect of social structure on individual and public health and has identified excessive mortality, shortening of life expectancy, rise of life-threatening risky behaviour and suicidality as major indicators of psycho-social stress. The fluctuations in suicide rates in the European Union and the former USSR countries have been aptly shown as supporting evidence to reflect the social and economic processes and transformations taking place in the country. By classifying the post-Soviet countries into two clusters – the one with high suicide rates and marked rise of suicides in response to stress and the other with with low suicide rates and blunted rise under the stress of transition – the author proves that suicide rates vary in different cultures under similar stressful conditions but this variation is not observed when mortality rates from cardiac infarction and cerebrovascular diseases are examined. In addition, he also analyses gender differences in suicide behaviour and other stress manifestations in these clusters. The interconnection between stress and alcohol consumption has also been reviewed and Rozanov proposes that national traditions and ethno-cultural peculiarities play an important role in determining variations in suicidal behaviour at the national level.

Revealing the suicide dynamics from another related point of view, in Chapter 7 Courtet and Olié trace a pathway to suicide running from social adversity to psychological pain and discuss the physiopathology of suicidal behaviour in the light of psychological pain. They describe suicide as a major social crisis in occidental countries and refer to the possible existence of an association between economic crisis and suicide. Describing the isolated elderly and prisoners as high risk populations, the authors attribute various social and economic factors to the spatial and temporal variation in suicide. Psycho-social stress, social vulnerability and social exclusion due to exposure to a harmful environment, such as sexual abuse, emotional neglect, disturbed relationship with parents or parental mental illness have been observed as carriers of negative emotions of dread, grief, shame, guilt, etc. and key precursors of social and psychological pain and thus, suicidal acts. Highlighting the need to avoid suicidal mortality and suicidal thoughts, the authors propose the use of analgesic drugs and also suggest prosocial pathways as protective factors for suicide.

The rise of modern communication systems, social networking and social media has resulted in an increase of clustering and contagion of suicidal behaviour. Research in this area is still in its nascent stage and Arensman and McAuliffe, in Chapter 8 of this volume, provide a review of the epidemiological, methodological, clinical and social issues in understanding the mechanism of suicide clustering. In addition to geographical clusters, the significance of time and space clustering among specific populations and settings, such as psychiatric inpatients, adolescents and young adults in community settings has been well explored. The authors worry about the recent rising trend of suicide clustering and contagion in older adults which was earlier found mostly in adolescents and young adults. Various approaches to assess clustering and contagion have been defined and the authors emphasize the need to establish relevant public health, health and bereavement support services for the needs of the people. The authors conclude the chapter with a call for better crisis response training and highlight the need to have a long-term programme of suicide risk reduction and community recovery.

Understanding suicidal behaviour remains incomplete without appreciating the interplay of various causal factors that lead to suicide. The goal of reducing suicides and suicidal behaviours can be accomplished only when the causes and correlates of suicide are identified and addressed with precise adequacy. The relative scantiness of empirical attention paid to understanding suicidal risk has mostly been the reason that has prevented clinicians and health scientists from achieving this goal. Part II, 'Varied research evidences and assessment perspectives' focuses on this very important aspect and brings to light the various precipitating factors of suicide in diverse societies and cultures and the resources required to deal effectively with suicide. This Part opens with Chapter 9 'Suicidal ideation and behaviour among sexual minority youth: correlates, vulnerabilities, and protective factors', wherein Samantha Pflum and her associates have tried to explore the relation of suicidal ideation among sexual minority youth by elucidating the mental health disparities of LGBTQ (lesbian, gay, bisexual, transgender, queer) youth. Depression, peer victimization and social isolation have been comprehensively elaborated as some of the important correlates of self-harm. Being specific to the correlative risk factors, the authors also provide recommendations for health practitioners, family, and school administrators to maximize protective factors and promote positive development and support.

Providing a detailed picturesque analysis of the global trends of various suicide-related factors, the volume proceeds in the next few chapters to discuss suicidal variations in different parts of the world including Hungary. In the tenth chapter, Rihmer, Gonda and Dome attempt to provide a clearer impetus on understanding the variations in suicidal behaviour by enunciating the spatial and temporal distribution of suicidal behaviour with a special focus on Hungary. In addition to psycho-social factors, genetic and biological contributions such as regional differences and geographical factors are identified and well elaborated upon as possible causes of the high suicide rates in Hungary. The authors report a positive correlation between psychiatric disorders and suicide rate and examine the effect of antidepressant treatments in reducing suicidal rates. To extend and illustrate the variations in suicide in the next chapter, Clemans and Bryan conceptualize suicide risk particularly for military personnel by deliberating on suicide in the United States military. Risk factors between the civilian and military populations are compared and the distinct culture of the United States military has been considered as the discriminating and contributing factor. Further, Fluid Vulnerability Theory has been adopted to conceptualize the risk of suicide among service members and provide a theoretical foundation to assess the risk level of military personnel. Illustrating the phases of the cognitive behavioural therapy model, the authors have suggested specific intervention strategies to mitigate the risk of suicide among service personnel.

Alcohol dependence ranks among the strongest suicide precursors and alcohol addicts have higher rates of attempted and completed suicides. Though the hypothetical relations are given consideration by the professionals, the origins of the close relationship between alcoholism and suicide have rarely been investigated and explored by researchers. Considering another global trend, Razvodovsky has extended the issue on similar lines in Chapter 12, 'Contribution of alcohol to suicide mortality in Eastern Europe' and he stresses that Eastern European countries constitute the highest suicide rates. Attributing alcohol as the most consistent predictor of suicide mortality and supporting his claim by highlighting several studies and experiments, the author argues that alcohol is a strong determinant of suicide both at the individual and population level. Drinking patterns and culture are examined and credited as important indicators of the alcohol–suicide association in spirits-drinking countries. Concluding his chapter, the author lists various natural experiments and empirical evidence to evaluate the efficacy of public health interventions and suggests that a restrictive alcohol policy can be considered an effective measure of suicide prevention in such countries.

The reporting and portrayal of suicide in the media have a significant influence on suicidal behaviour and the need for the proper depiction of media content and a proper understanding of its influence on suicide contagion urge further research in this area. Cheng and Yip delve in this emerging area of research in Chapter 13 and provide a critical review of media content representation of suicide in various societies, wherein they demonstrate the ways that media representation differs in various societies and the factors that influence these variations. Rather than focusing on the quantitative representation of suicide issues, the authors critically examine the content of non-fictional suicide reports in their study. They present a systematic meta-analytic literature review process and propose that traditional media representation possesses some common features but these are a result of common patterns of media's selective reporting that create myths in the readers' mind. Certain communalities observed were in terms of suicide victims' background, the method of suicide and the attributes leading to suicide. They also report how celebrity and youth suicides using violent methods were more appealing to the media. On the other hand, the authors optimistically state that online representation of suicide showed an inclination towards publishing anti-suicide information. Revealing the global trends on this issue, they very aptly report a cross-cultural study of suicide reports in Hungary, Japan, the United States, Germany, Austria and Finland to comprehensively demonstrate the cultural variations of media representation in these countries. The authors emphasize the importance of the implementation of media guidelines and the involvement of professionals to steer the development of media representation towards preventing suicidal behaviour.

After discussing various factors contributing to suicidality, the scope of the volume further extends to include the concept of suicide assessment and prevention. Elaborating upon the formal assessment of suicide risk, Bruce Bongar and colleagues in Chapter 14 examine the significance of formal risk assessment in the mental health care system and describe a comprehensive psychological and psychiatric evaluation based on the Risk Management Foundation of the Harvard Medical Institution (RMFHMI). The authors summarize the clinician's critical areas of exploration across the five domains of clinical diagnosis, history of suicidal behaviours, client strengths and vulnerabilities, risk factors of self-harm, and protective factors. Based on these critical areas, the authors theorize that strong religious beliefs, fear of social disapproval, a positive social support group, positive coping abilities and a positive family structure would restrain individuals from suicide attempts. The authors' critical review of the formal assessment of suicide risk in three distinct mental health care settings of Veterans' Affair Hospitals, general hospitals and community mental health gives a broad perspective to identify at-risk patients and suggests specific training protocols and step-by-step evaluation measures not only to identify risk factors but also to educate health professionals in the proper diagnosis of a suicidal individual. Maintaining the line of significance assigned to suicide risk assessment but slightly shifting the focus to the cultural identity of groups and individuals, Kugel and his associates in Chapter 15 bring forward the aspects of suicide risk in culturally diverse populations in their chapter 'Culturally competent suicide assessment'. The authors describe how the various constructs of suicide such as suicidal ideation, suicide method and risk and protective factors vary between ethnicities, gender and sexual orientation and express a concern about the need to develop and validate measures to recognize the unique factors to assess accurate risk levels across culturally diverse populations. Furthermore, the authors explain the CARS (Cultural Assessment of Risk for Suicide) measure based on the four categories of the Cultural Model of Suicide – cultural sanctions, idioms of distress, minority stress and social discord – to address the risk and cultural disparities in suicide among four diverse cultural minority populations of Asian Americans, Latino/a Americans, African Americans, and sexual minorities.

As the volume moves towards the end, it is important to discuss the best practices that must be undertaken in dealing with suicidal behaviour. In the last chapter of the volume, 'Ethical and legal issues in dealing with suicidal behaviour', Mukherjee and Kumar provide an overview of the prevalent dilemmas and the ethical and legal considerations in the process of suicide assessment and suicide prevention. Describing ethics as aspirational standards a counsellor should strive to attain, the authors highlight the moral dilemma involved in accepting the act of suicide as rational or irrational. The authors elaborate upon the general principles for constituting ethical standards in counselling. Beneficence and non-maleficience, fidelity and responsibility, integrity, justice and respect for people's rights and dignity have been listed as the important principles that are crucial for building a healthy client–counsellor relationship. The authors provide a legal perspective to the issue by delving into the case of India in particular. The chapter concludes by underlining the need for a legal and ethical framework and proposes professional guidelines for understanding the client and creating an environment for the healthy existence of humanity.

The theoretical underpinnings revealed in the first part along with a thorough understanding of the causal factors and assessment procedures elaborated in the second part of the volume present a comprehensive coverage of suicide-related issues and widen the horizon of the readers to think beyond the epidemiological perspective. The varied dynamics explored from a multidimensional viewpoint give a panoptic description of the problem and variants of suicidality. The focus on evolution, assessment and prevention of suicidal behaviour in a cross-cultural milieu presented in this volume is an attempt to provide scope for researchers and professionals working in this area across the globe to fully delve into each aspect and cater to each community separately so that the stigma of suicide can be effectively controlled and arrested.

Editing a volume on such a vast area of research is undoubtedly an arduous task and I express my gratitude to one and all who contributed to the extensive work and provided constant support. I am deeply indebted to the authors for the time and effort they have given to the project. Their outstanding work significantly contributed to a quality, informative and a professional product. I also wish to acknowledge with thanks the kindness of my colleagues at the Defence Institute of Psychological Research, Defence Research and Development Organisation, New Delhi, for their patience and cooperation in successfully completing the volume on suicidal behaviour in a short span of time. I hope this volume will serve as a pivotal reference point for the health care professionals and research scientists and will generate new ideas of research for the continual advancement of studies on suicidal behaviour in the service of mankind.

Part I
Theoretical underpinnings

1 Conceptualizing suicidal behaviour

Understanding and prevention

Hardeep Lal Joshi, Vijay Parkash and Updesh Kumar

Suicide is one of the major causes of death among people in the West and now the suicidal cases are rising in the Eastern countries as well (World Health Organization (WHO), 2012). WHO (1999) has estimated that approximately 1.53 million people will die from suicide, and ten to twenty times more people will attempt suicide across the world by the year 2020. These estimates indicate that on average one death will occur every 20 seconds and one attempt will be carried out every one to two seconds. Although of low predictive value, in these estimates the presence of psychopathology is perhaps the single most important predictor of suicide (Gvion and Apter, 2012).

According to another WHO estimate, every year about 170,000 deaths by suicide occur in India (as cited by Patel *et al.*, 2012). As per a decade-old estimate, every year, of the half million people dying by suicide across the world, 20 per cent were Indians (Singh and Singh, 2003) of the 17 per cent of the world population. In the past two decades the suicide rate has escalated from below 8 to above 10 per 100,000 (Vijayakumar, 2007). In a recent study published in the *Lancet* in June 2012, it was estimated that about 187,000 suicides occurred in 2010 (Patel *et al.*, 2012). These estimates show that suicide is fast becoming a menace to human life and therefore it calls for urgent action that can lead to finding ways to curb this growing tendency among people.

The aftermaths of suicide are often massive because not only does it annihilate a person's existence but also leaves his family and friends in the lurch, thrusting upon them emotional, mental and physical stress. A person who attempts suicide, essentially, needs medical help and treatment and therefore it is necessary to broaden the knowledge regarding suicide and carry out extensive research in this field.

Ancient understanding

Strikingly, in ancient times, the act of suicide was not considered disagreeable and was instead regarded as a good method to avoid life's frustrating circumstances. Ancient Romans before the fourth century deemed the quality of life to be of greater value than its longevity. Seneca, the first-century Roman philosopher, acknowledged suicide as a decent way to end life's misery. Even the Christian Church began denouncing suicide as sinful only in the fourth century which then proclaimed that the act of suicide is in violation of the Sixth Commandment – Thou shalt not kill – and therefore began viewing it as a crime. Later on, the Italian philosopher St Thomas Aquinas, in the thirteenth century, declared that suicide is a mortal sin because it invades God's power over human life. Since suicide began to be considered a crime against God, in Christianity, for a long time people committing suicide were debarred from burial in a Christian graveyard. It is interesting to note that suicide continued to be a criminal offence in the United Kingdom until 1961, where Christianity is the major religion.

Like the European countries, the concept of suicide was grappled with by Asian countries as well. From 1200 to the 1600s, suicide – hara-kiri in Japanese – was viewed as a dignified means of departing from life's disgraceful state of affairs. In ancient India too, suicide was preferred as a better option to death from disease. Considering the Confucianist views, the act of suicide is not condemnable. In Confucian opinion, the act of suicide is seen in relation to the events that lead up to it, and can therefore, depending on the circumstances, be seen as something honourable or dishonourable. In China, where Confucianism is followed widely, suicide is also seen as a passionate protection of one's honour or integrity and as a spirited resistance against something bad. In Confucian cultural tradition, suicide in general is seen as something negative but it can sometimes be justified if it is for a noble purpose. 'Confucius would see suicide as an option for protecting one's virtue and integrity, but that more can be gained by doing well in life instead of killing oneself' (Van Tuan, 2010, p. 5).

From the Buddhist point of view, it is a common belief that life is a transitory abode while death would be a long-lasting subsistence. However, in Buddhism, it is believed that the next life depends on the way one lives one's present life and suicide is condemned because running away from this life by means of 'death' cannot prevent the anxieties of the next life. It shows that Buddhist beliefs are close to the existential model of thinking (Van Tuan, 2010, p. 5). Similarly in Islamic countries, suicide is regarded as an unholy act because the Quran, the religious text of Islam, considers it to be one of the most horrible sins that obstructs man's spiritual path. This is one of the reasons why in most Muslim countries suicide is still considered as a crime. Although some countries do consider suicide a crime, individual suicide has been decriminalized in the Western world. In the United States of America, it is not illegal to commit suicide but the person can be penalized for an attempt. It is interesting to note that at present, no European country considers attempted suicide a crime (McLaughlin, 2007), whereas, in India, attempted suicide is a punishable offence.

Conceptualizing suicide

Many psychologists regard suicidal ideation as a form of mental illness and suicide as an outcome of this illness and, therefore, an extensive body of work has been done to study the various aspects and dimensions of suicide and suicidal behaviour. Sigmund Freud (1917) in his essay, 'Mourning and Melancholy', postulated that the life-instinct 'Eros' and the death-instinct 'Thanatos' are the two instincts that drive individuals. Researchers believe that Freud's conceptualization of the

> 'death instinct behaviors reflecting self-destructive tendencies, guilt feelings, suicide, melancholia, masochism and sadism are furnished with a motivational force of their own, as well as with a specific mechanism of action, that is the repetition compulsion. The death instinct drives man to the ultimate state of quiescence – death through the urge inherent in organic life to restore an earlier state of things'
>
> (Orbach, 2007, pp. 266, 267)

Freud used to believe that these self-destructive processes lead to depression and suicide. He further posited that most individuals struggle between the two instincts and suicide results when Thanatos wins over Eros. Although there have been many scholars who have contributed enormously to the field of suicidal behaviour research, major work in the conception of suicide was carried out by American psychologist Edwin S. Shneidman in the 1950s. Around six decades ago he co-founded the Los Angeles Suicide Prevention Center in 1958, for the better understanding of suicide. Shneidman neologized various terms like psychache, suicidology, psychological autopsy and postvention. As Shneidman pioneered the research in this field he is often referred to as the father of contemporary suicidology (Leenaars, 2010; Shneidman, 1993).

Derived from the Latin words 'sui' (of oneself) and 'caedere' (to kill) the word 'suicide' was first used in the seventeenth century by Sir Thomas Browne. He introduced this term in his published book *Religio Medici* in 1643. In 1903 the first 'International Classification of Diseases and Causes of Death' was adopted which included 'suicide' in the section related to morbidity and mortality due to external factors. Thinkers like Emile Durkheim and Sigmund Freud in their respective studies pointed out the effect of external factors on suicide and therefore led to the encompassing of sociological and psychological aspects in the definition of suicide. But before proceeding to the discussion of the definition of suicide, it is essential to understand that the term 'suicide' is often used only for those reported cases where the attempt to kill oneself has resulted in death which apparently makes it quite a restricted term in the sense that it does not cover all the other related aspects of the act. This often leads to flawed estimation of the cases. Therefore, the term 'suicidal behaviour' is used to refer to the multidimensional nature of suicide and the acts related to it. Though the nomenclature of suicidal behaviours too has been an issue of international debate among experts as well as there being variations involved in those cases where the attempts do not lead to lethal outcomes, the term 'suicidal behaviour' is generally used as a more inclusive term (Silverman *et al.*, 2007a, b; Van Orden *et al.*, 2010).

We all know readily what suicide means whenever it is mentioned in everyday life. But technically, the word suicide does not simply mean 'killing oneself'. It is a much more complex concept and as mentioned above, the complexity arises from the fact that suicidal behaviour is used to describe a varied gamut of results, one of them being suicide. Basically, three categories of suicidal behaviour have been suggested: completed suicide, suicide attempt, and suicidal ideas (Beck *et al.*, 1972).

It may be noted that not every act of killing oneself can be classed as suicide. In order to be so, it is essential that the person must intentionally initiate the act, in the full knowledge or anticipation of its lethal results. On the other hand, there is much variation among the terms used for suicidal behaviours without lethal results so those acts of terminating one's own life which have non-fatal results are designated as suicidality, attempted suicide, suicide attempts, act of intentional self-harm or para-suicide (WHO, 1998). The International Classification of Diseases, (ICD-10; WHO, 1992) too has created a separate class of 'Intentional Self Harm' stating that it comprises 'purposely self inflicted poisoning or injury suicide (attempted)' (p. 1013).

Researchers have contended that there is a continuum from suicidal ideation to gesture to attempt to complete which depicts suicidal behaviour (Crosby *et al.*, 1999; Garland and Zigler, 1993; Silverman and Maris, 1995). Suicidal behaviour generally begins with ideation which includes thoughts about desire and method to commit suicide (Beck *et al.*, 1988). The person here thinks of or wishes to die, this then is reflected in his or her gestures, further transmuting into an attempt and finally might be resulting into completion. Hence it can be said that 'suicidal behavior is a set of noncontinuous and hetero-geneous spectra of behaviors, such that suicidal ideation, suicidal threats, gestures, self-cutting, low lethal suicide attempts, interrupted suicide attempts, near-fatal suicide attempts, and actual suicide' (Bursztein and Apter, 2009, as cited by Amitai and Apter, 2012, p. 986). Giving a nomenclature to major suicide-related behaviours, O'Carroll *et al.* (1996) described suicidal ideation as 'any self-reported thoughts of engaging in suicide-related behavior'; non-suicidal self-injury as 'direct, deliberate destruction of body tissue without lethal inten-tion'; and a suicide attempt as a 'potentially self-injurious behavior with a non-fatal outcome, for which there is evidence (explicit or implicit) that the person intended at some level to kill himself/herself' (cited by Amitai and Apter, 2012, p. 986). These behaviours differ on the scale of rescuability and lethality. In fact, rescuability and fatality are the factors that actually distinguish between suicidal gestures and attempts. Rescuability is high and fatality is low in suicidal gestures or parasuicide where the person concerned does not actually intend to die yet he/she commits the act of self-directed violence. In the absence of the intention to die as in the present context, the term 'self-harm' is used. But when there is a presence of intent to die, the rescuability is low and the chances of fatality become high. It may be noted that the applicability of the conceptualization of suicidal behaviour on a continuum for every individual is still to be proved (Silverman and Maris, 1995).

The attributes of lethal suicidal behaviour or suicide are quite different from non-lethal suicidal behaviour. Shneidman (1985) theorized that suicide resulted due to an intense emotional and psychological pain called 'psychache', which ultimately becomes unbearable and cannot be abated by previously successful coping patterns. Suicidal death thus, in a sense, is an escape from this pain. This notion of escape from unbearable experiences has also been endorsed by another researcher, Baumeister (1990). He regards the act of suicide as an escape from self, or at least self-awareness. An individual attains a state of 'cognitive deconstruction' in this attempt which involves both irrationality and disinhibition, such that drastic action becomes logical. Some other researchers have asserted that in most cases suicide is associated with negative events which lead to a sense of meaninglessness of life and hopelessness about future (Beck *et al.*, 1985; Eyman and Eyman, 1992), which create, independently or in combination, a psychological state that perceives suicide as a promising way out. Still other researchers proposed that hopelessness about the future may be a better long-term predictor of suicide (say, one or two years later) than it is for the short term (weeks or months) (Clark, 1995).

Defining suicide

Over the years, several pioneers and researchers have defined suicide in their own way, however, there still remains a need to have a single globally accepted definition. Although there seems to be an inherent communality among different definitions, some of the popular but differing definitions of suicide are as follows:

- 'All cases of death resulting directly or indirectly from a positive or negative act of the victim himself, which he knows will produce this result' (Durkheim, 1897/1951, p. 44).
- 'All behaviour that seeks and finds the solution to an existential problem by making an attempt on the life of the subject' (Baechler, 1979, p. 11).
- 'Suicide is a conscious act of self-induced annihilation, best understood as a multidimensional malaise in a needful individual who defines an issue for which suicide is perceived as the best solution' (Shneidman, 1985, p. 203).
- 'Suicide is an act with a fatal outcome which the deceased, knowing or expecting a fatal outcome had initiated and carried out with the purpose of provoking the changes he desired' (WHO, 1986).
- 'A fatal willful self-inflicted life-threatening act without apparent desire; implicit are two basic components lethality and intent' (Davis, 1988, p. 38, as cited by Maris *et al.*, 2000, p. 30).
- 'Death arising from an act inflicted upon oneself with the intention to kill oneself' (Rosenberg *et al.*, 1988, as cited by Maris *et al.*, 2000, p. 30).
- 'The definition of suicide has four elements: (1) a suicide has taken place if death occurs; (2) it must be of one's own doing; (3) the agency of suicide can be active or passive; (4) it implies intentionally ending one's own life' (Mayo, 1992, pp. 92, 95).

The above-cited definitions make it obvious that there is a lack of overall agreement among researchers on which key aspects to be included in the definition of suicide. Despite much debate, the researchers have still not reached consensus about it but over time, certain common elements have emerged from these different definitions. These elements include: the result of the behaviour, the intent to die to attain a different status, the agency of the act, the consciousness of results, the effect of a theoretical orientation and the influences of culture. The WHO Working Group thus later adopted a standard definition of suicide which not only includes all the above-stated elements but is also theoretically neutral, free of value judgement and one that is culturally normative. WHO (1998) defined suicide as the 'act of killing oneself, deliberately initiated and performed by the person concerned, in the full knowledge or expectation of its fatal outcome'.

Apparently, in any definition of suicide the intent to die is the central element. However, it may be noted that it is hard to be absolutely certain of the thought pattern of the deceased unless he has made his intention to die clear by way of a suicide-note or diary or a prior conversation. Then there are many attempts made impulsively during brief critical circumstances and are thus hardly planned. Besides, there are cases where people who think of committing suicide often have an ambivalent attitude towards killing themselves. In all such cases establishing a correlation between intent and outcome can be quite challenging (Carson *et al.*, 2004; WHO, 2002). Therefore, a slightly modified version of the above definition has recently been proposed to make it even more comprehensive and universally acceptable.

> Suicide is an act with fatal outcome, which the deceased, knowing or expecting a potentially fatal outcome, has initiated and carried out with the purpose of bringing about wanted changes.
>
> (De Leo *et al.*, 2006, p. 5)

Suicide is a multifaceted phenomenon and it often occurs as a result of mutual or reciprocal actions of various factors. Although many extensive studies have been made in this field, there are still some problems which remain unsolved such as the standard definitions of different subtypes and phenotypes of suicidal behaviour and associated factors like aggression and impulsivity (Gvion and Apter, 2012). The psychologists, therefore, still have a number of questions to answer.

Theoretical perspectives

Though suicide is considered a behaviour related to modern society, it is not necessarily so. Great philosophers also described suicide in one way or the other. At that time, no theory was proposed because of less interest in this topic, yet almost all the great philosophers gave their opinion on suicide. In the Classical Greek era, suicide was always viewed negatively. Pythagoras proposed that suicide leads to imbalance because it is unnatural. Plato and Socrates also described suicide as wrong and against the state. Aristotle proposed punishment for committing suicide, considering it negative for mankind. It was in Classical Rome, that the opinion regarding suicide changed. In this era, suicide was not considered negative, or wrong, rather it was seen as a way to find freedom from problems. Around 1500, the writers and philosophers started changing their views regarding suicide. The main insight into the topic was provided by the French philosopher Rousseau who tried to free suicide from evil. According to Rousseau, the individual should not be blamed for suicide, it is society, which is compelling him to commit this act. David Hume described suicide apart from the concept of sin. Later on Immanuel Kant preserved the earlier Stoic stance, calling suicide unjust. Goethe presents the opposite view to Kant's, calling for right to death. In history, views regarding suicide are never unidimensional, some consider it negative whereas others stand at the opposite pole and justify its rationality.

Theoretically, suicide and suicidal behaviour are a complex and multi-dimensional phenomenon. It is difficult to study this topic because in order to compose a general theory, very large samples are required and in the general population, fewer suicide attempts and deaths are found. Second, people who actually attempt suicide are excluded from clinical trials, and those who die because of suicide are never available for assessment. Although research concerning suicidal behaviour has been conducted in an atheoretical context, different theoretical models have been proposed to describe it. Major approaches describing suicidal behaviour include biological, psychological and sociological perspectives.

Biological theories

There is a fair amount of research evidence that biological factors play an important role in suicide. It is found that the suicide rate is higher in monozygotic-twins as compared to dizygotic twins. It is also found that the suicide rate is higher among biological relatives of suicide attempters as compared to normal pro-bounds. Biological theorists also proposed that suicidal behaviour results from the presence of biologically-based diathesis. According to recent research (Mann, 2003; Van Pragg, 2001), the dysregulation of the serotonergic system in the ventromedial prefrontal cortex leads to a higher suicidal risk. Considering the role of biological factors along with other psychological and social factors, Kinderman (2005) proposed the biopsychosocial model wherein he suggested that biological factors, social factors and other environmental or life events lead to mental health problems through their conjoint effects on mental psychological processes, and these are the final common pathways to mental ill-health which may ultimately lead to suicidal behaviour in many untreated cases.

Psychological perspectives

Various psychological interpretations of suicide have been proposed by psychologists. Freud (1917) was the front runner among those experts. Freud suggested that suicide is motivated by unconscious intentions. According to Freud, the root cause of suicide was the loss or rejection of a significant object. The suicide attempter turns a death wish towards the person himself which has been directed against someone else. Freud considered it a type of self-punishment. The suicidal persons feel a sense of guilt and criticize themselves for each and everything and start developing prohibition towards harshness. In this way, the suicidal person is unable to organize his experiences in a coherent way which ultimately results in suicide. Freud's theory of instinctual self-destructive behaviour was further elaborated upon by Menninger (1938). He explained the three primary dynamics underlying suicidal behaviour. These dynamics included the wish to kill (ego – aggression turned inward); the wish to be killed (superego – self-aggression stemming from guilt), and the wish to die. Although the wish to kill is expressed against oneself by means of suicidal acts, the inherent aggression in that wish is intended for an ambivalently valued person. Menninger further proposes that the wish to be killed stems from intense superego guilt for outlawed sexual and aggressive unconscious id desires. He asserts that the wish to die represents the strength of the unconscious death instinct rather than representing a conscious (ego) wish to kill or a superego self-punishment. The wish to die indicates an id desire to revisit the prior birth tranquillity and it is manifested in non-fatal self-destructive acts and in self-exposure to dangerous activities. Because of the innate intensity of the death instinct, the wish to die is thus a form of playing with death (Menninger, 1938, as cited by Orbach, 2007, p. 267).

The other perspective on suicidal behaviour is given by cognitive behaviour psychologists. According to this perspective, depression is the main cause of suicide in which hopelessness is the main factor. The suicidal person views himself, the future and the environment as negative and this negative evaluation along with some cognitive errors and distortion pushes him to suicidal ideation and suicidal acts. The final outcome, that is, suicide is the result of cognition the person has developed. According to some cognitive behavioural psychologists, it is the cognitive schema, and according to some it is the irrational beliefs which are crucial factors in the development of negativity which is the main cause of suicide among suicidal people (Beck *et al.*, 1985).

Learning psychologists explained suicide as a learned behaviour. According to them, it is the forces of environment that shape the suicidal behaviour which is reinforced by the environment. Some psychologists like Bandura (1977) explained suicidal behaviour in terms of social learning. Suicide is committed by the person, as he observed it in the environment. The social learning theory points out the role of imitation, gives indirect insights about suicide contagion, and posits that a number of environmental factors such as suggestion on television, stories in the newspapers and observing others, that is, modelling may be some of the factors related to suicide.

Other researchers working in this area provide different types of explanations. Baumeister (1990) propounded 'escape theory' and explained suicidal behaviour in terms of motivations to escape from aversive self-awareness. He described a causal sequence of six primary steps or escapist events leading to suicidal behaviour.

The causal chain begins with events that make a person feel they are falling severely short of standards and/or expectations. The failure so perceived is attributed internally to the self and it makes self-awareness painful. This painful self-awareness of one's own inadequacies results in the generation of negative affect; and, consequently, a desire emerges to escape from that painful self-awareness and the associated affect. In the efforts to escape an individual attempts to achieve a state of cognitive deconstruction and the deconstructed state brings irrationality and disinhibition, making drastic self-harmful steps appear acceptable. It is at that point of time when suicide may be viewed as the ultimate step in the effort to escape from self and the world (Baumeister, 1990).

Williams (1997, 2001) expanded on the escape theory of Baumeister (1990) by putting forth the 'cry of pain' model to explain suicidal behaviour. Williams and colleagues (Williams, 1997; Williams and Pollock, 2000) contended that engaging in suicidal behaviour is not a cry for help, but it is a cry of pain due to a situation that is trapping a defeated individual. They proposed that suicidal behaviour emerges as a painful reaction to a situation involving defeat and where no avenues to escape or rescue are to be found. When these three conditions are unavoidably present in a situation, it activates the helplessness and hopelessness mode of behaviour, which may lead to suicidal behaviour (Williams and Pollock, 2000). Williams and Pollock (2000) explain that rather than the defeat itself, it is the state of entrapment in that situation that poses a danger for an individual to be involved in suicidal behaviour, because the sense of entrapment blocks the motivation to escape a situation in other ways than by ending one's life.

A more recent theory propounded by Joiner and associates (Joiner, 2005; Van Orden *et al.*, 2010) is known as the 'interpersonal theory' of suicidal behaviour and is based on thwarted belongingness, perceived burdensomeness, and acquired capability to withstand fear of death and perform lethal self-injury. This model asserts that an individual may have a desire to end his own life when he feels disconnected from others and feels that he is a burden on his significant others. This theory further states the acquisition of the ability to lethally injure oneself is a preliminary requirement for an at-risk individual to attempt or commit suicide; and without this lethal ability one would not be able to attempt suicide.

Another more recent explanation of suicidal behaviour can be seen in O'Connor's (2011) 'Integrated Motivational-Volitional (IMV) Model' that conceptualizes suicidal behaviour as being determined by a complex interaction of proximal and distal factors grouped into three phases: the pre-motivational, the motivational and the volitional phase. The pre-motivational phase includes background factors and triggering events; the motivation phase includes the generation of suicide ideation and intention formation; and the final volitional phase includes behavioural enactment and suicide attempt. One's intention to engage in suicidal behaviour is the key proximal predictor of suicidal behaviour. Taking Williams' (2001) assertions as the basis, this model also posits that suicidal intention results primarily from feelings of entrapment, which are triggered by defeat/humiliation appraisals. The IMV model describes some specific moderators that explain the transition from defeat/humiliation to entrapment, from entrapment to suicidal ideation/intent, and from suicidal ideation/intent to suicidal behaviour (Meissner, 2013).

There is another perspective to explain suicidal behaviour which looks upon suicide not as a uni-dimensional phenomenon but as a multi-dimensional one. This view gives consideration to the probability of mixed causal sequences as explained by the different perspectives above. According to this view, the suicidal person experiences unbearable psychological pain and finds no way to escape from it. The situation is traumatic. The suicidal person thinks that death is the only solution for all the problems and he is in a heightened state of disturbance explained by rejection, harassment, hopelessness and helplessness. The internal attitude of the person is ambivalent, showing acceptance and rejection at the same time. Simultaneously, many conflicts occupy the brain. The cognitive state of the person is restricted showing only one direction in thinking. Volitional motivational forces make the person take the drastic step of attempting suicide, the lethality of which is determined by the ability to self-harm and the intensity of the volitional force and accordingly it may result in completed suicide.

The sociological perspective

The major sociological interpretation of the problem of suicide was made by French sociologist, Emile Durkheim (1897/1951). He argued that suicide had less to do with the individual's own decisions and it was mainly the outcome of the societal influence on a person. In an attempt to explain suicidal behaviour by means of particular patterns of tensions between the individual and society, Durkheim categorized four types of suicide – Egoistic, Altruistic, Anomic and Fatalistic. Egoistic suicide is committed when a person has fewer ties with people. These people feel alienated from others; they enjoy less social support which is important for a person to function as a social being. Egoistic suicide is believed to occur among those people who feel socially excluded, with poor social support and lack of integration with society which results in sense of personal failure and worthlessness (O'Connor and Sheehy, 2001). Sociologists explain that fewer suicides take place among married people because of their ties with family members. Altruistic suicide is opposite to egoistic suicide as it is found among the individuals who are actually overly integrated into society. Durkheim opined that altruistic suicide is committed because of societal demands. It was described as a response to cultural expectation. Earlier in India, the Sati pratha was practised, a custom in which the widow in India threw herself on her dead husband's funeral pyre.

Anomic suicide was explained as linked with societal regulation or deregulation and it is initiated because of a sudden change in a person's relation with society. He explained anomie as a sense of disorientation which could show great vulnerability for suicide. This occurs when the societal rules guiding the lives of people do not remain appropriate and individuals become redundant. This leads to instability and alienation and, in some cases, suicide. According to Durkheim's opinion, the fatalistic suicide is considered to be prevalent in the case of excessive societal regulation where people feel that they have lost all direction in life and have no control over their own destiny (O'Connor and Sheehy, 2001). Although this sociological framework is as applicable today as it was over a hundred years ago, experts from other areas do not agree with Durkheim because the people who undergo some problems because of the sudden change in life also commit suicide. Also, Durkheim's postulations found rare empirical support and they fail to explain why a specific individual commits suicide.

Although the models proposed by a large group of researchers in this field have been discussed, there exist many other models that attempt to explain the process of suicidal behaviour in various ways but lack evidential support. However, the fact that remains common to all models is their focus on reflecting the suicidal process from initiation to attempt. The importance of understanding suicidal behaviour from multiple viewpoints lies in the basis it formulates for taking appropriate preventive measures so that human lives can be saved from such unnatural endings.

Preventing suicides

The relatively stable rates of suicide and suicidal behaviour over time highlight the need for greater attention to prevention and intervention efforts. Effective suicide prevention requires a thorough understanding of the suicidal process, which we have tried to present in the preceding sections. The extent to which we understand the dynamics underlying suicidal behaviour will help us to better identify the people at risk. Effective strategies for the prevention of suicidal behaviour should target eliminating the dynamics that perpetuate the engagement of an individual in suicidal acts. It can be seen that restricting access to lethal means and training health care professionals to identify and manage depression and suicidal behaviour are likely to contribute somehow to reducing suicide rates. Although effective prevention programmes do exist, the need for greater dissemination of information and the further development of prevention efforts is underscored by the fact that many people engaging in suicidal behaviour do not receive treatment of any kind (Nock *et al.*, 2008).

With the overall increase in suicidal behaviour, the need for effective interventions cannot be overstated. Intervention, also known as secondary prevention, refers to the healing and care of the suicidal crisis. Suicide is an event with biological (including biochemical), sociocultural, interpersonal, psychological, neuro-psychological and personal philosophical or existential aspects. Since suicide is not exclusively a medical problem, it does not always require a medical professional to save a life; a layperson too can sometimes serve as a rescuer. Even so, other professionals such as psychologists, psychiatrists, social workers, psychiatric nurses, can play a major role in suicide intervention (Leenaars *et al.*, 1994). The fundamental principle of crisis intervention programmes for suicide across the world is the belief that suicidal action is generally the product of a temporary, reversible, ambivalent state of mind (Stillion and McDowell, 1996). Suicidal behaviour involves numerous possible risk factors and most of the interventions originate from an understanding of such factors. There are several techniques for suicide intervention that are briefly outlined henceforth.

Crisis intervention

The main focus of suicide prevention efforts is on crisis intervention. The chief aim of crisis intervention is to help an individual deal with an immediate life crisis. In the case of a suicide attempt, the first step is to provide emergency medical help to the individual at a general hospital or in a clinical setting. When an individual who is considering suicide is ready to talk about his problem at a suicide prevention centre, it becomes easier to prevent an actual suicide attempt. At a crisis intervention centre, the main goal is to assist such an individual to regain his ability to cope with his immediate problems at the earliest. Emphasis is usually laid on: (1) maintaining contact with the individual over a brief period of time; (2) helping the individual understand that the acute distress is negatively affecting his capacity to evaluate the circumstances correctly and to choose from possible options; (3) helping the individual realize that other means of dealing with the crisis are present and are better than committing suicide; (4) taking a directive and supportive position; and (5) helping the individual see that the current distress and emotional turmoil will not continue forever (Carson *et al.*, 2004).

Treatment of mental disorders

The majority of those who attempt suicide suffer from a treatable mental disorder such as depression, schizophrenia, substance abuse, or borderline personality disorder. Studies and clinical experience have shown that the early identification and appropriate treatment of such disorders are an important technique to prevent suicide. In this respect, educating health care professionals to diagnose and treat mood disorder patients can help in lowering suicide rates among those who are at high risk.

Behavioural approaches

Another tradition in suicide prevention is that which concentrates on the particular characteristics of suicidal people, rather than focusing on mental disorder. Such an approach directly aims at the behaviour (Linehan, 1997). A variety of interventions have been developed, based on this approach, some of which are discussed below.

Behavioural interventions

Behavioural interventions involve a mental health worker conducting therapy sessions with the patient, and discussing prior and present suicidal behaviour and suicidal ideation, and trying to ascertain associations with possibly underlying causal factors (Linehan, 1997). A study was conducted by Salkovskis, Atha and Storer (1990) on patients at high risk of multiple suicide attempts, who had been admitted to an emergency ward because of taking an antidepressants overdose. The patients were given either the standard treatment for suicide attempts or the standard treatment along with a brief 'problem-oriented' intervention – a form of short-term psychotherapy that centred on the problem which was found to be bothering the patient most. The study found a significant advantage for those receiving the intervention along with the standard treatment six months after treatment, in terms of a reduction in their rates of repeated suicide attempts. Another study conducted by Linehan, Heard and Armstrong (1993) investigated the efficacy of dialectical behaviour therapy with those patients who exhibited borderline personality disorders, multiple behavioural dysfunction, significant mental disorders and a history of multiple suicide attempts. The findings revealed a positive outcome during the first year among patients who had received the therapy as compared to those who received standard treatment. In another study, MacLeod and colleagues (MacLeod *et al.*, 1998) showed the effectiveness of manual-assisted cognitive behaviour therapy in achieving significant improvements in suicidal patients with a history of attempting suicide and displaying a deficit in positive future thinking.

Quick help interventions

Recently some new programmes have been developed to provide immediate help to the individual who is showing any hint of suicidal behaviour. In this type of intervention, the patient or client is given an opportunity to be in touch with any medical or other professionals at a difficult time. The Green card technique is one of them. In the Green card intervention, the clients are given a card, carrying a direct and immediate access to a variety of options, such as an on-call psychiatrist or hospitalization. It has been shown that the Green card is beneficial for those considering suicide for the first time (Cotgrove *et al.*, 1995; Morgan *et al.*, 1993). The Tele-Help/Tele-Check service for the elderly operating in Italy is another intervention technique which is based on the tenet of availability of help and easy access (De Leo *et al.*, 1995). Tele-Help is an alarm system that the client can activate to call for help. The Tele-Check service keeps in touch with the clients and calls them twice a week to check on their needs and provide emotional support. This intervention technique has been also found to be quite effective by means of promoting faster help availability (De Leo *et al.*, 1995).

Relationship-based approaches

It is known that social relationships play an important role in determining the vulnerability to suicide: the more social relationships a person has in his life, the less he is vulnerable to suicide (Litman and Wold, 1976). Many interventions aim to increase social relationships so as to lessen repeated suicidal behaviour as bringing about an improvement in social ties is regarded as vital by the therapist. Such interventions improve in social relationships, which in turn serves as available help for the person under crisis. A particular outreach method, known as 'continuing relationship maintenance' (CRM) has been found to be effective by Litman and Wold (1976). This approach involves an active reaching out to the patient by the counsellor who strives to keep a regular connection with him. The improvements resulting from this method included reduced loneliness, more satisfactory intimate relationships, less depression and greater confidence in using community services. The efficacy of 'task-centred casework' – a problem-solving method that lays stress on the collaboration between a patient and a social worker over matters related to daily living was shown by Gibbons *et al.* (1978) and a greater improvement in handling social problems was shown by the group that received task-centred casework. In another study conducted by Hawton *et al.* (1987), a significant proportion of the out-patient group who received counselling focused on relationship building showed improvements in social adjustment, marital adjustment and relationships with their families.

Community-based efforts

It is observed that instead of treatment of suicide-related behaviour of the individual, the emphasis should be on the whole community so that this menace is prevented at a broader level rather than treated at a narrower level. Some of the community-based interventions that may prove vital to help curb the suicide problem may be as discussed in the following sections.

Suicide prevention centres

Apart from the intervention techniques discussed above, there is also specific community mental health services for individuals who exhibit suicidal behaviour. There are suicide prevention centres intended to serve as crisis centres that offer instant help, often over the telephone, but programmes with face-to-face counselling and outreach work are also used. In a study conducted by Lester (1997), 14 studies that examined the effectiveness of suicide prevention centres on suicide rates were reviewed. Seven out of these studies offered some confirmation for a preventive effect of these centres.

School-based interventions

In an attempt to train school staff, community members and health care providers to identify those at risk from suicide and refer them to appropriate mental health services, various programmes have been designed. The training varies from programme to programme, but in every case a strong link to local mental health services is necessary. It may be noted that the importance of mental health professionals cannot be undermined despite the training of school staff members, parents and others involved in school programmes. Yet, health care facilities solely cannot fulfil all the demands of young people, and thus school-based interventions play an important role in suicide prevention.

Multi-systemic approach

Multi-systemic therapy was initially designed for adolescents with conduct disorder, but has been modified later for adolescents with severe mental health problems, including attempted suicide (Henggeler *et al.*, 2002). This therapy involves assessment of the risk of suicide, followed by intensive family therapy to improve family support along with individual skills training for adolescents to assist them develop mood-regulation and social problem-solving skills, along with intervention in the wider school and interagency network to lower stress and improve support for the adolescent. The technique also involves regular, frequent, home-based family and individual therapy sessions, with additional sessions in the school or community settings, for over a period of three–six months. It has been found that multisystemic therapy was considerably more successful in lowering rates of attempted suicide at one-year follow-up as compared to emergency hospitalization and treatment by a multidisciplinary psychiatric team (Huey *et al.*, 2004).

Societal approaches

Experts in social sciences are of the view that the concentration should not only be on the individual but also on the social environment in which the problem behaviour is occurring. They propose some changes in the environment so that the undesired behaviour should not occur.

Restricting access to means

Restricting access to the means of suicide can play an important role in preventing suicide. This was first shown in Australia by Oliver and Hetzel (1972), who found that suicide rates lowered when access to sedatives – mainly barbiturates, which are lethal in high doses – was restricted. Besides, there is also evidence of a decline in suicide rates when access to other toxic substances such as pesticides is restricted. Gas detoxification – the removal of carbon monoxide from domestic gas and from car exhausts – has proved effective in decreasing the rates of suicide. Soon after carbon monoxide was removed from domestic gas, suicides from poisoning with domestic gas began to decline in England (Kreitman, 1972) and subsequently in many other countries (Lester, 1998). The link between the presence of handguns at home and suicide rates has also been observed (Carrington and Moyer, 1994; Kellermann *et al.*, 1992). There are numerous approaches to lowering gun-injuries, by means of restricting access to them. These often focus on legislation on sales and ownership of guns and on gun safety. Gun safety measures include education and training, different practices of gun storage (like separate storage of guns and ammunition, and keeping guns unloaded and in locked places) and trigger-blocking devices. Restrictions on the ownership of firearms have been linked with a decrease in their use for suicide in some countries such as Canada, the United States and Australia (Carrington and Moyer, 1994; Lester, 1998). Hence, societal measures may also help in adopting suicide preventive measures.

Conclusion

Suicide is a behavioural and social problem which is affecting each and every society. The clear understanding of the nature of the dynamics underlying suicidal behaviour is of paramount importance when designing effective preventive mechanisms. Suicide is a multidimensional phenomenon and different theoretical perspectives provide crucial insights to find the roots of the huge problem of suicide. Undoubtedly suicide is a problem not only for the person who commits it but also for the family, other relatives and the entire society. There is the utmost requirement to put adequate preventive measures in place to deal with this social menace. There is a need for continued dedicated research efforts to explore further, and social scientists along with medical professionals need to work in collaboration to prevent and treat this menace.

References

Amitai, M. and Apter, A. (2012). Social aspects of suicidal behavior and prevention in early life: A review. *International Journal of Environmental Research and Public Health*, 9(3), 985–994.

Baechler, J. (1979). *Suicides*. New York: Basic Books.

Bandura, A. (1977). *Social Learning Theory*. Englewood Cliffs, NJ: Prentice Hall.

Baumeister, R. F. (1990). Suicide as an escape from self. *Psychological Review*, 97(1), 90–113.

Beck, A. T., Davis, J. H., Frederick, C. J., Perlin, S., Pokorny, A. D., Schulman, R. E. *et al.* (1972). Classification and nomenclature. In H. L. P. Resnik and B. C. Hathorne (Eds), *Suicide Prevention in the Seventies* (pp. 7–12). Washington, DC: Government Printing Office.

Beck, A. T., Steer, R. A., Kovacs, M. M., and Garrison, B. (1985). Hopelessness and eventual suicide: A 10-year prospective study of patients hospitalized with suicidal ideation. *American Journal of Psychiatry*, 142(5), 559–563.

Beck, A. T., Steer, R. A., and Ranieri, W. (1988). Scale for suicide ideation: Psychometric properties of a self-report version. *Journal of Clinical Psychology*, 44(4), 499–505.

Bursztein, C., and Apter, A. (2009). Adolescent suicide. *Current Opinion in Psychiatry*, 22(1), 1–6.

Carrington, P. J., and Moyer, M. A. (1994). Gun control and suicide in Ontario. *American Journal of Psychiatry*, 151(4), 606–608.

Carson, R. C., Butcher, J. M., and Mineka, S. (2004). *Abnormal Psychology and Modern Life* (11th edn). Delhi: Pearson Education, Inc.

Clark, D. C. (1995). Epidemiology, assessment, and management of suicide in depressed patients. In E. E. Beckham and W. R. Leber (Eds), *Handbook of Depression* (2nd edn) (pp. 526–538). New York: Guilford.

Cotgrove, A., Zirinsky, L., Black, D., and Weston, D. (1995). Secondary prevention of attempted suicide in adolescence. *Journal of Adolescence*, 18(5), 569–577.

Crosby, A. E., Cheltenham, M. P., and Sacks, J. J. (1999). Incidence of suicidal ideation and behavior in the United States, 1994. *Suicide and Life-Threatening Behavior*, 29(2), 131–140.

De Leo, D., Burgis, S., Bertolote, J. M., Kerkhof, A. J., and. Bille-Brahe, U. (2006). Definitions of suicidal behavior: Lessons learned from the WHO/EURO Multicentre Study. *Crisis: The Journal of Crisis Intervention and Suicide Prevention*, 27(1), 4–15.

De Leo, D., Carollo, G., and Dello Buono, M. (1995). Lower suicide rates associated with a tele-help/tele-check service for the elderly at home. *American Journal of Psychiatry*, 152(4), 632–634.

Durkheim, E. (1897/1951). *Suicide: A Study in Sociology* (J. A. Spaulding and G. Simpson, Trans. Eds). London: The Free Press.

Eyman, J. R., and Eyman, S. K. (1992). Psychological testing for potentially suicidal individuals. In B. Bongar (Ed.), *Suicide: Guidelines for Assessment, Management and Treatment* (pp. 127–143). New York: Oxford University Press.

Freud, S. (1917). *Mourning and Melancholia XVII* (2nd edn.). New York: Hogarth Press.

Garland, A. F., and Zigler, E. (1993). Adolescent suicide prevention: Current research and social policy implications. *American Psychologists*, 48(2), 169–182.

Gibbons, J. S., Butler, J., Urwin, P., and Gibbons, J. L. (1978). Evaluation of a social work service for self-poisoning patients. *British Journal of Psychiatry*, 133(2), 111–118.

Gvion. Y., and Apter, A. (2012). Suicide and suicidal behavior. *Public Health Reviews*, 34(1), 1–20.

Hawton, K., McKeown, S., Day, A., Martin, P., O'Connor, M., and Yule, J. (1987). Evaluation of outpatient counseling compared with general practitioner care following overdoses. *Psychological Medicine*, 17(3), 751–761.

Henggeler, S. W., Schoenwald, S. K., Rowland, M. D., and Cunningham, P. B. (2002). *Serious Emotional Disturbance in Children and Adolescents: Multisystemic Therapy*. New York: Guilford Press.

Huey, S. J., Jr., Henggeler, S. W., Rowland, M. D., Halliday-Boykins, C. A., Cunningham, P. C., Pickrel, S. G., and Edwards, J. (2004). Multisystemic therapy effects on attempted suicide by youths presenting psychiatric emergencies. *Journal of the American Academy of Child and Adolescent Psychiatry*, 43(2), 183–190.

Joiner, T. (2005). *Why People Die by Suicide*. Cambridge, MA: Harvard University Press.

Kellermann, A. L., Rivara, F. P., Somes, G., Reay, D. T., Francisco, J., Banton J. G., *et al.* (1992). Suicide in the home in relation to gun ownership. *New England Journal of Medicine*, 327(7), 467–472.

Kinderman, P. (2005). A psychological model of mental disorder. *Harvard Review of Psychiatry*, 13(4), 206–217.

Kreitman, N. (1972). The coal gas history: United Kingdom suicide rates, 1960–1971. *British Journal of Preventive and Social Medicine*, 30(2), 86–93.

Leenaars, A. A. (2010). Edwin S. Shneidman on suicide. *Suicidology Online*, 1(1), 5–18.

Leenaars, A. A., Maltsberger, J. T., and Neimeyer, R. A. (1994). *Treatment of Suicidal People*. New York: Routledge.

Lester, D. (1997). The effectiveness of suicide prevention centres: A review. *Suicide and Life-Threatening Behaviour*, 27(3), 304–310.

Lester, D. (1998). Preventing suicide by restricting access to methods for suicide. *Archives of Suicide Research*, 4(1), 7–24.

Linehan, M. M. (1997). Behavioural treatments of suicidal behaviours: Definitional obfuscation and treatment outcomes. In D. M. Stoff and J. J. Mann (Eds), *The Neurobiology of Suicide: From the Bench to the Clinic* (pp. 302–328). New York: New York Academy of Sciences.

Linehan, M. M., Heard, H. L., and Armstrong, H. E. (1993). Naturalistic follow-up of a behavioural treatment for chronically parasuicidal borderline patients. *Archives of General Psychiatry*, 50(12), 971–974.

Litman, R. E., and Wold, C. I. (1976). Beyond crisis intervention. In E. S. Schneidman (Ed.), *Suicidology, Contemporary Developments* (pp. 528–546). New York: Grune & Stratton.

MacLeod, A. K., Tata, P., Evans, K., Tyrer, P., Schmidt, U., Davidson, K., *et al.* (1998). Recovery of positive future thinking within a high-risk parasuicide group: Results from a pilot randomised controlled trial. *British Journal of Clinical Psychology*, 37(4), 371–379.

Mann, J. J. (2003). Neurobiology of suicidal behaviour. *Nature Reviews Neuroscience*, 4(10), 819–828.

Maris, R. W., Berman, A. L., and Silverman, M. M. (2000). *Comprehensive Textbook of Suicidology*. New York: The Guilford Press.

Mayo, D. J. (1992). What is being predicted? The definition of 'suicide.' In R. Maris, A. Berman, J. Maltsberger, and R. Yufit (Eds), *Assessment and Prediction of Suicide*, (pp. 88–101). New York: Guilford.

McLaughlin, C. (2007). *Suicide-related Behavior Understanding, Caring and Therapeutic Responses*. Chichester: John Wiley & Sons.

Meissner, B. L. (2013). Attitudes, beliefs and myths about suicidal behaviour: A qualitative investigation of South African male students. Master of Science thesis. Stellenbosch University, South Africa.

Menninger, K. (1938). *Man against Himself.* New York: Harcourt, Brace.

Morgan, H. G., Jones, E. M., and Owen, J. H. (1993). Secondary prevention of non-fatal deliberate self-harm: The Green Card Study. *British Journal of Psychiatry*, 163(1), 111–112.

Nock, M. K., Borges, G., Bromet, E. J., Cha, C. B., Kessler, R. C., and Lee, S. (2008). Suicide and suicidal behavior. *Epidemiologic Reviews*, 30(1), 133–154.

O'Carroll, P. W., Berman, A. L., Maris, R. W., Moscicki, E. K., Tanney, B. L., and Silverman, M. M. (1996). Beyond the Tower of Babel: A nomenclature for suicidology. *Suicide and Life Threatening Behaviour*, 26(3), 237–252.

O'Connor, R. C. (2011). Towards an integrated motivational-volitional model of suicidal behaviour. In R. C. O'Connor, S. Platt and J. Gordon (Eds), *International Handbook of Suicide Prevention: Research, Policy and Practice* (pp. 181–198). Chichester: John Wiley & Sons Ltd.

O'Connor, R. C., and Sheehy, N. P. (2001). Suicidal behaviour. *The Psychologist*, 14(1), 20–24.

Oliver, R. G., and Hetzel, B. S. (1972). Rise and fall of suicide rates in Australia: Relation to sedative availability. *Medical Journal of Australia*, 2(17), 919–923.

Orbach, I. (2007). Self-destructive processes and suicide. *Israel Journal of Psychiatry and Related Sciences*, 44(4), 266–279.

Patel, V., Ramasundarahettige, C., Vijayakumar, L., Thakur, J. S., Gajalakshmi, V., Gururaj, G., *et al.* (2012). Suicide mortality in India: A nationally representative survey. *Lancet*, 379(9834), 2343–2351.

Rosenberg, M. L., Davidson, L. E., Smith, J. C., Berman, A. L., Buzbee, H., Gantner, G., *et al.* (1988). Operational criteria for the determination of suicide. *Journal of Forensic Sciences*, 33(6), 1445–1456.

Salkovskis, P. M., Atha, C., and Storer, D. (1990). Cognitive behavioural problem-solving in the treatment of patients who repeatedly attempt suicide: A controlled trial. *British Journal of Psychiatry*, 157(6), 871–876.

Shneidman, E. S. (1985). *Definition of Suicide*. Northvale, NJ: Jason Aronson Incorporated.

Shneidman, E. S. (1993). *Suicide as Psychache: A Clinical Approach to Self-destructive Behavior*. Lanham, MD: Jason Aronson Incorporated.

Silverman, M. M., and Maris, R. W. (1995). The prevention of suicidal behaviors: An overview. *Suicide and Life-Threatening Behavior*, 25(1), 10–21.

Silverman, M. M., Berman, A. L., Sanddal, N. D., O'Carroll, P. W., and Joiner, T. E (2007a). Rebuilding the Tower of Babel: A revised nomenclature for the study of suicide and suicidal behaviors: Part 1: Background, rationale, and methodology. *Suicide and Life-Threatening Behavior*, 37(3), 248–263.

Silverman, M. M., Berman, A. L., Sanddal, N. D., O'Carroll, P. W., and Joiner, T. E (2007b). Rebuilding the Tower of Babel: A revised nomenclature for the study of suicide and suicidal behaviors: Part II: Suicide-related ideations, communications and behaviors. *Suicide and Life-Threatening Behavior*, 37(3), 264–277.

Singh, A. R., and Singh, S. A. (2003). Preface, Towards a suicide-free society: Identify suicide prevention as public health policy. *Mens Sana Monographs*, 2, 0–1.

Stillion, M., and McDowell, E. E. (1996). *Suicide across the Life Span* (2nd edn). Washington, DC: Taylor & Francis.

Van Orden, K. A., Witte, T. K., Cukrowicz, K. C., Braithwaite, S. R., Selby, E. A., and Joiner, T. E. Jr. (2010). The Interpersonal theory of suicide. *Psychological Review*, 117(2), 575–600.

Van Pragg, H. M. (2001). Suicide and aggression: Are they biologically two sides of the same coin? In D. Lester (Ed.), *Suicide Prevention: Resources for the New Millennium* (pp. 45–64). Philadelphia, PA: Brunner-Routledge.

Van Tuan, N. (2010). *Mental Disorders and Attempted Suicides in Vietnam*. Stockholm: Karolinska Institute.

Vijayakumar, L. (2007). Suicide and its prevention: The urgent need in India. *Indian Journal of Psychiatry*, 49(2), 81–84.

Williams, J. M. G. (1997). *The Cry of Pain*. London: Penguin.

Williams, J. M. G. (2001). *Suicide and Attempted Suicide. Understanding the Cry of Pain*. London: Penguin.

Williams, J. M. G., and Pollock, L. R. (2000). The psychology of suicidal behaviour. In K. Hawton and K. van Heeringen (Eds), *The International Handbook of Suicide and Attempted Suicide* (pp. 79–93). Chichester: John Wiley & Sons.

World Health Organization (1986). *Summary Report, Working Group in Preventative Practices in Suicide and Attempted Suicide.* Copenhagen: WHO Regional Office for Europe.

World Health Organization (1992). *International Classification of Diseases – 10.* Geneva: World Health Organization.

World Health Organization (1998). *Primary Prevention of Mental, Neurological and Psychosocial Disorders.* Geneva: World Health Organization.

World Health Organization (1999). *Figures and Facts about Suicide.* Geneva: World Health Organization.

World Health Organization (2002). Self-directed violence. In E. G. Krug, L. L. Dahlberg, J. A. Mercy, A. B. Zwi, and R. Lozano (Eds), *World Report on Violence and Health* (pp. 183–212). Geneva: World Health Organization.

World Health Organization (2012). Country reports and charts available. Geneva: World Health Organization. Retrieved from www.who.int/mental_health/prevention/suicide/country_reports/en/index.html

2   Genetics of suicidal behavior

Marco Sarchiapone and Miriam Iosue

Suicidal behavior represents one of the most complex human behaviors, influenced by the action of several biological, psychological and social factors. To try to explain this complexity, the stress–diathesis model was proposed, suggesting that the vulnerability to suicide is determined by a variety of predisposing (distal) risk factors on which stressful life events and other potentiating (proximal) factors act as triggers (Mann *et al.*, 1999; Mościcki, 1997). In this sense, the person's genetic make-up constitutes one of the most important predisposing factors contributing to the suicide vulnerability.

It is now well established that suicide clusters in families and that genetic factors seem to play a role in 30 percent–50 percent of cases with suicidal behavior (McGuffin *et al.*, 2001; Roy *et al.*, 1995). The inheritance of suicidal behavior seems to be linked to two main components: the predisposition to psychiatric disorders and the predisposition to impulsiveness–aggressiveness traits. However, the presence of genetic risk factors does not imply a deterministic mechanism since the inheritance of suicidal behavior is related to the interaction of multiple genes and the influences of the environment.

Family, adoption and twin studies

The aim of family studies on suicidal behavior is to compare its rates in the relatives of subjects who showed or did not show this behavior. It is now well established that suicidal behavior aggregates within families and that individuals with a family history of suicidal behavior are at increased risk of both attempting and committing suicide when compared with individuals without such a family history.

In 1982, Murphy and Wetzel collected the family history of suicidal behaviors (suicide, attempted suicide, and suicide threats) of 127 patients hospitalized after a suicide attempt. They found that 16 percent of patients with a diagnosis of primary affective disorder had a family history of suicide and 17 percent had a family history of suicide attempts (Murphy and Wetzel, 1982). In 1983, Roy studied patients with a wide variety of diagnoses, such as schizophrenia, unipolar and bipolar affective disorders, depressive neurosis, and personality disorders. Almost half (48.6 percent) of the patients with a family history of suicide had attempted suicide. Comparing these patients with patients without a family history of suicide, Roy found that a family history of suicide significantly increased the risk for suicide attempt (Roy, 1983). In the same year, Tsuang studied the risk of suicide in the first-degree relatives of schizophrenic, manic-depressive and depressive patients in comparison with relatives of surgical controls, finding an almost eight time higher risk of suicide among relatives of psychiatric patients. Moreover, relatives of psychiatric patients who had committed suicide, when compared with the relatives of patients who didn't, showed a four-fold higher risk of suicide (Tsuang, 1983).

Egeland and Sussex (1985) ascertained suicides for a 100-year period (1880 to 1980) in the Amish community in Lancaster County, Pennsylvania, showing that suicides cluster in pedigrees. Indeed, of the 26 people who had committed suicide, 19 (73 percent) were clustered in four primary pedigrees, containing a heavy loading for affective disorders and suicide. They concluded that this clustering of suicides followed the distribution of affective disorders in the kinship, thus suggesting the role of inheritance. However, they also found family pedigrees with heavy loadings for affective disorders but without suicides suggesting that their presence was not in itself a predictor for suicidal behavior.

Similar results were reported not only among psychiatric patients (Powell, 2000; Tsai et al., 2002), but also among adolescents and young people (Shafii et al., 1985) and in the general population (Kim et al., 2005; Qin et al., 2002; Qin, 2003; Runeson and Asberg, 2003). For example, Runeson and Asberg (2003) found that the rate of suicide was twice as high in the families of suicide victims than in the families of comparison subjects who died of other causes and that, despite the strong connection between suicide and mental disorder, a family history of suicide was a significant risk factor independent of severe mental disorder.

All these findings demonstrated that a familial transmission of suicide exists and that it is at least partly distinct from the familial transmission of psychiatric disorders often associated with suicidal behavior. Moreover, as noted by Brent and Mann (2005), these studies showed how suicide attempt and completion are linked to the transmission of a unique clinical phenotype of suicidal behavior, since the rate of suicide is elevated in the families of attempters, and the rate of attempted suicide is elevated in the families of suicide completers.

Nevertheless, family studies can only prove that there is a familial aggregation of suicidal behavior but they are not able to distinguish how much this transmission is due to genetic or environmental factors (Brent and Mann, 2005). Stronger evidence of a genetic susceptibility to suicidal behavior came from adoption and twin studies. Adoption studies are designed to evaluate genetic and environmental influences on phenotype through the study of first-degree relatives reared in different families and environments. One of the first studies was performed in Denmark by Schulsinger et al. (1979) using the Danish adoption registry. They compared the rates of suicide among the biological and adoptive relatives of 57 adoptees who committed suicide and among the biological and adoptive relatives of 57 matched living adoptees. They found a six-fold higher rate of suicidal behavior in the biological relatives of adoptees who committed suicide. Moreover, none of the adoptive relatives of both suicide and control cases committed suicide. Since 50 percent of the biological relatives of suicide subjects had never had contact with psychiatric services, it was possible to suppose that they did not suffer any psychiatric disorder thus confirming that suicidal behavior is at least partially independent of the presence of psychiatric disorders. Using the same adoption registry, Wender *et al.* (1986) compared biological and adoptive relatives of adult adoptees with and without mood disorder. The biological relatives of the adoptees with mood disorder showed a 15-fold increase of suicide, and this was particularly true for adoptees with a diagnosis of 'affective reaction' which includes the inability to control impulsive behavior.

Twin studies compare the similarity of monozygotic (MZ) and dizygotic (DZ) twins. Monozygotic twins share the same genes, instead dizygotic twins share only 50 percent of them, for this reason if the trait similarity of monozygotic twins is significantly higher than the similarity of dizygotic twins, this indicates that genes play an important role in this trait.

Several studies demonstrated that MZ twin pairs have significantly greater concordance for suicidal behavior than DZ twin pairs (Kallmann and Anastasio, 1947; Roy *et al.*, 1991; Segal, 2009). Roy, Segal and Sarchiapone (1995) investigated suicide attempts among 35 living co-twins whose twin had committed suicide, finding that 10 of the 26 living MZ co-twins had themselves attempted suicide, compared with 0 of the 9 living DZ co-twins ($p < 0.04$). Statham *et al.* (1998) studied a very large sample of 5,995 Australian twins. The concordance rates were higher for both suicidal thoughts and for serious suicide attempts in the MZ twins than in the DZ twins. After controlling for other risk factors for suicide, such as psychiatric disorder, traumatic events and neuroticism, a history of suicide attempts or persistent thoughts in the respondent's co-twin remained a powerful predictor in MZ pairs (odds ratio = 3.9), but was not consistently predictive in DZ pairs. The authors concluded that, overall, genetic factors accounted for approximately 45 percent of the variance in suicidal thoughts and behavior.

Even if adoption and twin studies demonstrate the existence of genetic risk factors for suicidal behavior, there are several methodological limitations in these approaches (Brent and Mann, 2005; Lester, 2002) and they are not able to identify what these genetic factors are which are being transmitted.

Candidate gene approach studies

Given the strong association with depression, the main focus of genetic studies on suicide was the serotonin system. Studies suggested a role of serotonin in suicide. Indeed, a low cerebrospinal fluid (CSF) concentration of 5-hydroxyindoleacetic acid (5-HLAA), which is the main metabolite of serotonin, was associated with increased impulsiveness, impaired control of aggressive behavior and suicide attempts (Asberg *et al.*, 1976; Linnoila and Virkkunen, 1992; Virkkunen *et al.*, 1995).

Tryptophan hydroxylase (TPH) studies

Tryptophan is an essential amino acid for serotonin synthesis and the tryptophan hydroxylase (TPH) is the initial and rate-limiting enzyme in the biosynthesis of serotonin. In humans there are two TPH isoenzymes encoded by two genes. TPH1 was the first to be identified and it is located on the short arm of chromosome 11 (11p15.3—p14). The second (TPH2) is located on the long arm of chromosome 12 (12q21.1). An association between suicidal behavior and TPH1 polymorphism was first reported by Nielsen (1994), investigating 56 impulsive and 14 non-impulsive, alcoholic, violent offenders and 20 healthy volunteers. They found a significant association between TPH genotype and CSF 5-HIAA concentration in the extreme impulsive group. In particular, the impulsive alcoholics with the LL or UL genotype showed the lowest CSF 5-HIAA concentrations. Since a history of suicide attempts was significantly associated with UL or LL genotype in all of the alcoholic offenders, the presence of the L allele may influence the predisposition to suicidal behavior. Most of the studies investigated the TPH1 intron 7 A218C single nucleotide polymorphism (SNP) finding conflicting results. Bellivier *et al.* (1998) compared the TPH intron 7 A218C polymorphism in DNA samples from 152 bipolar disorder patients and 94 normal controls. They found that the risk of bipolar disorder was increased by the presence of at least one copy of the TPH A allele, and the risk was higher for TPH A–homozygous subjects. Nevertheless this TPH polymorphism was not associated with a history of suicide attempts. Lalovic and Turecki (2002) conducted a meta-analysis on 17 publications concluding that the association between suicidal behavior and an intron 7 polymorphism of the TPH1 gene was not demonstrated. However, the studies on this polymorphism continued and more recent meta-analyses confirmed its association with suicidal behavior (Li and He, 2006; Rujescu *et al.*, 2003). Galfalvy *et al.* (2009) published a perspective study of 343 patients with a Major Depressive Episode who were monitored for suicide attempts for up to one year. The patients were genotyped for polymorphisms A218C in intron 7 and A-6526G in the promoter region of TPH1. Both the AA genotype on intron 7 and the AA genotype on the promoter predicted suicide attempts during the one-year follow-up and were associated with past attempts at high medical lethality. Baud *et al.* (2009) offered a possible explanation of the role of TPH1 genotype in the predisposition to suicidal behavior. In their study, suicide attempters carrying the AA genotype in intron 7 showed reduced capacity to control anger, which is one of the most important risk factor for suicide ideation and attempt.

After the identification of the second gene encoding for TPH (TPH2), the focus of research shifted to this gene, especially because it is highly expressed in the brain regions. Zill *et al.* (2004) reported an association of SNPs and a haplotype with completed suicide, even if these findings were not confirmed by De Luca *et al.* (2005) in schizophrenic patients. Recently, Fudalej *et al.* (2010) showed a higher frequency of the TT genotype in the TPH2 SNP (rs1386483) in suicide victims than controls, and this difference was particularly higher for those with a history of repeated suicide attempts.

Serotonin transporter (5-HTT) studies

The serotonin transporter (5-HTT) regulates the serotonergic transmission, since it is involved in the reuptake of serotonin from the synaptic gap. Mann *et al.* (2000) collected postmortem brain samples from 220 individuals and found that binding to 5-HTT was lower in the ventral prefrontal cortex of suicides compared with nonsuicides. This alteration of 5-HTT binding in suicidal individuals could be explained by differences in the 5-HTT gene. The most studied is a polymorphism in the promoter region of the serotonin transporter gene (5-HTTLPR) due to a 44 base pair deletion (SS)/insertion (LL) (Heils *et al.*, 2002). The homozygote (SS) and heterozygote (SL) short forms of the 5-HTTLPR locus are associated with fewer binding sites than in the long form homozygote (LL). Bondy *et al.* (2000) compared Caucasian suicide victims and healthy controls and reported a highly significant increased frequency of one or two short alleles in suicide victims, independent of the clinical diagnosis. On the contrary, Mann *et al.* (2000) reported that the 5-HTTLPR genotype was associated with major depression but not with suicide or 5-HTT binding. A meta-analysis (Lin and Tsai, 2004) supported the association of the short allele of 5-HTTLPR polymorphism especially with violent suicidal behavior in the psychiatric population. Similarly, Wasserman *et al.* (2007) reported a higher occurrence of the S allele among suicide attempters with a high medical damage.

5-HT receptors studies

A number of studies investigated the link between serotonin receptors and suicidal behavior, finding conflicting results. A recent meta-analysis concerning 5-HTR1A concluded that the SNP C-1019G variant (rs6295) was not associated with suicidal behavior (González-Castro *et al.*, 2013). Similarly, a significant association between the HTR1B G861C polymorphism and suicidal behavior was not confirmed (Kia-Keating *et al.*, 2007). Turecki *et al.* (1999) demonstrated that 5-HTR2A binding was greater in the prefrontal cortex of suicide victims. They also investigated two polymorphisms of the 5-HTR2A gene (T102C and A-1438G) which significantly affected the receptor's binding, even if no interaction between suicidal behavior and this locus was observed. Saiz and colleagues (2008) compared suicide attempters and controls, reporting no differences between the two groups in the genotype and allele distributions of two 5-HT2A polymorphism, A-1438G (rs6311) and T102C (rs6313). Nevertheless, they found an excess of the −1438A allele in nonimpulsive suicide attempts. Turecki and colleagues (2003) investigated variation in genes that code for seven serotonin receptors (5-HTR1B, 5-HTR1Dα, 5-HTR1E, 5-HTR1F, 5-HTR2C, 5-HTR5A and 5-HTR6) and observed no differences in allelic or genotypic distributions between suicide victims and controls.

The small sample sizes of the studies may have affected their power for detection of genetic effects, moreover other 5-HT receptors were not sufficiently investigated (Anguelova *et al.*, 2003; Wasserman *et al.*, 2009).

Monoamine oxidase (MAO) studies

Monoamine oxidases (MAO) are enzymes involved in the catabolism of amines (serotonin, noradrenaline and dopamine). In humans there are two MAO isoforms (MAO-A and MAO-B). The gene for MAO-A is located on the X chromosome (Xp11.23) and the promoter of the gene contains a functional polymorphism consisting of a 30-bp repeated sequence present in 3, 3.5, 4, or 5 copies. Alleles with 3.5 or 4 copies of the repeat sequence are transcribed 2–10 times more efficiently than those with 3 or 5 copies of the repeat (Sabol *et al.*, 1998). Genetic studies in mice linked deficiencies in MAO-A gene function to increased aggression (Cases *et al.*, 1995), which is an important risk factor for suicide (Gvion and Apter, 2011; Linnoila and Virkkunen, 1992). Caspi (2002) found that male maltreated children with a genotype conferring high levels of MAO-A expression were less likely to develop antisocial problems in adulthood. Prichard *et al.* (2008) did not find an association between the MAO-A genotype and antisocial behavior, while Weder *et al.* (2009) reported a significant inter-action between moderate levels of trauma exposure and the 'low-activity' MAOA genotype in conferring risk for aggression. The literature concerning the associa-tion of this polymorphism with suicidal behavior showed conflicting results. Ho *et al.* (2000) reported that MAOA polymorphism was associated with history of suicide attempts in bipolar subjects, especially females. Ono and colleagues (2002) did not find evidence of association with completed suicides. Courtet *et al.* (2005) did not confirm an association with suicide attempts, even if an excess of high-activity MAO-A gene promoter alleles was associated with violent methods of suicide attempt. A recent meta-analysis (Hung *et al.*, 2012) concluded that there is no association between the polymorphism and suicidal behaviors.

Catechol-O-methyltransferase (COMT) studies

The catechol-O-methyltransferase (COMT) is an enzyme involved in the catecholamines' inactivation. A functional polymorphism in the COMT gene (COMT-V158M) was described as associated with lower enzymatic activity (Weinshilboum *et al.*, 1999). Rujescu *et al.* (2003) linked this polymor-phism to suicidal behavior and anger-related traits. Ono *et al.* (2004) found that the frequency of the Val/Val genotype, a high-activity COMT genotype, was significantly less in suicide completers than in controls, but only in males. Zalsman *et al.* (2008) excluded an association between the polymorphism and suicidal behavior in mood disorder patients. A meta-analysis (Kia-Keating *et al.*, 2007) suggested an association between COMT and suicidal behavior and highlighted possible gender differences. However, a further meta-analysis (Tovilla-Zárate *et al.*, 2011) did not confirm these results, suggesting that additional studies are needed.

Neutrophins studies

Neurotrophins are a family of polypeptide growth factors, present in all vertebrate species, which influence the proliferation, differentiation, and survival of neuronal cells. The Brain Derived Neurotrophic Factor (BDNF) is a neutrophin involved in neuronal and plasticity of serotonergic and dopaminergic neurons. The BDNF gene lies on the reverse strand of chromosome 11p13 and encodes a precursor peptide pro-BDNF. The tyrosine kinase B (TrkB) is the BDNF receptor. Dwivedi *et al.* (2003) reported a significant reduction in the mRNA levels of BDNF and TrkB in both the prefrontal cortex and hippocampus of suicide subjects compared with nonpsychiatric healthy controls. Similar results were described also for teenage suicide victims (Pandey *et al.*, 2008). Karege *et al.* (2005) reported a significant decrease in BDNF levels in the hippocampus and PFC but not in the entorhinal cortex, of suicide victims, suggesting that a decrease in BDNF may be specific only to certain brain areas.

A single nucleotide polymorphism in the BDNF gene, leading to a valine (Val) to methionine (Met) substitution at codon 66 in the prodomain (BDNFMet), was identified. Kim *et al.* (2008) showed a 4.9-fold higher risk of suicide attempts in bipolar patients with the Met/Met genotype compared those with the Val/Val genotype. We genotyped 170 depressed patients for the BDNF Val66Met polymorphism (Sarchiapone *et al.*, 2008), finding a significant association between this polymorphism and suicidal behavior, even if a further analysis on 512 subjects did not confirm this result (Zarrilli *et al.*, 2009). However, GXE and epigenetic studies provided additional evidence of the role of BDNF in the pathogenesis of suicidal behavior.

Corticotropin-releasing hormone (CRH) studies

Hyperactivity of the hypothalamic-pituitary-adrenal (HPA) axis seems to be linked to suicidal behavior (Jokinen and Nordström, 2009). The HPA axis is responsible for stress response and it is regulated by the corticotrophin-releasing hormone (CRH). CRH is a hypothalamic factor that stimulates the pituitary gland, binding two receptors, CRHR1 and CRHR2. Wasserman *et al.* (2008) analyzed SNPs in the CRHR1 gene in 542 family trios with suicide attempter offspring. They found a significant association of a SNP (rs4792887) with suicide attempters exposed to low levels of stress, among whom most males were depressed. They conducted a further investigation (Wasserman *et al.*, 2009) and, besides confirming previous results, they found other two risk SNPs (rs110402 and rs12936511) which were associated and linked with depression scores among suicidal males. De Luca *et al.* (2007) analyzed three CRHR2 polymorphisms, CRHR2(CA), CRHR2(GT), and CRHR2(GAT), in 312 families where at least one subject had bipolar disorder. Even if there was no difference in the distribution of the alleles for all three markers, an association between haplotype 5–2–3 and higher severity of suicide-related traits was found.

In summary, the research on the CRH and HPA axis represents a new field of interest in the genetics of suicide showing promising results.

Gene–environment interaction studies

A further step in our knowledge on genetics of suicidal behavior comes from Gene–Environment interaction (GxE) studies. The most famous study in this field was conducted by Caspi *et al.* (2003). They found that a genetic polymorphism in the promoter of the serotonin transporter gene affects the likelihood of life stresses precipitating depression. Moreover, the occurrence of stressful life events predicted the onset of newly diagnosed depression or suicidal ideation and attempts among subjects with the short promoter but not among subjects with the long promoter. Roy *et al.* (2007) demonstrated how childhood trauma may interact with low expressing 5-HTTLPR genotypes to increase the risk of suicidal behavior among patients with substance dependence. Our studies on male prisoners identified an interaction between childhood emotional abuse and the AA 5-HT2A genotype in increasing suicidal risk (Sarchiapone and Vladmir, 2010). Brezo and colleagues (2009) performed a longitudinal cohort study showing how HTR2A variants (rs6561333, rs7997012 and rs1885884) were involved in suicide attempts through interactions with histories of sexual and physical abuse.

Perroud *et al.* (2008) investigated the interaction between BDNF Val66Met and childhood trauma in 615 non-violent and 198 violent suicide attempters. They found that childhood sexual abuse was associated with violent suicide attempts in adulthood only among Val/Val individuals. This interaction between BDNF polymorphism and childhood trauma was not confirmed by the previous cited study by Sarchiapone *et al.* (2008).

As described before, GxE effects were detected by Wasserman *et al.* (2008, p. 1) in relation to the CRHR1 gene. They also described two other GxE effects in suicide attempters: one among females, between 5′-SNP rs7209436 and childhood/adolescence physical assault; the second, male-specific, between 3′-SNP rs16940665 and adulthood physical assault exposure. Roy *et al.* (2010) investigated the FKBP5, an HPA-axis regulating gene, suggesting that childhood trauma and variants of the FKBP5 gene may interact to increase the risk of attempting suicide.

These studies confirmed the genetic liability for suicidal behavior, which can also be modulated by environmental factors as well as by psychological and personality characteristics. Taking into account all these variables represents one of the biggest challenges of future studies.

Future perspectives: genome-wide association studies and epigenetics

Genome-wide association studies (GWAS) have demonstrated a great potential for individuating new genes associated with suicidal behavior. The main advantage of these studies is that they examine a large set of gene polymorphisms without selecting one from an artificial hypothesis.

The first genome-wide scan of suicidal behavior was performed by Hesselbrock *et al.* (2004). Significant evidence of linkage was found on chromosome 2 for the phenotype suicide attempts. They also analyzed a 'suicidality index' related to lifetime suicidal thoughts and behavior. This index showed modest evidence for linkage to chromosomes 1 and 3, but these results did not reach statistical significance. Willour *et al.* (2007) confirmed these results showing a covariate-based linkage signal on 2p12 at marker D2S1777. Willour *et al.* (2011) extended their analysis, finding an association signal on 2p25 (rs300774) at the threshold of genome-wide significance. Perlis *et al.* (2010) analyzed data on lifetime suicide attempts from genome-wide association studies of bipolar and major depressive disorder providing suggestive evidences for different loci, while Galfalvy *et al.* (2013) recently identified 58 SNPs. Nevertheless, how these polymorphisms can be implicated in pathways leading to suicidal behavior needs further clarification.

Epigenetics is often defined as the study of heritable changes in genome function that occur without a change in DNA sequence. Sequeira *et al.* (2006) identified a role for the SSAT342 locus in the regulation of gene expression of SSAT, the rate-limiting enzyme in the catabolism of polyamines. Indeed they found a higher frequency of the SSAT342C allele among suicide victims compared to controls. McGowan *et al.* (2008) found a hypermethylation of the rRNA throughout the promoter and 5′ regulatory region in the brain of suicide subjects, consistent with reduced rRNA expression in the hippocampus. Another study (McGowan *et al.*, 2009) also reported decreased levels of glucocorticoid receptor mRNA, as well as mRNA transcripts bearing the gluco-corticoid receptor 1_F splice variant and increased cytosine methylation of a neuron-specific glucocorticoid receptor (NR3C1) promoter in the hippocampus of suicide victims with a history of childhood abuse.

In the study conducted by Poulter *et al.* (2008), the DNA methyltransferase (DNMT) gene transcript's expression was altered in the frontopolar cortex, the amygdala, and the paraventricular nucleus of the hypothalamus of suicide victims. Furthermore, within the frontopolar cortex, three cytosine/guanosine sites in the gamma-aminobutyric acid (GABA)(A) receptor alpha1 subunit promoter region were hypermethylated relative to control subjects.

The already cited study by Dwivedi *et al.* (2003) reported a reduced expression of BDNF and TrkB in postmortem brain in suicide subjects. We compared 44 suicide completers with 33 non-suicidal controls, describing a hyper-methylation of BDNF promoter/exon IV in the Wernicke area of the postmortem brain of suicide subjects. Ernst *et al.* (2009) showed a decreased expression of TrkB.T1 in the frontal cortex (Brodmann areas 8 and 9) of suicide completers and associated this downregulation with the methylation state of the promoter region, while, in the same sample of the previous study, we found that the TrkB and TrkB-T1 expression and promoter methylation in Wernicke area did not correlate with suicidal behavior, confirming that the expression and methylation state of suicide-related genes, even belonging to the same pathway, may be specific for brain area.

The results of epigenetic studies are promising and are important to clarify the mechanisms of DNA expression, improving our knowledge on the mutual links that exist between life events, DNA sequence, gene expression and protein synthesis.

Conclusion

All the discussed findings seem to confirm the important role of genetics in the pathogenesis of suicidal behavior, also showing how the inheritance of suicide risk factors is at least partially independent of the inheritance of psychiatric disorders. As well as for other psychopathological traits, suicidal behavior inheritance could result from the contribution of multiple genes with small effect size. Nevertheless, genetics is only one of several factors which affect the suicidal threshold and maybe only when specific combinations of genes meet specific combinations of life events is suicide more likely to occur.

References

Agerbo, E., Nordentoft, M., and Mortensen, P. B. (2002). Familial, psychiatric, and socioeconomic risk factors for suicide in young people: Nested case-control study. *BMJ (Clinical Research Ed.)*, 325(7355), 74.

Anguelova, M., Benkelfat, C., and Turecki, G. (2003). A systematic review of association studies investigating genes coding for serotonin receptors and the serotonin transporter: II. Suicidal behavior. *Molecular Psychiatry*, 8(7), 646–653.

Asberg, M., Träskman, L., and Thorén, P. (1976). 5-HIAA in the cerebrospinal fluid: A biochemical suicide predictor? *Archives of General Psychiatry*, 33(10), 1193–1197.

Baud, P., Perroud, N., Courtet, P., Jaussent, I., Relecom, C., Jollant, F., and Malafosse, A. (2009). Modulation of anger control in suicide attempters by TPH-1. *Genes, Brain and Behavior*, 8(1), 97–100.

Bellivier, F., Leboyer, M., Courtet, P., Buresi, C., Beaufils, B., Samolyk, D., *et al.* (1998). Association between the tryptophan hydroxylase gene and manic-depressive illness. *Archives of General Psychiatry*, 55(1), 33–37.

Bondy, B., Erfurth, A., de Jonge, S., Krüger, M., and Meyer, H. (2000). Possible association of the short allele of the serotonin transporter promoter gene polymorphism (5-HTTLPR) with violent suicide. *Molecular Psychiatry*, 5(2), 193–195.

Brent, D. A., Bridge, J., Johnson, B. A., and Connolly, J. (1996). Suicidal behavior runs in families: A controlled family study of adolescent suicide victims. *Archives of General Psychiatry*, 53(12), 1145–1152.

Brent, D. A., and Mann, J. J. (2005). Family genetic studies, suicide, and suicidal behavior. *American Journal of Medical Genetics. Part C, Seminars in Medical Genetics*, 133C(1), 13–24.

Brezo, J., Bureau, A., Mérette, C., Jomphe, V., Barker, E. D., Vitaro, F., *et al.* (2009). Differences and similarities in the serotonergic diathesis for suicide attempts and mood disorders: A 22-year longitudinal gene–environment study. *Molecular Psychiatry*, 15(8), 831–843.

Cases, O., Seif, I., Grimsby, J., Gaspar, P., Chen, K., Pournin, S., *et al.* (1995). Aggressive behavior and altered amounts of brain serotonin and norepinephrine in mice lacking MAOA. *Science*, 268(5218), 1763–1766.

Caspi, A. (2002). Role of genotype in the cycle of violence in maltreated children. *Science*, 297(5582), 851–854.

Caspi, A., Sugden, K., Moffitt, T. E., Taylor, A., Craig, I. W., Harrington, H., *et al.* (2003). Influence of life stress on depression: Moderation by a polymorphism in the 5-htt gene. *Science,* 301(5631), 386–389.

Courtet, P., Jollant, F., Buresi, C., Castelnau, D., Mouthon, D., and Malafosse, A. (2005). The monoamine oxidase A gene may influence the means used in suicide attempts. *Psychiatric Genetics,* 15(3), 189–193.

De Luca, V., Tharmalingam, S., and Kennedy, J. L. (2007). Association study between the corticotropin-releasing hormone receptor 2 gene and suicidality in bipolar disorder. *European Psychiatry: The Journal of the Association of European Psychiatrists,* 22(5), 282–287.

De Luca, V., Voineskos, D., Wong, G. W. H., Shinkai, T., Rothe, C., Strauss, J., and Kennedy, J. L. (2005). Promoter polymorphism of second tryptophan hydroxylase isoform (TPH2) in schizophrenia and suicidality. *Psychiatry Research,* 134(2), 195–198.

Dwivedi, Y., Rizavi, H. S., Conley, R. R., Roberts, R. C., Tamminga, C. A., and Pandey, G. N. (2003). Altered gene expression of brain-derived neurotrophic factor and receptor tyrosine kinase B in postmortem brain of suicide subjects. *Archives of General Psychiatry,* 60(8), 804–815.

Egeland, J. A. and Sussex, J. N. (1985). Suicide and family loading for affective disorders. *JAMA: The Journal of the American Medical Association,* 254(7), 915–918.

Ernst, C., Deleva, V., Deng, X., Sequeira, A., Pomarenski, A., Klempan, T., *et al.* (2009). Alternative splicing, methylation state, and expression profile of tropomyosin-related kinase B in the frontal cortex of suicide completers. *Archives of General Psychiatry,* 66(1), 22–32.

Fudalej, S., Ilgen, M., Fudalej, M., Kostrzewa, G., Barry, K., Wojnar, M., *et al.* (2010). Association between tryptophan hydroxylase 2 gene polymorphism and completed suicide. *Suicide and Life-Threatening Behavior,* 40(6), 553–560.

Galfalvy, H., Huang, Y., Oquendo, M. A., Currier, D., and Mann, J. J. (2009). Increased risk of suicide attempt in mood disorders and TPH1 genotype. *Journal of Affective Disorders,* 115(3), 331–338.

Galfalvy, H., Zalsman, G., Huang, Y.-Y., Murphy, L., Rosoklija, G., Dwork, A. J., *et al.* (2013). A pilot genome-wide association and gene expression array study of suicide with and without major depression. *The World Journal of Biological Psychiatry,* 14(8), 574–582.

González-Castro, T. B., Tovilla-Zárate, C. A., Juárez-Rojop, I., Pool García, S., Genis, A., Nicolini, H., and López Narváez, L. (2013). Association of 5HTR1A gene variants with suicidal behavior: Case-control study and updated meta-analysis. *Journal of Psychiatric Research,* 47(11), 1665–1672.

Gould, M. S., Fisher, P., Parides, M., Flory, M., and Shaffer, D. (1996). Psycho-social risk factors of child and adolescent completed suicide. *Archives of General Psychiatry,* 53(12), 1155–1162.

Gvion, Y., and Apter, A. (2011). Aggression, impulsivity, and suicide behavior: A review of the literature. *Archives of Suicide Research,* 15(2), 93–112.

Heils, A., Teufel, A., Petri, S., Stöber, G., Riederer, P., Bengel, D., and Lesch, K. P. (2002). Allelic variation of human serotonin transporter gene expression. *Journal of Neurochemistry,* 66(6), 2621–2624.

Hesselbrock, V., Dick, D., Hesselbrock, M., Foroud, T., Schuckit, M., Edenberg, H., *et al.* (2004). The search for genetic risk factors associated with suicidal behavior. *Alcoholism: Clinical and Experimental Research*, 28(s1), 70S–76S.

Ho, L. W., Furlong, R. A., Rubinsztein, J. S., Walsh, C., Paykel, E. S., and Rubinsztein, D. C. (2000). Genetic associations with clinical characteristics in bipolar affective disorder and recurrent unipolar depressive disorder. *American Journal of Medical Genetics*, 96(1), 36–42.

Hung, C.-F., Lung, F.-W., Hung, T.-H., Chong, M.-Y., Wu, C.-K., Wen, J.-K., and Lin, P.-Y. (2012). Monoamine oxidase A gene polymorphism and suicide: An association study and meta-analysis. *Journal of Affective Disorders*, 136(3), 643–649.

Jokinen, J., and Nordström, P. (2009). HPA axis hyperactivity and attempted suicide in young adult mood disorder inpatients. *Journal of Affective Disorders*, 116(1–2), 117–120.

Kallmann, F. J. and Anastasio, M. M. (1947). Twin studies on the psychopathology of suicide. *The Journal of Nervous and Mental Disease*, 105(1), 40–55.

Karege, F., Vaudan, G., Schwald, M., Perroud, N., and La Harpe, R. (2005). Neurotrophin levels in postmortem brains of suicide victims and the effects of antemortem diagnosis and psychotropic drugs. *Brain Research. Molecular Brain Research*, 136(1–2), 29–37.

Kia-Keating, B. M., Glatt, S. J., and Tsuang, M. T. (2007). Meta-analyses suggest association between COMT, but not HTR1B, alleles, and suicidal behavior. *American Journal of Medical Genetics Part B: Neuropsychiatric Genetics*, 144B(8), 1048–1053.

Kim, B., Kim, C. Y., Hong, J. P., Kim, S. Y., Lee, C., and Joo, Y. H. (2008). Brain-derived neurotrophic factor Val/Met polymorphism and bipolar disorder. Association of the Met allele with suicidal behavior of bipolar patients. *Neuropsychobiology*, 58(2), 97–103.

Kim, C. D., Seguin, M., Therrien, N., Riopel, G., Chawky, N., Lesage, A. D., and Turecki, G. (2005). Familial aggregation of suicidal behavior: A family study of male suicide completers from the general population. *The American Journal of Psychiatry*, 162(5), 1017–1019.

Lalovic, A. and Turecki, G. (2002). Meta-analysis of the association between tryptophan hydroxylase and suicidal behavior. *American Journal of Medical Genetics*, 114(5), 533–540.

Lester, D. (2002). Twin studies of suicidal behavior. *Archives of Suicide Research*, 6(4), 383–389.

Li, D. and He, L. (2006). Further clarification of the contribution of the tryptophan hydroxylase (TPH) gene to suicidal behavior using systematic allelic and genotypic meta-analyses. *Human Genetics*, 119(3), 233–240.

Lin, P.-Y., and Tsai, G. (2004). Association between serotonin transporter gene promoter polymorphism and suicide: Results of a meta-analysis. *Biological Psychiatry*, 55(10), 1023–1030.

Linnoila, V. M. and Virkkunen, M. (1992). Aggression, suicidality, and serotonin. *The Journal of Clinical Psychiatry*, 53 Suppl, 46–51.

Mann, J. J., Huang, Y., Underwood, M. D., Kassir, S. A., Oppenheim, S., Kelly, T. M., *et al.* (2000). A serotonin transporter gene promoter polymorphism (5-HTTLPR) and prefrontal cortical binding in major depression and suicide. *Archives of General Psychiatry*, 57(8), 729–738.

Mann, J. J., Waternaux, C., Haas, G. L., and Malone, K. M. (1999). Toward a clinical model of suicidal behavior in psychiatric patients. *The American Journal of Psychiatry*, 156(2), 181–189.

McGowan, P. O., Sasaki, A., D'Alessio, A. C., Dymov, S., Labonté, B., Szyf, M., *et al.* (2009). Epigenetic regulation of the glucocorticoid receptor in human brain associates with childhood abuse. *Nature Neuroscience*, 12(3), 342–348.

McGowan, P. O., Sasaki, A., Huang, T. C. T., Unterberger, A., Suderman, M., Ernst, C., *et al.* (2008). Promoter-wide hypermethylation of the ribosomal RNA gene promoter in the suicide brain. *PLoS ONE*, 3(5), e2085.

McGuffin, P., Marušič, A., and Farmer, A. (2001). What can psychiatric genetics offer suicidology? *Crisis: The Journal of Crisis Intervention and Suicide Prevention*, 22(2), 61–65.

Mościcki, E. K. (1997). Identification of suicide risk factors using epidemiologic studies. *The Psychiatric Clinics of North America*, 20(3), 499–517.

Murphy, G. E. and Wetzel, R. D. (1982). Family history of suicidal behavior among suicide attempters. *The Journal of Nervous and Mental Disease*, 170(2), 86–90.

Nielsen, D. A. (1994). Suicidality and 5-hydroxyindoleacetic acid concentration associated with a tryptophan hydroxylase polymorphism. *Archives of General Psychiatry*, 51(1), 34–38.

Ono, H., Shirakawa, O., Nishiguchi, N., Nishimura, A., Nushida, H., Ueno, Y., and Maeda, K. (2002). No evidence of an association between a functional monoamine oxidase a gene polymorphism and completed suicides. *American Journal of Medical Genetics*, 114(3), 340–342.

Ono, H., Shirakawa, O., Nushida, H., Ueno, Y., and Maeda, K. (2004). Association between catechol-O-methyltransferase functional polymorphism and male suicide completers. *Neuropsychopharmacology: Official Publication of the American College of Neuropsychopharmacology*, 29(7), 1374–1377.

Pandey, G. N., Ren, X., Rizavi, H. S., Conley, R. R., Roberts, R. C., and Dwivedi, Y. (2008). Brain-derived neurotrophic factor and tyrosine kinase B receptor signalling in post-mortem brain of teenage suicide victims. *The International Journal of Neuropsychopharmacology*, 11(8), 1047–1061.

Perlis, R. H., Huang, J., Purcell, S., Fava, M., Rush, A. J., Sullivan, P. F., *et al.* (2010). Genome-wide association study of suicide attempts in mood disorder patients. *American Journal of Psychiatry*, 167(12), 1499–1507.

Perroud, N., Courtet, P., Vincze, I., Jaussent, I., Jollant, F., Bellivier, F., *et al.* (2008). Interaction between BDNF Val66Met and childhood trauma on adult's violent suicide attempt. *Genes, Brain, and Behavior*, 7(3), 314–322.

Poulter, M. O., Du, L., Weaver, I. C. G., Palkovits, M., Faludi, G., Merali, Z., *et al.* (2008). GABAA receptor promoter hypermethylation in suicide brain: implications for the involvement of epigenetic processes. *Biological Psychiatry*, 64(8), 645–652.

Powell, J. (2000). Suicide in psychiatric hospital in-patients: Risk factors and their predictive power. *The British Journal of Psychiatry*, 176(3), 266–272.

Prichard, Z., Mackinnon, A., Jorm, A. F., and Easteal, S. (2008). No evidence for interaction between MAOA and childhood adversity for antisocial behavior. *American Journal of Medical Genetics Part B: Neuropsychiatric Genetics*, 147B(2), 228–232.

Qin, P. (2003). Suicide risk in relation to socioeconomic, demographic, psychiatric, and familial factors: A national register-based study of all suicides in Denmark, 1981–1997. *American Journal of Psychiatry*, 160(4), 765–772.

Qin, P., Agerbo, E., and Mortensen, P. B. (2002). Suicide risk in relation to family history of completed suicide and psychiatric disorders: A nested case-control study based on longitudinal registers. *The Lancet*, 360(9340), 1126–1130.

Roy, A. (1983). Family history of suicide. *Archives of General Psychiatry*, 40(9), 971–974.

Roy, A., Gorodetsky, E., Yuan, Q., Goldman, D., and Enoch, M.-A. (2010). Interaction of FKBP5, a stress-related gene, with childhood trauma increases the risk for attempting suicide. *Neuropsychopharmacology*, 35(8), 1674–1683.

Roy, A., Hu, X.-Z., Janal, M. N., and Goldman, D. (2007). Interaction between childhood trauma and serotonin transporter gene variation in suicide. *Neuropsychopharmacology*, 32(9), 2046–2052.

Roy, A., Segal, N. L., Centerwall, B. S., and Robinette, C. D. (1991). Suicide in twins. *Archives of General Psychiatry*, 48(1), 29–32.

Roy, A., Segal, N. L., and Sarchiapone, M. (1995). Attempted suicide among living co-twins of twin suicide victims. *The American Journal of Psychiatry*, 152(7), 1075–1076.

Rujescu, D., Giegling, I., Gietl, A., Hartmann, A. M., and Möller, H.-J. (2003). A functional single nucleotide polymorphism (V158M) in the COMT gene is associated with aggressive personality traits. *Biological Psychiatry*, 54(1), 34–39.

Rujescu, D., Giegling, I., Sato, T., Hartmann, A. M., and Möller, H. J. (2003). Genetic variations in tryptophan hydroxylase in suicidal behavior. *Biological Psychiatry*, 54(4), 465–473.

Runeson, B., and Asberg, M. (2003). Family history of suicide among suicide victims. *The American Journal of Psychiatry*, 160(8), 1525–1526.

Sabol, S. Z., Hu, S., and Hamer, D. (1998). A functional polymorphism in the monoamine oxidase A gene promoter. *Human Genetics*, 103(3), 273–279.

Saiz, P. A., García-Portilla, M. P., Paredes, B., Arango, C., Morales, B., Alvarez, V., *et al.* (2008). Association between the A-1438G polymorphism of the serotonin 2A receptor gene and nonimpulsive suicide attempts. *Psychiatric Genetics*, 18(5), 213–218.

Sarchiapone, M., Carli, V., Roy, A., Iacoviello, L., Cuomo, C., Latella, M. C., *et al.* (2008). Association of polymorphism (Val66Met) of brain-derived neurotrophic factor with suicide attempts in depressed patients. *Neuropsychobiology*, 57(3), 139–145.

Sarchiapone, M. and Vladmir, C. (2010). S18–02- Gene-environment interaction: 5-HT2A AA genotype and childhood emotional abuse upturn suicide risk in male prisoners. *European Psychiatry*, 25(Suppl. 1), 37.

Schulsinger, F., Kety, S., Rosenthal, D., and Wender, P. (1979). A family study of suicide. In M. Schou and E. Stromgren (Eds), *Origin, Prevention and Treatment of Affective Disorders* (pp. 277–287). London: Academic Press.

Segal, N. L. (2009). Suicidal behaviors in surviving monozygotic and dizygotic co-twins: Is the nature of the co-twin's cause of death a factor? *Suicide and Life-Threatening Behavior*, 39(6), 569–575.

Sequeira, A., Gwadry, F. G., Ffrench-Mullen, J. M. H., Canetti, L., Gingras, Y., Casero, R. A., *et al.* (2006). Implication of SSAT by gene expression and genetic variation in suicide and major depression. *Archives of General Psychiatry*, 63(1), 35–48.

Shafii, M., Carrigan, S., Whittinghill, J. R., and Derrick, A. (1985). Psychological autopsy of completed suicide in children and adolescents. *The American Journal of Psychiatry*, 142(9), 1061–1064.

Statham, D. J., Heath, A. C., Madden, P. A., Bucholz, K. K., Bierut, L., Dinwiddie, S. H., *et al.* (1998). Suicidal behaviour: An epidemiological and genetic study. *Psychological Medicine*, 28(4), 839–855.

Tovilla-Zárate, C., Juárez-Rojop, I., Ramón-Frias, T., Villar-Soto, M., Pool-García, S., Medellín, B., *et al.* (2011). No association between COMT val158met polymorphism and suicidal behavior: Meta-analysis and new data. *BMC Psychiatry*, 11(1), 151.

Tsai, S.-Y. M., Kuo, C.-J., Chen, C.-C., and Lee, H.-C. (2002). Risk factors for completed suicide in bipolar disorder. *The Journal of Clinical Psychiatry*, 63(6), 469–476.

Tsuang, M. T. (1983). Risk of suicide in the relatives of schizophrenics, manics, depressives, and controls. *The Journal of Clinical Psychiatry*, 44(11), 396–400.

Turecki, G., Brière, R., Dewar, K., Antonetti, T., Lesage, A. D., Séguin, M., *et al.* (1999). Prediction of level of serotonin 2A receptor binding by serotonin receptor 2A genetic variation in postmortem brain samples from subjects who did or did not commit suicide. *American Journal of Psychiatry*, 156(9), 1456–1458.

Turecki, G., Sequeira, A., Gingras, Y., Seguin, M., Lesage, A., Tousignant, M., *et al.* (2003). Suicide and serotonin: Study of variation at seven serotonin receptor genes in suicide completers. *American Journal of Medical Genetics*, 118B(1), 36–40.

Virkkunen, M., Goldman, D., Nielsen, D. A., and Linnoila, M. (1995). Low brain serotonin turnover rate (low CSF 5-HIAA) and impulsive violence. *Journal of Psychiatry and Neuroscience: JPN*, 20(4), 271–275.

Wasserman, D., Geijer, T., Sokolowski, M., Frisch, A., Michaelovsky, E., Weizman, A., *et al.* (2007). Association of the serotonin transporter promotor polymorphism with suicide attempters with a high medical damage. *European Neuropsychopharmacology*, 17(3), 230–233.

Wasserman, D., Sokolowski, M., Rozanov, V., and Wasserman, J. (2008). The CRHR1 gene: A marker for suicidality in depressed males exposed to low stress. *Genes, Brain, and Behavior*, 7(1), 14–19.

Wasserman, D., Sokolowski, M., Wasserman, J., and Rujescu, D. (2009). Neurobiology and the genetics of suicide. In D. Wasserman and C. Wassermann (Eds) *Oxford Textbook of Suicidology and Suicide Prevention* (pp. 165–182). New York: Oxford University Press.

Wasserman, D., Wasserman, J., Rozanov, V., and Sokolowski, M. (2009). Depression in suicidal males: Genetic risk variants in the *CRHR1* gene. *Genes, Brain and Behavior*, 8(1), 72–79.

Weder, N., Yang, B. Z., Douglas-Palumberi, H., Massey, J., Krystal, J. H., Gelernter, J., and Kaufman, J. (2009). MAOA genotype, maltreatment, and aggressive behavior: The changing impact of genotype at varying levels of trauma. *Biological Psychiatry*, 65(5), 417–424.

Weinshilboum, R. M., Otterness, D. M., and Szumlanski, C. L. (1999). Methylation pharmacogenetics: Catechol O-methyltransferase, thiopurine methyltransferase, and histamine N-methyltransferase. *Annual Review of Pharmacology and Toxicology*, 39(1), 19–52.

Wender, P. H., Kety, S. S., Rosenthal, D., Schulsinger, F., Ortmann, J., and Lunde, I. (1986). Psychiatric disorders in the biological and adoptive families of adopted individuals with affective disorders. *Archives of General Psychiatry*, 43(10), 923–929.

Willour, V. L., Seifuddin, F., Mahon, P. B., Jancic, D., Pirooznia, M., Steele, J., *et al.* (2011). A genome-wide association study of attempted suicide. *Molecular Psychiatry*, 17(4), 433–444.

Willour, V. L., Zandi, P. P., Badner, J. A., Steele, J., Miao, K., Lopez, V., *et al.* (2007). Attempted suicide in bipolar disorder pedigrees: Evidence for linkage to 2p12. *Biological Psychiatry*, 61(5), 725–727.

Zalsman, G., Huang, Y., Oquendo, M. A., Brent, D. A., Giner, L., Haghighi, F., *et al.* (2008). No association of COMT Val158Met polymorphism with suicidal behavior or CSF monoamine metabolites in mood disorders. *Archives of Suicide Research*, 12(4), 327–335.

Zarrilli, F., Angioliollo, A., Castaldo, G., Chiariotti, L., Keller, S., Sacchetti, S., *et al.* (2009). Brain derived neurotrophic factor (BDNF) genetic polymorphism (Val66Met) in suicide: a study of 512 cases. *American Journal of Medical Genetics. Part B, Neuropsychiatric Genetics: The Official Publication of the International Society of Psychiatric Genetics*, 150B(4), 599–600.

Zill, P., Büttner, A., Eisenmenger, W., Möller, H.-J., Bondy, B., and Ackenheil, M. (2004). Single nucleotide polymorphism and haplotype analysis of a novel tryptophan hydroxylase Isoform (TPH2) gene in suicide victims. *Biological Psychiatry*, 56(8), 581–586.

3 Suicidality and personality

Linking pathways

Vijay Parkash and Updesh Kumar

The high incidence of suicidal deaths make it an issue of grave concern and a potentially dangerous public health predicament as it is among the leading causes of death among youths across the globe. Suicide is considered to account for over one million deaths per year making it one of the ten leading causes of death (Hawton and van Heeringen, 2009). Regardless of rigorous efforts, successful prophecy and protective strategies have remained obscure; and it is suggestive of the fact that our comprehension of the interplay of factors that lead to various kinds of suicidal behaviour still remains deficient. Psychological autopsy-based studies of suicide victims have revealed that individuals who commit suicide have had several contributing factors, including some specific personality traits and even mental disorders (Pompili *et al.*, 2004). Some of the associated risk factors for suicide include age, sex, unemployment, other specific sociodemographic characteristics such as religious affiliations, and presence of various psychiatric problems (Hawton and van Heeringen, 2009; Mann *et al.*, 2005).

A growing body of evidence has established a link between certain personality factors and suicidality (Brezo *et al.*, 2006). Personality traits characterize emotional, behavioural, motivational, interpersonal, experiential and cognitive styles which help us to cope with the environment. Given the perceptible significance of personality to the development of suicidality, the dilemma remains as to which direction one should look to identify the personality features that may be termed as contributory. It is evident that there is not a straightforward causal link between personality traits and suicidality. A more likely and realistic picture is that certain personality features intermingle with eliciting stimuli along the intricate chain of development of suicidal behaviour. However, the existing literature attempting to explain the role of different individual concepts of personality in isolation remains relatively deficient about arriving at definite conclusions about the influence of personality traits on suicidality (Brezo *et al.*, 2006). In light of this, in the present chapter we attempt to concisely bring together the major research findings linking personality and suicidality, so as to try to make the reader wholistically conversant with the significance borne by different personality-related factors in influencing suicidal behaviour. Depending on different models, these personality factors have been named as neuroticism, agreeableness, openness to experience, conscientiousness and extroversion (Costa and McCrae, 1988); extroversion, psychoticism and neuroticism (Eysenck, 1990); harm avoidance, novelty seeking, reward dependence and persistence (Cloninger *et al.*, 1993); or emotional instability, compulsivity, antagonism and inhibition (Livesley *et al.*, 1998) and so on. Although some of the specific determinants of suicidality will be discussed in detail in subsequent chapters of this volume, in the following sections we will attempt to establish a broader linkage of the various personality factors explained by different models with the varied aspects of suicidality.

The five-factor model of personality and suicidality

Keeping in view the trait-based descriptions of personality, the five-factor model is considered the most comprehensive and widely accepted model to explain personality (Costa and McCrae, 1992; McCrae and Costa, 1987). The five personality dimensions explained by the five-factor model show clear innate characteristics (Jang *et al.*, 1996; Terracciano *et al.*, 2010) and have been found to be linked with varied psychiatric problems such as anxiety, depression, substance use, and personality disorders (Hayward *et al.*, 2013; Koorevaar *et al.*, 2013; Kotov *et al.*, 2010; Weber *et al.*, 2012).

Brezo and colleagues (2006) conducted a systematic analysis of the linkage between personality traits and risk of indulgence in suicidal behaviour and found that the two major dimensions of the five-factor model – neuroticism and extraversion – were the most consistently replicated personality traits linked with suicide-related behaviours. As anticipated, neuroticism-borne positive association and extraversion were found to have a negative relationship with suicidal behaviour. Higher levels of neuroticism were found to be positively linked with suicidal behaviours including suicidal ideation, suicide attempts and completed suicide; whereas extraversion was found to serve as a protective factor against suicidality (Brezo *et al.*, 2006, as cited by Blüml *et al.*, 2013). Heisel and colleagues (Heisel *et al.*, 2006) conducted a study on depressed older adults and concluded that higher scores of neuroticism and openness dimensions of personality were significantly correlated with suicidal ideation. Other studies on suicidal ideation reveal that high scores on neuroticism and low scores on extraversion, agreeableness and conscientiousness in a college student sample were associated with increased suicidal ideation (Kerby, 2003); whereas, in another study on university students, neuroticism emerged as a significant predictor for suicide ideation (Chioqueta and Stiles, 2005). Blüml *et al.* (2013) put forth that researches in this area also signify gender differences and conclude that gender plays an important role in determining the influence of personality traits on suicidality (Rozanov and Mid'ko, 2011). In another study on suicide ideation among young adults, Velting (1999) reported that neuroticism was found in association with suicidal ideation in females, while among male participants conscientiousness was found to be negatively correlated with suicidal ideation.

Going from ideation to suicide attempts, similar findings were reported by Useda *et al.* (2004) for the association between various facets underlying the Big Five personality dimensions and suicide attempts among another sample of depressed older adults. Giving consideration to personality factors associated with completed suicides, a study conducted by Fang, Heisel, Duberstein and Zhang (2012, as cited by Blüml *et al.*, 2013) in an adult sample in rural China concluded that a personality style characterized by a blend of high neuroticism and low extraversion was found to be associated with increased suicide risk. In a more recent study conducted on 2427 adult German participants by Blüml and colleagues (2013), it was observed that the personality factors, extraversion, conscientiousness, neuroticism and openness, and the presence of depression were significantly associated with suicidality. Specifically, neuroticism and openness were found to have significant direct association with suicide risk, whereas extraversion and conscientiousness were found to be inversely associated and serve as protective factors against suicide risk.

It has been seen in many studies that increased risk for suicidality is found persistently linked to neuroticism (Brezo *et al.*, 2006; Chioqueta and Stiles, 2005; Fang *et al.*, 2012; Heisel *et al.*, 2006; Kerby, 2003; Useda *et al.*, 2004), which is often associated with negative affectivity and maladaptive coping styles (DeNeve and Cooper, 1998; Gunthert *et al.*, 1999). Hence, it can be said that the linking pathway between neuroticism and increased suicidality passes through negative affect and maladaptive coping. As opposed to high levels of neuroticism, low levels of extraversion are associated with a negative perspective on life and hopelessness; whereas higher extraversion tends to promote positive affectivity (DeNeve and Cooper, 1998; Duberstein *et al.*, 2001), a pathway that often links extraversion with reduced suicidal behaviour (Brezo *et al.*, 2006; Kerby, 2003; Fang *et al.*, 2012).

Although neuroticism and extraversion are frequently linked with suicidality, there is relatively less confirmation regarding the influence of the other personality factors on suicidality. Though Heisel *et al.* (2006) found openness to be associated with suicide ideation among depressed older adults, they pointed out that, on the one hand, openness may enhance the probability of reporting suicide ideation as tapped by self-report measures and, on the other hand, by means of timely reporting of suicidality and thereby enhancing the chances of clinical interventions, openness may also reduce the actual risk of suicidal deaths (Heisel *et al.*, 2006). The linking pathways between openness and suicidal behaviours can be traced in the findings which report a linkage of high levels of openness with cognitive distortion, lack of insight and impulsivity (Piedmont *et al.*, 2009, 2012). As has been reported by a few studies, low levels of conscientiousness are related with increased suicidal ideation (Kerby, 2003; Velting, 1999), the path that leads from conscientiousness to suicidality may be manifest in the linkage of low levels of conscientiousness with impulsive tendencies, substance abuse and deficits in active coping strategies (Hayward *et al.*, 2013; Manuck *et al.*, 1998; Watson and Hubbard, 1996), which are the probable risk factors for suicidal behaviours.

The Big Three personality dimensions and suicidality

Other than the currently popular five-factor model, researchers have also tried to explore the relationship of Eysenck's (1990) Big Three personality dimensions with suicidal behaviours. Based on one such endeavour, Kumar (1990) found that higher levels of psychoticism were positively associated with suicidal ideation among a sample of university students. Some recent studies also confirm this finding and assert that psychoticism is significantly related with suicidal behaviour (Kerby, 2003; Singh and Joshi, 2008). In a study conducted on 250 college students, Singh and Joshi found significant associations of suicidal behaviour with extraversion and psychoticism dimensions of Eysenck's personality model. In their study suicidal ideation was significantly predicted by depression and the linking pathways between personality and suicidality emerged through the medium of development of depression which was predicted by neuroticism and psychotic personality dimensions. There are many other researchers who have found suicidality related to childhood temperament (Caspi *et al.*, 1996) and personality characteristics such as neuroticism and psychoticism (Dyck, 1991; Nordstrom *et al.*, 1995). Among the Eysenckian personality descriptors, neuroticism, toughmindedness and social non-conformity have been found to be significant correlates of persistent suicidal thoughts (Singh and Joshi, 2008; Statham *et al.*, 1998). Extending support to the notions of other researchers, Kumar *et al.* (2013) have shown the linkage of the Big Three personality factors with suicidal attempts by finding significant associations of the narrower traits of impulsivity, violence and loneliness with increased likelihood of suicide attempts.

There are many other researchers supporting this notion that some personality characteristics (Akiskal *et al.*, 2003; Heisel *et al.*, 2006; Kochman *et al.*, 2005) seem to have the most important role. Supporting the linking pathways between personality and suicidality, it has frequently been observed that impulsivity and aggressiveness type of personality features (Mann *et al.*, 2005; Rihmer, 2007), impaired problem-solving capacity, a high level of neuroticism, and low openness (Heisel *et al.*, 2006; Stankovic *et al.*, 2006) serve as risk factors for both attempted and completed suicide. While the linkage of neuroticism with suicidality flows through its underlying traits such as anxiousness, depressiveness, and mood lability (Eysenck, 1987; Miller and Pilkonis, 2006), impulsive and aggressive personality make-up directly prompts an individual to take extreme steps like suicide. Though impulsivity and aggression are among the most crucial personality factors linked to suicidal inclination, we will not discuss them in this chapter as Gvion and Apter will be specifically deliberating on their role in Chapter 5 of this volume.

Temperament

Taking the genetically determined side of personality make-up, temperament is considered as a constellation of structural behavioural characteristics that individuals have in their nature from birth and are relatively stable for the whole of life (Yumru *et al.*, 2008). It has been seen that temperamental traits are found to be associated with suicidality in clinical samples as well as the general population. In the case of suicide attempters, of the temperamental traits described by

Cloninger *et al.* (1993), harm avoidance is found generally higher, and self-directedness and cooperativeness are found to be lower (Calati *et al.*, 2008; Rothenhausler *et al.*, 2006). Yumru and associates have found that suicide attempters had higher impulsiveness, harm avoidance, reward dependence and self-transcendence (Yumru *et al.*, 2008). They reported that in suicide attempters harm avoidance and self-transcendence scores were higher and reward dependence was lower as compared to non-attempters; also, a negative correlation was found between reward dependence and number of suicide attempts. Indicating the linkage through the medium of hopelessness, they found that harm avoidance had a positive correlation with hopelessness among the suicide attempters. Justifying it and in line with other researchers (e.g., Calati *et al.*, 2008; Rothenhausler *et al.*, 2006), in suicide attempters, the harm avoidance score was significantly higher and the self-directedness score was significantly lower than normal controls (Yumru *et al.*, 2008).

Another linking pathway can be traced due to the fact that, according to Cloninger's theory, a low level of self-directedness is a harbinger of personality disorder and the likely presence of personality disorders among the suicide attempters with a low level of self-directedness may be acting as an underlying cause of suicidal behaviour (Yumru *et al.*, 2008). Some other researchers also assert that individuals with a high level of harm avoidance and a low level of self-directedness are considered to have a 'weak' personality (Le Bon *et al.*, 2004) that might not be able to withstand the strains and may break down. Based on a more recent study, Perroud *et al.* (2013) commented on the direct association of severity of suicidal behaviour with higher levels of harm avoidance and novelty-seeking. They concluded that besides impulsivity and anger-related traits, harm avoidance was the only temperamental trait independently associated with a history of suicide attempts. Indicating the suicidal pathways through harm avoidance, self-directedness, impulsivity and anger control, they suggested that early detection of subjects displaying risk factors such as high harm avoidance and low self-directedness, associated with high impulsivity and poor anger control, may help the health care professionals to prevent suicidal behaviours (Perroud *et al.*, 2013).

Other models of temperament also mention such temperamental traits that may be linked to an individual's increased vulnerability to suicidal behaviour. Using Strelau's (1983) regulative temperaments as a focus of study, Parkash (2010) found that the temperamental traits briskness and endurance correlate negatively with maladaptive coping, hopelessness and depression and thereby may be considered as protective factors, however, another temperamental trait perseveration correlates positively with anger, hopelessness and depression which may be considered as the linking pathways to suicidal thoughts.

Considering other temperament models, many recent studies have focused on affective temperaments and revealed a strong association between some specific affective temperament types and suicidal behaviour (Akiskal *et al.*, 2003). In a comparative study on cyclothymic and non-cyclothymic bipolar-II patients, Akiskal *et al.* found that cyclothymic individuals reported notably more frequent suicide attempts and experienced more current hospitalization for sui-cidal risk. In another study on juvenile inpatients with current major depressive episode, Kochman *et al.* (2005) found that cyclothymic-hypersensitive tempera-ment at baseline significantly forecast suicidal behaviour. Young *et al.* (1994/1995) also reported similar findings that bipolar patients with cyclothymic history reported a significantly higher number of prior suicide attempts. Henry and col-leagues (1999) while studying the depressive and hyperthymic temperament in relation to suicidal behaviour among bipolar patients, found that patients with high depressive temperament scores had a history of significantly more frequent suicide attempts (cited by Rihmer *et al.*, 2009).

While investigating the affective temperament profile of consecutively hospital-ized Italian psychiatric patients, Pompili and colleagues (2008) found the major-ity of them with unipolar major depressive or bipolar disorder, and a significant number (more than 60 out of 150) were a suicide risk at admission. They reported that, compared to the non-suicidal patients, the suicidal psychiatric patients were found to be significantly higher on depressive, cyclothymic, irritable and anxious, and significantly lower on hyperthymic subscales of the TEMPS-A (Temperament Evaluation of Memphis, Pisa, Paris and San Diego-Autoquestionnaire version). Cloninger *et al.* (1998) had similarly concluded that rates of current depression and prior suicide attempts were the highest among persons with cyclothymic and depressive personality types.

Studying affective temperament among non-violent suicide attempters, Rihmer *et al.* (2009) reported that depressive, cyclothymic, irritable and anxious temperaments were significantly more frequent and common among suicide attempters. The pathways running from temperament types to suicidality can be traced to the findings that the different affective temperament types such as depressive, cyclothymic, hyperthymic, irritable and anxious are trait-related man-ifestations and usually the predecessors of the major depressive and mood disor-ders (Akiskal and Pinto, 1999; Kochman *et al.*, 2005; Rihmer *et al.*, 2009). This provides significant suggestive input on the affective temperaments serving as probable predictors of suicidal behaviour.

Self-esteem

Going beyond the typical personality models, research evidence reveals that a common variable and related personality factor linked to suicide is self-esteem (Overholser *et al.*, 1995). Self-esteem is considered to be linked to sense of worthfulness. According to Overholser *et al.*, individuals with high self-esteem tend to be positive in their attitudes about themselves and are generally found content with their lives. On the other hand, people who have low self-esteem are considered to have feelings of incompetence and worthlessness, and a negative view of themselves. As a link with suicidality it can be inferred that when a person has a pessimistic and worthless view of himself or herself, then there becomes a general likelihood of increased suicidal tendencies (Overholser *et al.*, 1995). In another study, Dori and Overholser (1999) also found low self-esteem as an indicator of suicidal ideation. They observed that, compared with their non-suicidal counterparts, suicide attempters had significantly lower self-esteem and higher levels of depression and hopelessness. Connecting the findings with self-esteem it was found that depressed and hopeless adolescents with adequate levels of self-esteem were less likely to demonstrate suicidal behaviours as compared to those with low self-esteem (Dori and Overholser, 1999). Rassmussen *et al.* (1997) had also found significant positive association of suicidal ideation with high depression and low self-esteem. Vella *et al.* (1996) found that suicidal ideation was inversely correlated with self-esteem among a college population. Suicidal ideation increases with declined self-esteem.

Personality disorders

Although the belief in 'suicidal personality' has by and large been discarded, there remains an opinion that personality factors are of significance in suicidal behaviours. The association between personality disorder and suicidal behaviour has been identified by the researchers in this field. Personality disorders play a role as significant risk factors for one's chance to get involved in suicidal behaviour. Psychological autopsy-based studies frequently show that individuals with personality disorders have a considerable probability of indulging in suicide attempts and they are found among suicide committers (Pompili *et al.*, 2004). Pompili and associates (2004) reviewed the empirically based literature from the years ranging from 1980 to 2004 and identified studies dealing with suicide and borderline personality disorder, narcissistic personality disorder, antisocial personality disorder, and risk factors for suicide in personality disorders. Their overview revealed that some personality disorders have a sturdy linkage to suicidal behaviours and that identification of certain specific personality-related risk factors may be used for the development of protective measures. Since personality disorders have a substantial prevalence rate, prediction and prevention of suicide among people with personality disorders are a major public health concern.

Personality disorders are psychiatric conditions which are characterized by an unceasing mould of internal experience and behaviour that are nonflexible and present in a variety of situations. These psychiatric conditions have a significant influence on patients' interpersonal relationships, and their functioning in social and occupational settings. As far as their etiology and clinical features are concerned, different personality disorders are heterogeneous in nature. It is the combination of genetically determined temperamental traits and different environmental events that determines the symptom complexes of personality disorders. Each specific disorder has a specific and varying relative contribution of genetic and environmental factors (Pompili *et al.*, 2004). Researchers believe that the estimated prevalence of personality disorders ranges from 6 to 13 per cent in the general population (Samuels *et al.*, 1994; Weissman, 1993). Seeing the prevalence of personality disorders among cases of attempted and completed suicides, researchers opine that up to 77 per cent of suicide attempters (Engstrom *et al.*, 1997; Ferreira de Castro *et al.*, 1998; Nimeus *et al.*, 1997; Suominen *et al.*, 1996)

and at least one-third (ranging from 31 to 62 per cent) of the victims of completed suicides (Brent *et al.*, 1994; Cheng *et al.*, 1997; Foster *et al.*, 1997; Lesage
et al., 1994) have suffered from personality disorders. It has also been found that
suicide attempters with personality disorders have the highest level of repetition
(Suominen *et al.*, 2000).

Serving as a significant risk factor for suicidal behaviour, personality
disorders have been found to predict completed suicides in the follow-up
(Allebeck *et al.*, 1988; Paris, 1993; Stone, 1989) In post-mortem retrospective
interview studies and multiaxial diagnostic assessment-based studies, personality
disorders have been found to be prevalent with almost 57 per cent of suicide
victims, generally young victims (Lesage *et al.*, 1994; Rich and Runeson, 1992).
It has also been found that there is a substantial likelihood of a history of suicidal
thoughts or attempts among subjects with personality disorders, and their
first- and second-degree relatives are also relatively likely to have indulged in
suicidal behaviours (Samuels *et al.*, 1994).

In a study of fatal and non-fatal suicidal behaviour among adolescents,
Marttunen *et al.* (1994) found that among the adolescents with non-fatal
suicidal behaviour, approximately 45 per cent males and 33 per cent females
behaved antisocially and 17 per cent of victims of fatal suicidal behaviour met the
criteria for conduct disorder or antisocial personality disorder. It has also been
found that the risk of a serious suicide attempt was almost four times higher
among individuals with antisocial personality disorder as compared with those
without the disorder; and this risk is almost nine times higher in men under the
age of 30 (Beautrais *et al.*, 1996).

Borderline personality disorder

Empirical evidence suggests that 9–33 per cent of all suicides are represented
by individuals with borderline personality disorder (Runeson and Beskow,
1991; Kullgren *et al.*, 1986). Peterson and Bongar (1990) found a link of
chronic suicidality and repetitive suicidal crises with the behaviours that met the
criteria of borderline personality disorder. The finding received support from
Paris and Zweig-Frank (2001) who indicated that the diagnosis of borderline
personality disorders is significantly correlated with increased risk of eventual
suicide. Young people under the age of 30 were found to be at higher risk
(Friedman and Corn, 1987). The higher rate of linkage between borderline personality disorders and suicidal behaviour is reflected in different forms including
recurrent suicidal behaviour, gestures, threats, or self-mutilating behaviour
(Pompili *et al.*, 2004).

Supporting a prevailing notion that considers borderline personality disorder
as the suicidal personality disorder, Mehlum *et al.* (1994) pointed out that the
features such as a lack of control of high intensity affects such as depression,
anxiety or anger, which may be the characteristic features of borderline personality disorder, may increase the tendency towards suicidal behaviour. Depression is
considered to be associated with suicidality in the majority of cases and the linking

pathways can be inferred in the fact that many researchers believe that in borderline personality disorder there is a high prevalence of comorbidity with major depression (Fyer *et al.*, 1988). Standing by the assertion that there is a strong link between borderline personality features and suicidality, Yen *et al.* (2004) pointed out the association between each DSM-IV (*Diagnostic and Statistical Manual* – IV) criterion of borderline personality disorder and aspects of suicidal behaviour. According to Yen and colleagues (2004), the criterion of the borderline personality disorder which is most strongly associated with suicidal behaviour is affective instability. Impulsivity assessed as a diagnostic criterion among patients with borderline personality disorder has also been found to be related to suicide attempts in many cases. If the assessed borderline personality disorder criteria also include hopelessness, then that is likely to increase the seriousness of suicidal intent. It is believed that self-harm or suicidal behaviour is central to the clinical picture of some personality disorders including borderline personality disorder (Pompili *et al.*, 2004).

Empirical studies have shown that among individuals having borderline personality disorder, older age, impulsivity, antisocial personality traits, depressive mood, and previous suicide attempts serve as risk factors for further suicidal behaviour (Brodsky *et al.*, 1997; Kjelsberg *et al.*, 1991; Paris *et al.*, 1989). Pompili *et al.* (2004) also found that many suicide attempters with personality disorders had a history of previous suicide attempts compared with those without personality disorders. In addition to the personality disorders, adverse life events may act as a catalyst to push high-risk individuals into actual suicidal crisis. Kelly *et al.* (2002) found that suicide attempters experience adverse life events such as stressful events at home, with the family or financially. It has been observed that changes in habits, sexual difficulties, separation from wife or girlfriend, problems with in-laws, and change in social activities are the events that occur relatively more often among the suicidal patients having borderline personality disorder (Lesage *et al.*, 1994). If we look at the linking personality factors, on the basis of derivations from clinical reports and longitudinal follow-up studies, Soloff *et al.* (1994) concluded that in borderline personality disorder the probable risk factors for suicidal behaviour include: (1) impulsivity, aggression, and hostility; (2) alcohol and substance abuse; (3) antisocial traits; (4) severity of borderline personality disorder; (5) comorbidity with affective disorder; and (6) repeated previous attempts.

Narcissistic personality disorder

In a psychological autopsy-based study conducted by Apter and his colleagues (1993), on a sample of 43 consecutive suicides that occurred among young Israeli males during compulsory military service, schizoid personality disorder was found to be the most common Axis II personality disorder (more than 37 per cent of victims having it) followed by narcissistic personality disorder (more than 23 per cent of victims found affected by it). Based on a 15-year comparative follow-up of psychiatric patients, Stone (1989) concluded that in comparison with the patients without narcissistic personality traits, the patients who suffered from narcissistic personality disorder had a significantly higher likelihood of having died by suicide. Stone further asserted that a heightened risk for suicide has been found associated with narcissistic features in borderline personalities. The pathway linking it to suicide may be traced in the hypothesis that narcissism might increase the suicidal vulnerability in people with intense self-pride (justifiable or inflated) as any sudden unexpected drop in social position may influence such a person more drastically than others and it might lead to suicidal behaviour in the efforts to avoid facing society.

Antisocial personality disorder

In the domain of personality disorders, antisocial personality disorder also tends to show a link with suicidality. Evidence exists to provide indications of linking pathways between antisocial personality traits and suicidal acts. Studies conducted on suicide attempters have shown that criminal behaviour or antisocial personality disorder is a significant predictor of subsequent suicide attempts (Bunglass and Horton, 1974; Morgan *et al.*, 1976). There are other researchers who confirm these associations of antisocial personality with suicidality. In a study conducted by Garvey and Spoden (1980) it was found that suicide was attempted by more than two-thirds of their patients having antisocial personality disorder. Another group of researchers (Woodruff *et al.*, 1971) reported that around a quarter of the outpatients diagnosed with antisocial personality disorder attempted suicide. A study conducted on a large group of people with sociopathic personality traits found that more than 10 per cent of them had attempted suicide (Robins, 1966). Pompili *et al.* (2004) opine that suicide attempters are found with generally more frequent social problems such as with marriage or love affairs. Garvey and Spoden's (1980) findings were similar, wherein they had reported that most of the non-serious suicide attempts were more or less solely associated to problems with some significant other. The finding in Garvey and Spoden's study showing the majority of suicide attempts by sociopaths as relatively safe and 'non-serious' provides evidence to support the notion that rather than killing oneself, suicide attempts are used by sociopaths to act out their frustration and to manipulate others (Pompili *et al.*, 2004).

It has been clear by the preceding discussion that while considering the associative linkage of suicidal behaviour with personality disorders, most of the existing studies focus on cluster B personality disorders of DSM-IV including borderline personality disorder, narcissistic personality disorder and antisocial personality disorder. There is a heavy representation of individuals with one or more cluster B personality disorders among those who attempt suicide, which may often result in death and completed suicide (Pompili *et al.*, 2004). According to DSM-IV criteria, impulsivity is a key symptom of the behaviour of cluster B personality disorder patients. These impulsive cluster B patients most of the time look for a quick and sweeping resolution of their disturbing impulses. Moreover, the need to be admired among the narcissistic individuals and the craving to manipulate others among the antisocial individuals increase the risk of indulgence in suicidal behaviours. Such individuals may use suicidality as an extreme whimper for help if they do not receive enough support from the environment to gratify their psychic needs.

Conclusion

Suicidal behaviour has long been a matter of research and scientific concern since more than a million people die by suicidal means every year. Any effort focused on suicide prevention requires a detailed in-depth understanding of all the factors associated with the risk of suicidal behaviour. The research on these factors provides a wide coverage including the genetic, biological, personological, social and environmental factors that may be associated with suicidality. Continuous efforts are being made to trace all the linking pathways of suicidality so that their identification can help guide the use of appropriate preventive measures centring on the causative factors. Analysis of different research on personality and suicidality has helped make certain linking pathways evident. Adequate personality assessment and the resultant identification of vulnerable personality traits like neuroticism, impulsivity, aggression, emotional reactivity, harm avoidance, self-directedness and the symptoms of various personality disorders are likely to prove the key to determine the most effective preventive measures to safeguard human lives against the maladaptive behaviour patterns of suicidality. Also, there seems to be a dire need for more dedicated research focusing on very specific narrower traits that are crucial to the understanding of suicidal dynamics. Future research, therefore, should concentrate on tracing the roots of suicidal behaviour rather than finding the surface-level triggering factors.

References

Akiskal, H. S., Hantouche, E. G., and Allilaire, J. F. (2003). Bipolar II with and without cyclothymic temperament: 'dark' and 'sunny' expressions of soft bipolarity. *Journal of Affective Disorders*, 73(1–2), 49–57.

Akiskal, H. S. and Pinto, O. (1999). The evolving bipolar spectrum: Prototypes I, II, III, and IV. *Psychiatric Clinics of North America*, 22(3), 517–534.

Allebeck, P., Allgulander, C., and Fisher, L. D. (1988). Predictors of completed suicide in a cohort of 50,465 young men: Role of personality and deviant behaviour. *British Medical Journal*, 297(6642), 176–178.

Apter, A., Bleich, A., King, R. A., Kron, S., Fluch, A., Kotler, M., and Cohen, D. J. (1993). Death without warning? A clinical postmortem study of suicide in 43 Israeli adolescent males. *Archives of General Psychiatry*, 50(2), 138–142.

Beautrais, A. L., Joyce, P. R , Mulder, R. T., Fergusson, D. M., and Deavoll, B. J., and Nightingale, S. K. (1996). Prevalence and comorbidity of mental disorders in persons making serious suicide attempts: A case control study. *American Journal of Psychiatry*, 153(8), 1009–1014.

Blüml, V., Kapusta, N. D., Doering, S., Brähler, E., Wagner, B., and Kersting, A. (2013). Personality factors and suicide risk in a representative sample of the German general population. *PLoS ONE*, 8(10), e76646.

Brent, D. A., Johnson, B. A., Perper, J., Connolly, J., Bridge, J., Bartle, S., and Rather, C. (1994). Personality disorder, personality traits, impulsive violence, and completed suicide in adolescents. *Journal of American Academy of Child and Adolescent Psychiatry*, 33(8), 1080–1086.

Brezo, J., Paris, J., and Turecki, G. (2006). Personality traits as correlates of suicidal ideation, suicide attempts, and suicide completions: A systematic review. *Acta Psychiatrica Scandinavica*, 113(3), 180–206.

Brodsky, B. S., Malone, K. M., Ellis, S. P., Dulit, R. A., and Mann, J. J. (1997). Characteristics of borderline personality disorder associated with suicidal behavior. *American Journal of Psychiatry*, 154(12), 1715–1719.

Bunglass, P., and Horton, J. (1974). The repetition of parasuicide: A comparison of three cohorts. *British Journal of Psychiatry*, 125(2), 168–174.

Calati, R., Giegling, I., Rujescu, D., Hartmann, A. M., Möller, H. J., De Ronchi, D., and Serretti, A. (2008). Temperament and character of suicide attempters. *Journal of Psychiatric Research*, 42(11), 938–945.

Caspi, A., Moffitt, T. E., Newman, D. L., and Silva, P. A. (1996). Behavioral observations at age 3 years predict adult psychiatric disorders. *Archives of General Psychiatry*, 53(11), 1033–1039.

Cheng, A. T., Mann, A. H., and Chan, K. A. (1997). Personality disorder and suicide: A case-control study. *British Journal of Psychiatry*, 170(5), 441–446.

Chioqueta, A. P., and Stiles, T. C. (2005). Personality traits and the development of depression, hopelessness, and suicide ideation. *Personality and Individual Differences*, 38(6), 1283–1291.

Cloninger, C. R., Bayon, C., and Svrakic, D. M. (1998). Measurement of temperament and character in mood disorders: A model of fundamental states as personality types. *Journal of Affective Disorders*, 51(1), 21–32.

Cloninger, C. R., Svrakic, D. M., and Przybeck, T. R. (1993). A psychobiological model of temperament and character. *Archives of General Psychiatry*, 50(12), 975–990.

Costa, P. T., Jr. and McCrae, R. R. (1988). From catalog to classification: Murray's needs and the five-factor model. *Journal of Personality and Social Psychology*, 55(2), 258–265.

Costa, P. T., Jr. and McCrae, R. R. (1992). Normal personality assessment in clinical practice: The NEO personality inventory. *Psychological Assessment*, 4(1), 5–13.

DeNeve, K. M. and Cooper, H. (1998). The Happy Personality: A meta-analysis of 137 personality traits and subjective well-being. *Psychological Bulletin*, 124(2), 197–229.

Dori, G. A. and Overholser, J. C. (1999). Depression, hopelessness, and self-esteem: Accounting for suicidality in adolescent psychiatric inpatients. *Suicide and Life-Threatening Behavior*, 29(4), 309–318.

Duberstein, P. R., Conner, K. R., Conwell, Y., and Cox, C. (2001). Personality correlates of hopelessness in depressed inpatients 50 years of age and older. *Journal of Personality Assessment*, 77(2), 380–390.

Dyck, M. J. (1991). Positive and negative attitudes mediating suicide ideation. *Suicide and Life-Threatening Behavior*, 21(4), 360–373.

Engstrom, G., Alling, C., Gustavsson, P., Oreland, L., and Traskman-Bendz, L. (1997). Clinical characteristics and biological parameters in temperamental clusters of suicide attempters. *Journal of Affective Disorders*, 44(1), 45–55.

Eysenck, H. J. (1987). The definition of personality disorders and the criteria appropriate for their description. *Journal of Personality Disorders*, 1(3), 211–219.

Eysenck, H. J. (1990). Genetic and environmental contributions to individual differences: The three major dimensions of personality. *Journal of Personality*, 58(1), 245–261.

Fang, L., Heisel, M. J., Duberstein, P. R., and Zhang, J. (2012). Combined effects of neuroticism and extraversion: Findings from a matched case control study of suicide in rural China. *Journal of Nervous and Mental Disease*, 200(7), 598–602.

Ferreira de Castro, F. E., Cunha, M. A., Pimenta, F., and Costa, I. (1998). Parasuicide and mental disorders. *Acta Psychiatrica Scandinavica*, 97(1), 25–31.

Foster, T., Gillespie, K., and McClelland, R. (1997). Mental disorders and suicide in Northern Ireland. *British Journal of Psychiatry*, 170(5), 447–452.

Friedman, R. C. and Corn, R. (1987). Suicide and the borderline depressed adolescent and young adult. *Journal of American Academy of Psychoanalysis*, 15(4), 429–448.

Fyer, M. R., Frances, A. J., Sullivan, T., Hurt, S. W., and Clarkin, J. (1988). Comorbidity of borderline personality disorder. *Archives of General Psychiatry*, 45(4), 348–352.

Garvey, M. J., and Spoden, F. (1980). Suicide attempts in antisocial personality disorder. *Comprehensive Psychiatry*, 21(2), 146–149.

Gunthert, K. C., Cohen, L. H., and Armeli, S. (1999). The role of neuroticism in daily stress and coping. *Journal of Personality and Social Psychology*, 77(5), 1087–1100.

Hawton, K., and van Heeringen, K. (2009). Suicide. *The Lancet*, 373(9672), 1372–1381.

Hayward, R. D., Taylor, W. D., Smoski, M. J., Steffens, D. C., and Payne, M. E. (2013). Association of five-factor model personality domains and facets with presence, onset, and treatment outcomes of major depression in older adults. *American Journal of Geriatric Psychiatry*, 21(1), 88–96.

Heisel, M. J., Duberstein, P. R., Conner, K. R., Franus, N., Beckman, A., and Conwell, Y. (2006). Personality and reports of suicide ideation among depressed adults 50 years of age or older. *Journal of Affective Disorders*, 90(2–3), 175–180.

Henry, C., Lacoste, J., Bellivier, F., Verdoux, H., Bourgeois, M. L., and Leboyer, M. (1999). Temperament in bipolar illness: Impact on prognosis. *Journal of Affective Disorders*, 56(2–3), 103–108.

Jang, K. L., Livesley, W. J., and Vernon, P. A. (1996). Heritability of the Big Five personality dimensions and their facets: A twin study. *Journal of Personality*, 64(3), 577–591.

Kelly, T. M., Cornelius, J. R., and Lynch, K. G. (2002). Psychiatric and substance use disorders as risk factors for attempted suicide among adolescents: A case control study. *Suicide and Life-Threatening Behavior*, 32(3), 301–312.

Kerby, D. S. (2003). CART analysis with unit-weighted regression to predict suicidal ideation from Big Five traits. *Personality and Individual Differences*, 35(2), 249–261.

Kjelsberg, E., Eikeseth, P. H., and Dahl, A. A. (1991). Suicide in borderline patients – predictive factors. *Acta Psychiatrica Scandinavica*, 84(3), 283–287.

Kochman, F. J., Hantouche, E. G., Ferrari, P., Lancrenon, S., Bayart, D., and Akiskal, H. S. (2005). Cyclothymic temperament as a prospective predictor of bipolarity and suicidality in children and adolescents with major depressive disorder. *Journal of Affective Disorders*, 85(1–2), 181–189.

Koorevaar, A. M. L., Comijs, H. C., Dhondt, A. D. F., van Marwijk, H. W. J., van der Mast, R. C., Naarding, P., *et al.* (2013). Big Five personality and depression diagnosis, severity and age of onset in older adults. *Journal of Affective Disorders*, 151(1), 178–185.

Kotov, R., Gamez, W., Schmidt, F., and Watson, D. (2010). Linking 'big' personality traits to anxiety, depressive, and substance use disorders: A meta-analysis. *Psychological Bulletin*, 136(5), 768–821.

Kullgren, G., Renberg, E., and Jacobsson, L. (1986). An empirical study of borderline personality disorder and psychiatric suicides. *Journal of Nervous and Mental Disease*, 174(6), 328–331.

Kumar, P. N. S., Rajmohan, V., and Sushil, K. (2013). An exploratory analysis of personality factors contributed to suicide attempts. *Indian Journal of Psychological Medicine*, 35(4), 378–384.

Kumar, U. (1990). A study of correlates of suicide ideation among homogeneous groups of psychoses-prone university students. Unpublished doctoral thesis. Department of Psychology, Panjab University, Chandigarh.

Le Bon, O., Basiaux, P., Streel, E., Tecco, J., Hanak, C., Hansenne, M., *et al.* (2004). Personality profile and drug of choice: A multivariate analysis using Cloninger's TCI on heroin addicts, alcoholics, and a random population group. *Drug and Alcohol Dependence*, 73(2), 175–182.

Lesage, A. D., Boyer, R., Grunberg, F., Vanier, C., Morissette, R., Menard-Buteau, C., and Loyer, M. (1994). Suicide and mental disorders: A case-control study of young men. *American Journal of Psychiatry*, 151(7), 1063–1068.

Livesley, W. J., Jang, K. L., and Vernon, P. A. (1998). Phenotypic and genetic structure of traits delineating personality disorder. *Archives of General Psychiatry*, 55(10), 941–948.

Mann, J. J., Apter, A., Bertolote, J., Beautrais, A., Currier, D., Hass, A., and Hendin, H. (2005). Suicide prevention strategies: A systematic review. *Journal of American Medical Association*, 294(16), 2064–2074.

Manuck, S. B., Flory, J. D., McCaffery, J. M., Matthews, K. A., Mann, J. J., and Muldoon, M. F. (1998). Aggression, impulsivity, and central nervous system serotonergic responsivity in a nonpatient sample. *Neuropsychopharmacology*, 19(4), 287–299.

Marttunen, M. J., Aro, H. M., Henriksson, M. M., and Lonnqvist, J. K. (1994). Antisocial behaviour in adolescent suicide. *Acta Psychiatrica Scandinavica*, 89(3), 167–173.

McCrae, R. R., and Costa, P. T. Jr. (1987). Validation of the Five-Factor model of personality across instruments and observers. *Journal of Personality and Social Psychology*, 52(1), 81–90.

Mehlum, L., Friis, S., Vaglum, P., and Karterud, S. (1994). The longitudinal pattern of suicidal behaviour in borderline personality disorder: A prospective follow-up study. *Acta Psychiatrica Scandinavica*, 90(2), 124–130.

Miller, J. D. and Pilkonis, P. A. (2006). Neuroticism and affective instability: The same or different? *American Journal of Psychiatry*, 163(5), 839–845.

Morgan, H. G., Barton, J., Pottle, S., and Pocock, H., and Burns-Cox, C. J. (1976). Deliberate self-harm: A follow-up study of 279 patients. *British Journal of Psychiatry*, 128(3), 361–368.

Nimeus, A., Traskman-Bendz, L., and Alsen, M. (1997). Hopelessness and suicidal behavior. *Journal of Affective Disorders*, 42(1–2), 137–144.

Nordstrom, P., Schalling, D., and Asberg, M. (1995). Temperamental vulnerability in attempted suicide. *Acta Psychiatrica Scandinavica*, 92(2), 155–160.

Overholser, J. C., Adams, D. M., Lehnert, K. L., and Brinkman, D. C. (1995). Self-esteem deficits and suicidal tendencies among adolescents. *Journal of the American Academy of Child and Adolescent Psychiatry*, 34(7), 919–928.

Paris, J. (1993). The treatment of borderline personality disorder in light of the research on its long-term outcome. *Canadian Journal of Psychiatry*, 38 (Suppl 1), s28–s34.

Paris, J., Nowlis, D., and Brown, R. (1989). Predictors of suicide in borderline personality disorder. *Canadian Journal of Psychiatry*, 34(1), 8–9.

Paris, J. and Zweig-Frank, H. (2001). A 27-year follow-up of patients with borderline personality disorder. *Comprehensive Psychiatry*, 42(6), 482–487.

Parkash, V. (2010). Emotional intelligence and temperament as moderators of reactions to stress. Unpublished doctoral thesis. Department of Psychology, Kurukshetra University, Kurukshetra.

Perroud, N., Baud, P., Ardu, S., Krejci, I., Mouthon, D., Vessaz, M., *et al.* (2013). Temperament personality profiles in suicidal behaviour: An investigation of associated demographic, clinical and genetic factors. *Journal of Affective Disorders*, 146(2), 246–253.

Peterson, L. G. and Bongar, B. (1990). Repetitive suicidal crises: Characteristics of repeating versus nonrepeating suicidal visitors to a psychiatric emergency service. *Psychopathology*, 23(3), 136–145.

Piedmont, R. L., Sherman, M. F., and Sherman, N. C. (2012). Maladaptively high and low openness: The case for experiential permeability. *Journal of Personality*, 80(6), 1641–1668.

Piedmont, R. L., Sherman, M. F., Sherman, N. C., Dy-Liacco, G. S., and Williams, J. E. G. (2009). Using the Five-Factor Model to identify a new personality disorder domain: The case for experiential permeability. *Journal of Personality and Social Psychology*, 96(6), 1245–1258.

Pompili, M., Rihmer, Z., Akiskal, H. S., Innamorati, M., Iliceto, P., Akiskal, K. K., *et al.* (2008). Temperament and personality dimensions in suicidal and nonsuicidal psychiatric inpatients. *Psychopathology*, 41(5), 313–321.

Pompili, M., Ruberto, A., Girardi, P., and Tatarelli, R. (2004). Suicidality in DSM-IV cluster B personality disorders. An overview. *Annali dell'Istituto superiore di sanità*, 40(4), 475–483.

Rassmussen, K. M., Negy, C., Carlson, R., and Burns, J. M. (1997). Suicide ideation and acculturation among low socioeconomic status Mexican American adolescents. *Journal of Early Adolescence*, 17(4), 390–407.

Rich, C. L. and Runeson, B. S. (1992). Similarities in diagnostic comorbidity between suicide among young people in Sweden and the United States. *Acta Psychiatrica Scandinavica*, 86(5), 335–339.

Rihmer, A., Rozsa, S., Rihmer, Z., Gonda, X., Akiskal, K. K., and Akiskal, H. S. (2009). Affective temperaments, as measured by TEMPS-A, among nonviolent suicide attempters. *Journal of Affective Disorders*, 116(1–2), 18–22.

Rihmer, Z. (2007). Suicide risk in mood disorders. *Current Opinion in Psychiatry*, 20(1), 17–22.

Robins, L. N. (1966). *Deviant Children Grown Up*. Baltimore, MD: Williams and Wilkins.

Rothenhausler, H. B., Stepan, A., and Kapfhammer, H. P. (2006). Soluble interleukin 2 receptor levels, temperament and character in formerly depressed suicide attempters compared with normal controls. *Suicide and Life-Threatening Behavior*, 36(4), 455–466.

Rozanov, V. A., and Mid'ko, A. A. (2011). Personality patterns of suicide attempters: Gender differences in Ukraine. *Spanish Journal of Psychology*, 14(2), 693–700.

Runeson, B., and Beskow, J. (1991). Borderline personality disorder in young Swedish suicides. *Journal of Nervous and Mental Disease*, 179(3), 153–156.

Samuels, J. F., Nestadt, G., Romanoski, A. J., Folstein, M. F., and McHugh, P. R. (1994). DSM-III personality disorders in the community. *American Journal of Psychiatry*, 151(7), 1055–1062.

Singh, R. and Joshi, H. L. (2008). Suicidal ideation in relation to depression, life stress and personality among college students. *Journal of Indian Academy of Applied Psychology*, 34(2), 259–265.

Soloff, P. H., Lis, J. A., Kelly, T., Cornelius, J., and Ulrich, R. (1994). Risk factors for suicidal behavior in borderline personality disorder. *American Journal of Psychiatry*, 151(9), 1316–1323.

Stankovic, Z., Saula-Marojevic, B., and Potrebic, A. (2006). Personality profile of depressive patients with a history of suicide attempts. *Psychiatria Danubina*, 18(3–4), 159–168.

Statham, D. J., Heath, A. C., Madden, P. A. F., Bucholz, K. K., Bierut, L., Dinwiddie, S. H., *et al.* (1998). Suicidal behaviour: An epidemiological and genetic study. *Psychological Medicine*, 28(4), 839–855.

Stone, M. H. (1989). Long-term follow-up of narcissistic/borderline patients. *Psychiatric Clinics of North America*, 12(3), 621–641.

Strelau, J. (1983). A regulative theory of temperament. *Australian Journal of Psychology*, 35(3), 305–317.

Suominen, K. H., Isometsa, E. T., Henriksson, M. M., Ostamo, A. I., and Lonnqvist, J. K. (2000). Suicide attempts and personality disorder. *Acta Psychiatrica Scandinavica*, 102(2), 118–125.

Suominen, K. H., Henriksson, M., Suokas, J., Isometsa, E., Ostamo, A., and Lonnqvist, J. (1996). Mental disorders and comorbidity in attempted suicide. *Acta Psychiatrica Scandinavica*, 94(4), 234–240.

Terracciano, A., Sanna, S., Uda, M., Deiana, B., Usala, G., Busonero, F., *et al.* (2010). Genome-wide association scan for five major dimensions of personality. *Molecular Psychiatry*, 15(6), 647–656.

Useda, J. D., Duberstein, P. R., Conner, K. R., and Conwell, Y. (2004). Personality and attempted suicide in depressed adults 50 years of age and older: A facet level analysis. *Comprehensive Psychiatry*, 45(5), 353–361.

Vella, M. L., Persic, S., and Lester, D. (1996). Does self-esteem predict suicidality after controls for depression? *Psychological Reports*, 79(3), 1178.

Velting, D. M. (1999). Suicidal ideation and the five-factor model of personality. *Personality and Individual Differences*, 27(5), 943–952.

Watson, D., and Hubbard, B. (1996). Adaptational style and dispositional structure: Coping in the context of the Five-Factor Model. *Journal of Personality*, 64(4), 736–774.

Weber, K., Giannakopoulos, P., Bacchetta, J. P., Quast, S., Herrmann, F. R., Delaloye, C., *et al.* (2012). Personality traits are associated with acute major depression across the age spectrum. *Aging and Mental Health*, 16(4), 472–480.

Weissman, M. M. (1993). The epidemiology of personality disorders: A 1990 update. *Journal of Personality Disorders*, 7(Suppl 1), 44–62.

Woodruff, R. A. Jr., Guze, S. B., and Clayton, P. J. (1971). The medical and psychiatric implications of antisocial personality (sociopathy). *Diseases of the Nervous System*, 32(6), 712–714.

Yen, S., Shea, M. T., Sanislow, C. A., Grilo, C. M., Skodol, A. E., Gunderson, J. G., *et al.* (2004). Borderline personality disorder criteria associated with prospectively observed suicidal behavior. *American Journal of Psychiatry*, 161(7), 1296–1298.

Young, L. T., Cooke, R. G., Robb, J. C., and Joffe, R. T. (1994/1995). Double bipolar disorder: A separate entity? *Depression*, 2(4), 223–225.

Yumru, M., Savas, H. A., Herken, H., and Kokacya, M. H. (2008). Suicide and personality. *Anatolian Journal of Psychiatry*, 9(4), 232–237.

4   Emotion dysregulation and suicidality

Michael D. Anestis

Suicidality is a complex construct and numerous theories have emerged to explain who is most vulnerable to suicidal desire and behavior and how those individuals develop that vulnerability. A number of such theories have posited that suicidal behavior serves at least in part as a method by which an individual can escape acute crises. In Baumeister's (1990) escape theory of suicide, he posited that suicidal behavior can best be conceptualized as an effort to escape from aversive self-awareness. He argued that, when in a state of aversive self-awareness, an individual's ability to resist impulses to engage in suicidal behavior diminishes, thereby increasing the odds of an attempt that emerges explosively in response to an acute affective state. Similarly, Mann *et al.* (1999) argued for a diathesis-stress model in which individuals with high levels of trait impulsivity (diathesis) encounter upsetting events (stress) and then respond to these acute states with attempts aimed at escaping aversive sensations. A commonality across these theories is the notion that, at times, suicidal behavior serves as a method to avoid acute affective states. Building on these ideas, the notion that emotion dysregulation might play an important role in suicidal behavior has become commonly accepted.

Emotion dysregulation is a multifaceted construct that involves deficits across a broad range of areas. These areas include the identification, understanding, and acceptance of emotional states, the ability to persist towards goals while upset, the ability to resist impulses while upset, and the degree to which an individual exhibits a range of adaptive strategies for managing his or her emotions (Gratz and Roemer, 2004). Numerous measures for assessing emotion dysregulation exist and numerous subcomponents of the larger construct (e.g., distress tolerance, negative urgency, affective lability) have been subject to a substantial amount of research and clinical attention. Indeed, difficulties with emotion dysregulation have been tied to a number of problematic outcomes, including binge eating, substance use, antisocial behavior, non-suicidal self-injury (NSSI), and risky sexual behavior (e.g., Anestis *et al.*, 2007, 2009; Buckner *et al.*, 2007; Glenn and Klonsky, 2010; Messman-Moore *et al.*, 2010; Tull *et al.*, 2012).

Psychiatric diagnoses characterized by difficulties with emotion dysregulation have also been routinely associated with increased rates of non-lethal and lethal suicidal behavior (e.g., borderline personality disorder; Paris and Zweig-Frank,

2001). Indeed, Dialectical Behavior Therapy (DBT; Linehan and Heard, 1992) and Emotion Regulation Group Therapy (ERGT; Gratz and Gunderson, 2006) have been demonstrated to be efficacious and/or effective psycho-social approaches to the treatment of suicidality (e.g., Gratz and Tull, 2011; Kliem *et al.*, 2010; Linehan *et al.*, 2006), thereby prompting an increasing belief in the potential robust and proximal role of emotion dysregulation in suicidal behavior. DBT and ERGT both teach broad emotion regulation and specific distress tolerance skills aimed at enabling suicidal individuals to weather difficult and upsetting moments rather than harming themselves. In this sense, the treatments are posited to influence suicide-related outcomes by enhancing an individual's capacity to effectively regulate their emotions in the moment and enabling them to opt to utilize means for regulation that are more effective and less costly than a suicide attempt. This point is further supported by research that has linked emotion dysregulation difficulties with suicidal ideation (e.g., Lynch *et al.*, 2004; Orbach *et al.*, 2007).

The relationship between emotion dysregulation and suicidality becomes more complex, however, when considering results from studies that have looked specifically at suicidal behavior rather than ideation or a broad measure of suicide risk. In a sample of depressed children, Tamas and colleagues (2007) reported that suicide attempters did not differ on any facet of emotion dysregulation relative to children with suicidal ideation and suicide plans, but no suicide attempts, children with only suicidal ideation, or children with no ideation but repeated thoughts of death. Such results seem to echo previous findings linking emotion dysregulation to suicidal ideation, but do not necessarily point to a direct and incrementally valid association with suicidal behavior. Similarly, in a sample of adolescent inpatients, Zlotnick *et al.* (1997) reported that attempters exhibited greater levels of emotion dysregulation, but that emotion dysregulation did not differentiate those with attempts from those with only ideation. In this sense, a robust relationship between emotion dysregulation and suicidal behavior (as opposed to ideation, which may in turn prompt behavior) does not appear to be supported by these data.

One theoretical framework that appears to have substantial value in terms of framing the complex relationship between emotion dysregulation and suicidality is the Interpersonal-Psychological Theory of Suicidal Behavior (IPTS; Joiner, 2005). The IPTS differs from other theories in that it differentiates between the *desire* for suicide and the *capability* for suicide. Desire is thought to be prompted by the joint presence of thwarted belongingness (an individual's sense that he or she lacks meaningful connections to others) and perceived burdensomeness (an individual's sense that he or she is a liability to others and more valuable dead). The capacity, on the other hand, is thought to be comprised of elevated pain tolerance and a diminished fear of death and bodily harm. Although a portion of this capacity appears to be genetic (Smith *et al.*, 2012), it is largely theorized to be acquired through repeated exposure to painful and/or provocative events, which lead to habituation to pain and fear. The vast majority of individuals with suicidal desire will not have the capability and the vast majority of those with the capability will not have desire. It is only in the relatively rare combination of suicidal desire and capability that serious or lethal suicidal behavior will emerge, thereby explaining why so many with ideation do not attempt and why so many who attempt do not die. The primary hypothesis of the theory – that both desire and capability must be present for serious suicidal behavior to occur – has been supported across multiple samples (e.g., Anestis and Joiner, 2011; Joiner *et al.*, 2009; see Van Orden *et al.* 2010, for a thorough review of the empirical evidence underlying the theory). The IPTS views suicidal behavior as a planned pursuit of death and an outcome that does not emerge suddenly in response to acute affect states. Emotion dysregulation is not viewed as irrelevant; however, the nature of its relationship to each component of suicide risk is thought to be nuanced.

Thus far, there has been limited research considering the association between emotion dysregulation and suicidality through the lens of the IPTS. Anestis *et al.* (2011) examined a sample of undergraduates and theorized that difficulties regulating negative emotions would predict elevated suicidal desire (burdensomeness and belongingness) but diminished acquired capability. They noted that the need to immediately avoid aversive states may not be consistent with the nature of suicidal behavior, in which pain and/or intense fear of death/bodily harm must be experienced in the pursuit of death. The authors examined two sub-components of emotion dysregulation – negative urgency (the tendency to act rashly in an effort to reduce the intensity of negative affective states; Whiteside and Lynam, 2001) and distress tolerance (the degree to which an individual can function while upset in a manner consistent with functioning during euthymic states; Simons and Gaher, 2005). Indeed, results from this study demonstrated that difficulties with emotion dysregulation predicted elevated suicidal desire and diminished acquired capability, measured both through self-report and a behavioral measure of physio-logical pain tolerance. The somewhat counter-intuitive finding between emotion dysregulation and the acquired capability has since been replicated using a behavioral measure of distress tolerance as well, increasing confidence that the effect is not spurious (Anestis and Joiner, 2011).

Although promising preliminary evidence, the above-mentioned findings were found exclusively in relatively healthy undergraduate samples, thereby leaving their external validity open to serious question. More recently, however, similar research has been conducted using clinical populations. For instance, in a sample of adults receiving residential treatment for substance use disorders, the relationships between suicidal behavior and both borderline personality disorder (BPD) and posttraumatic stress disorder (PTSD) were found to increase at higher levels of distress tolerance (Anestis *et al.*, 2012a, b). Neither disorder exhibited a significant association with suicidal desire at low levels of distress tolerance (greater difficulties with emotion dysregulation), but as an individual's ability to tolerate distress increased, so did the magnitude of the relationship between disorder and suicide attempts. Furthermore, these effects held for attempts with ambiguous intent to die, attempts with clear intent to die, and medically serious attempts.

Although the acquired capability was not measured directly, when considered alongside the previously reported positive association between distress tolerance and the acquired capability, these findings speak to the notion that individuals vulnerable to suicidal desire (e.g., those with BPD or PTSD) are more likely to engage in suicidal behavior when they have developed the capacity to do so. As noted before, the IPTS conceptualizes suicidal behavior as an experience requiring a purposeful confrontation with fear (of death and/or severe bodily harm) and either the presence or threat of physiological pain. In this sense, the behavior is unlikely to yield the primary outcome desired by an emotionally dysregulated individual in a moment of crisis: an immediate decrease in the intensity of an aversive affective state. This stands in direct contrast to behaviors such as binge eating and NSSI, which have been shown to be motivated primarily by the drive to experience immediate relief (e.g., Smyth *et al.*, 2007; Nock and Prinstein, 2005). In this sense, such evidence indicates that suicidal behavior may be, in some ways, qualitatively different than other problematic behavior, not only in its greater potential for lethality, but also in the mental and physical obstacles that impact the motives, function, and probability of the behavior.

A reasonable concern when reading about findings like those from Anestis and Joiner (2012) is that individuals with BPD or PTSD are unlikely to exhibit high distress tolerance. The rareness, however, can be easily seen as strength of the model. Although it is true that such individuals do not typically exhibit high distress tolerance, they also do not typically engage in suicidal behavior. Suicidal behavior is certainly elevated in these populations relative to others; however, it remains a low base rate phenomenon, so it seems reasonable to assume that the typical presentation of either disorder would not be the most robust path towards suicidal behavior.

Building on these findings, Anestis *et al.* (2013a) examined a sample of adults receiving inpatient treatment for substance use disorders and found that distress tolerance moderated the relationship between NSSI and suicide potential, with the relationship becoming stronger at higher levels of distress tolerance. The authors conceptualized suicide potential as a continuum extending from no prior suicidal behavior, to one or more low lethality attempts, to a history of high lethality suicidal behavior. The findings thus point towards the notion that even NSSI, a robust predictor not only of past suicidal behavior (e.g., Nock *et al.*, 2006) but also future attempts (e.g., Cooper *et al.*, 2005), may not be enough on its own to facilitate suicidal behavior.

Taking this a step further, however, Anestis *et al.* (2013b) reported that low distress tolerance (greater difficulties with emotion dysregulation) predicted a greater number of lifetime suicide attempts, but that this relationship was mediated by lifetime NSSI frequency. Put another way, the relationship between a component of emotion dysregulation and suicidal behavior was explained by the impact of a specific painful and provocative event (NSSI) frequently engaged in by emotionally dysregulated individuals. This finding mirrored that of Anestis *et al.* (2012), who found that the relationships between negative urgency (a subcomponent of emotion dysregulation) and both the acquired capability and suicidal behavior were mediated by lifetime exposure to painful and/or provocative events. In this sense, it appears as though it is not the emotion dysregulation itself, but rather the behaviors engaged in by a subset of emotionally dysregulated individuals, that explain the elevated rates of suicidal behavior in emotionally dysregulated populations.

Such findings are entirely consistent with the IPTS framework. Data indicate that the most frequently endorsed function of NSSI is intrapersonal negitive reinforcement in the form of immediate reductions in the intensity of negitive affect (e.g., Nock and Prinstein, 2005). Furthermore, data indicate that engaging in NSSI may truly offer such affective relief (e.g., Bresin and Gordon, 2013) and that engaging in a greater number of episodes and/or methods of NSSI is associated with a greater level of pain tolerance (e.g., Franklin *et al.*, 2012; Hooley *et al.*, 2010; McCoy *et al.*, 2010; Russ *et al.*, 1999; Russ *et al.*, 1992). Such findings indicate that emotionally dysregulated individuals may engage in NSSI to manage negative emotions. Because the behavior is effective in producing the desired result, it becomes a common practice in distressing moments. Although the individuals' emotion dysregulation is initially associated with a lower capacity to engage in lethal self-harm, over time the repeated episodes of NSSI increase pain tolerance levels and provide practice with the notion of inflicting harm upon one's own body. As such, if and when suicidal desire becomes present – a distinct possibility in emotionally dysregulated individuals – the capacity becomes more likely to be present as well, thereby increasing the odds of serious or lethal suicidal behavior.

Although no studies to my knowledge have directly tested this proposition, it seems entirely plausible to me that this same path exists for any painful and/or provocative experience utilized regularly as an emotion regulation strategy. Something moderately threatening and/or painful is engaged in repeatedly and, over time, the individual habituates to the fear and pain. The result is then twofold: the individual must engage in the behavior more often or with greater severity to get the same effect (affective relief) and the individual becomes bolder with respect to pain and fear. In this sense, there could be an infinite number of paths from emotion dysregulation to suicidal behavior, some more robust than others (e.g., NSSI versus excessive exercise), but the path would always involve specific behaviors facilitating suicidal behavior over an extended period of time.

In many ways, this model is counterintuitive. If emotionally dysregulated individuals attempt and die by suicide at greater rates than non-emotionally dysregulated individuals, how can I argue that emotion dysregulation itself is only an indirect risk factor for suicidal behavior and, in fact, an obstacle for certain aspects of risk? Here again, I'd point to the discrepancies between the frequency of suicidal ideation versus suicide plans versus non-lethal suicidal behavior versus death by suicide. With each step in that chain, the sample grows smaller. Most who think of suicide do not make a plan. Most who make a plan do not make an attempt. Most who make an attempt do not die. As such, it seems entirely plausible that this painful and frightening behavior that runs in direct contrast to the evolutionary imperative of self-preservation might be difficult and that the few who ultimately engage in it acquire the capacity to do so with great effort over an extended period of time. The data indicate that at least certain components of emotion dysregulation serve as an obstacle to the acquired capability for suicide even as they predict greater levels of suicidal desire. The model thus posits that many emotionally dysregulated individuals will desire, and maybe even plan, for suicidal behavior, but will not engage in the behavior itself. That being said: a subset of those individuals will engage in emotion regulatory behaviors that are painful and/or provocative (e.g., NSSI) and, over time, those individuals will develop the capacity for lethal self-harm, eventually transitioning from ideation and plans to behavior. Their discomfort with aversive affective sensations initially placed them at a disadvantage for the acquired capability relative to the general population, but that same emotion dysregulation led some of them to repeatedly engage in behaviors that altered their relationships with death and pain and made the notion of a suicide attempt less difficult. In the meantime, the general population engaged in fewer of these behaviors and exhibited lower levels of suicidal desire, leading to a lower rate of suicidal behavior, despite their initial advantage on one aspect of risk.

Conclusion and future directions

Many aspects of this model remain untested empirically and the evidence base that exists is in many ways preliminary. As such, it is important to consider the findings within that context. Furthermore, some potential sources of confusion should be clarified. It seems plausible that some may read this chapter and assume that the message is that effective regulation of affect and the ability to tolerate distress are harmful. This is not my argument. As is the case with many variables, context is pivotal. In most environments, effective emotion regulation is a path towards health and well-being. It is simply when this capacity – or at least parts of it (e.g., distress tolerance) – is paired with suicidal desire that it becomes potentially problematic. Indeed, the success of DBT in the treatment of suicidal behavior (e.g., Kliem *et al.*, 2010; Linehan *et al.*, 2006) and numerous findings linking effective emotion regulation to increased well-being (e.g., Quoidbach *et al.*, 2010) are strong evidence that the capacity to regulate aversive states is in no way iatrogenic.

In this sense, the proposed model emphasizes the importance of nuance when considering risk factors for a complex construct like suicidality as well as the importance of empirically dispelling prominent myths regarding suicidal behavior (Joiner, 2010). What makes an individual vulnerable to one aspect of suicide risk (e.g., suicidal desire) does not necessarily make that same individual vulnerable to other aspects of suicide risk (e.g., capacity for suicide). Similarly, although some variables (e.g., emotion dysregulation) may in some ways serve as an obstacle to certain aspects of risk (e.g., capacity for suicide), this is not to say that individuals with elevation in that variable cannot overcome that obstacle. Ultimately, the strength in a model such as this is that it aligns well with the fact that such a small percentage of those with ideation make attempts and so few of those who attempt die by suicide. There are many aspects to risk and that path to lethal self-harm is not simple.

References

Anestis, M. D., Anestis, J. C., and Joiner, T. E. (2009). Affective considerations in antisocial behavior: An examination of negative urgency in primary and secondary psychopathy. *Personality and Individual Differences*, 47(6), 668–670.

Anestis, M. D., Bagge, C. L., Tull, M. T., and Joiner, T. E. (2011). Clarifying the role of emotion dysregulation in the interpersonal-psychological theory of suicidal behavior in an undergraduate sample. *Journal of Psychiatric Research*, 45(5), 603–611.

Anestis, M. D., Fink, E. L., Bender, T. W., Selby, E. A., Smith, A. R., Witte, T. K., and Joiner, T. E. (2012a). Re-considering the association between negative urgency and suicidality. *Personality and Mental Health*, 6(2), 138–146.

Anestis, M. D., Gratz, K. L., Bagge, C.L., and Tull, M. T. (2012b). The interactive role of distress tolerance and borderline personality disorder in suicide attempts among substance users in residential treatment. *Comprehensive Psychiatry*, 53(8), 1208–1216.

Anestis, M. D., and Joiner, T. E. (2011). Examining the role of emotion in suicidality: Negative urgency as an amplifier of the relationship between components of the interpersonal-psychological theory of suicidal behavior and life-time number of suicide attempts. *Journal of Affective Disorders*, 129(1–3), 261–269.

Anestis, M. D., and Joiner, T. E. (2012). Behaviorally-indexed distress tolerance and suicidality. *Journal of Psychiatric Research*, 46(6), 703–707.

Anestis, M. D., Knorr, A. N., Tull, M. T., Lavender, J. M., and Gratz, K. L. (2013a). The importance of high distress tolerance in the relationship between non-suicidal self-injury and suicide potential. *Suicide and Life-Threatening Behavior*, 43(6), 663–675.

Anestis, M. D., Pennings, S. M., Lavender, J. M., Tull, M. T., and Gratz, K. L. (2013b). Low distress tolerance as an indirect risk factor for suicidal behavior: Considering the explanatory role of non-suicidal self-injury. *Comprehensive Psychiatry*, 54(7), 996–1002.

Anestis, M. D., Selby, E.A., and Joiner, T. E. (2007). The role of urgency in maladaptive behaviors. *Behaviour Research and Therapy*, 45(12), 3018–3029.

Anestis, M. D., Tull, M. T., Bagge, C. L., and Gratz, K. L. (2012c). The moderating role of distress tolerance in the relationship between posttraumatic stress disorder symptom clusters and suicidal behavior among trauma-exposed substance users in residential treatment. *Archives of Suicide Research*, 16(3), 198–211.

Baumeister, R. F. (1990). Suicide as escape from self. *Psychological Review*, 97(1), 90–113.

Bresin, K., and Gordon, K. H. (2013). Changes in negative affect following pain (vs. nonpainful) stimulation in individuals with and without a history of nonsuicidal self-injury. *Personality Disorders*, 4(1), 62–66.

Buckner, J. D., Keough, M. E., and Schmidt, N. B. (2007). Problematic alcohol and cannabis use among young adults: The roles of depression and discomfort and distress tolerance. *Addictive Behaviors*, 32(9), 1957–1963.

Cooper, J., Kapur, N., Webb, R., Lawlor, M., Guthrie, E., Mackway-Jones, K., and Appleby, L. (2005). Suicide after deliberate self-harm: A 4 year cohort study. *American Journal of Psychiatry*, 162(2), 297–303.

Franklin, J. C., Aaron, R. V., Arthur, M. S., Shorkey, S. P., and Printsein, M. J. (2012). Non-suicidal self-injury and diminished pain perception: The role of emotion dysregulation. *Comprehensive Psychiatry*, 53(6), 691–700.

Glenn, C. R., and Klonsky, E. D. (2010). A multimethod analysis of impulsivity in non-suicidal self-injury. *Personality Disorders*, 1(1), 67–75.

Gratz, K. L., and Gunderson, J. G. (2006). Preliminary data on an acceptance-based emotion regulation group intervention for deliberate self-harm among women with borderline personality disorder. *Behavior Therapy*, 37(1), 25–35.

Gratz, K. L., and Roemer, L. (2004). Multidimensional assessment of emotion regulation and dysregulation: Development, factor structure, and initial validation of the difficulties in Emotion Regulation Scale. *Journal of Psychopathology and Behavioral Assessment*, 26(1), 41–54.

Gratz, K. L. and Tull, M. T. (2011). Extending research on the utility of an adjunctive emotion regulation group therapy for deliberate self-harm among women with borderline personality pathology. *Personality Disorders*, 2(4), 316–326.

Hooley, J. M., Ho, D. T., Slater, J., and Lockshin, A. (2010). Pain perception and non-suicidal self-injury: A laboratory investigation. *Personality Disorders*, 1(3), 170–179.

Joiner, T. E. (2005). *Why People Die by Suicide*. Cambridge, MA: Harvard University Press.

Joiner, T. E. (2010). *Myths about Suicide*. Cambridge, MA: Harvard University Press.

Joiner, T. E., Van Orden, K. A., Witte, T. K., Selby, E. A., Ribeiro, J., Lewis, R., and Rudd, M. D. (2009). Main predictions of the Interpersonal-Psychological Theory of suicidal behavior: Empirical tests in two samples of young adults. *Journal of Abnormal Psychology*, 118(3), 634–646.

Kliem, S., Kroger, C., and Kosfelder, J. (2010). Dialectical behavior therapy for borderline personality disorder: A meta-analysis using mixed-effects modeling. *Journal of Consulting and Clinical Psychology*, 78(6), 936–951.

Linehan, M. M., Comtois, K. A., Murray, A. M., Brown, M. Z., Gallop, R. J., Heard, H. L., *et al.* (2006). Two-year randomized controlled trial and follow-up of dialectical behavior therapy vs therapy by experts for suicidal behaviors and borderline personality disorder. *Archives of General Psychiatry*, 63(7), 757–766.

Linehan, M. M., and Heard, H. L. (1992). Dialectical behavior therapy for borderline personality disorder. In J. F. Clarkin, E. Marziali, and H. Munroe-Blum (Eds), *Borderline Personality Disorder: Clinical and Empirical Perspective* (pp. 248–267). New York: Guilford Press.

Lynch, T. R., Cheavens, J. S., Morse, J. Q., and Rosenthal, M. Z. (2004). A model predicting suicidal ideation and hopelessness in depressed older adults: The impact of emotion inhibition and affect intensity. *Aging and Mental Health*, 8(6), 486–497.

Mann, J. J., Waternaux, C., Haas, G. L., and Malone, K. M. (1999). Toward a clinical model of suicidal behavior in psychiatric patients. *American Journal of Psychiatry*, 156(2), 181–189.

McCoy, K., Fremouw, W., and McNeil, D. W. (2010). Thresholds and tolerance of physical pain among young adults who self-injure. *Pain Research and Management*, 15(6), 371–377.

Messman-Moore, T. L., Walsh, K. L., and DiLillo, D. (2010). Emotion dysregulation and risky sexual behavior in revictimization. *Child Abuse and Neglect*, 34(12), 967–976.

Nock, M. K., Joiner, T. E., Gordon, K. H., Lloyd-Richardson, E., and Prinstein, M. J. (2006). Non-suicidal self-injury among adolescents: Diagnostic correlates and relation to suicide attempts. *Psychiatry Research*, 111(1), 65–72.

Nock, M. K. and Prinstein, M. J. (2005). Contextual features and behavioral functions of self-mutilation. *Journal of Abnormal Psychology*, 114(1), 140–146.

Orbach, I., Blomenson, R., Mikulincer, M., Gilboa-Schechtman, E., Rogolsky, M., and Retzoni, G. (2007). Perceiving a problem-solving task as a threat and suicidal behavior in adolescents. *Journal of Social and Clinical Psychology*, 26(9), 1010–1034.

Paris, J. and Zweig-Frank, H. (2001). A 27 year follow-up of patients with borderline personality disorder. *Comprehensive Psychiatry*, 42(6), 482–487.

Quoidbach, J., Berry, E. V., Hansenne, M., and Mikolajczak, M. (2010). Positive emotion regulation and well-being: Comparing the impact of eight savoring and dampening strategies. *Personality and Individual Differences*, 49(5), 368–373.

Russ, M. J., Campbell, S. S., Kakuma, T., Harrison, K., and Zanine, E. (1999). EEG theta activity and pain insensitivity in self-injurious borderline patients. *Psychiatry Research*, 89(3), 201–214.

Russ, M. J., Roth, S. D., Lerman, A., and Kakuma, T. (1992). Pain perception in self-injurious patients with borderline personality disorder. *Biological Psychiatry*, 32(6), 501–511.

Simons, J. R. and Gaher, R. M. (2005). The Distress Tolerance Scale: Development and validation of a self-report measure. *Motivation and Emotion*, 29(2), 83–102.

Smith, A., Ribeiro, J., Mikolajewski, A., Taylor, J., Joiner, T., and Iacono, W. (2012). An examination of environmental and genetic contributions to the determinants of suicidal behavior among male twins. *Psychiatry Research*, 197(1–2), 60–65.

Smyth, J. M., Wonderlich, S. A., Heron, K. E., Sliwinski, M. J., Crosby, R. D., Mitchell, J. E., and Engel, S. G. (2007). Daily and momentary mood and stress are associated with binge eating and vomiting in bulimia nervosa patients in the natural environment. *Journal of Consulting and Clinical Psychology*, 75(4), 629–638.

Tamas, Z., Kovacs, M., Gentzler, A. L., Tepper, P., Gadoros, J., Kiss, E., Kapornai, K., and Vetro, A. (2007). The relations of temperament and emotion self-regulation with suicidal behaviors in a clinical sample of depressed children in Hungary. *Journal of Abnormal Child Psychology*, 35(4), 640–652.

Tull, M. T., Weiss, N. H., Adams, C. E., and Gratz, K. L. (2012). The contribution of emotion regulation difficulties to risky sexual behavior within a sample of patients in residential substance abuse treatment. *Addictive Behaviors*, 37(10), 1084–1092.

Van Orden, K. A., Witte, T. K., Cukrowicz, K. C., Braithwaite, S. R., Selby, E. A., and Joiner, T. E. (2010). The interpersonal theory of suicide. *Psychological Review*, 117(2), 575–600.

Whiteside, S. P., and Lynam, D. R. (2001). The five factor model and impulsivity: Using a structural model of personality to understand impulsivity. *Personality and Individual Differences*, 30(4), 669–689.

Zlotnick, C., Donaldson, D., Spirito, A., and Pearlstein, T. (1997). Affect regulation and suicide attempts in adolescent inpatients. *Journal of the American Academy of Child and Adolescent Psychiatry*, 36(6), 793–798.

5 Role of aggression and impulsivity in suicide attempts and in suicide completion

Yari Gvion and Alan Apter

Suicide is the tenth leading cause of death worldwide, accounting for 1.5 percent of all deaths in the Western world (Hawton and van Heeringen, 2009). About 25 suicide attempts occur for every fatal suicide (Simon, 2008). Approximately 90 percent of individuals who commit suicide meet the criteria for a psychiatric disorder (Cavanagh *et al.*, 2003). However, despite the fact that most suicide attempters suffer from psychopathology, most persons with psychiatric disorders do not attempt suicide. Therefore other factors over and above psychopathology must be involved. Predictors of suicidal behavior and risk factors include a history of previous suicide attempts, certain demographic variables, clinical symptoms, traits and states and issues related to medical and social support (Hawton and van Heeringen, 2009; Gvion and Apter, 2012). So it seems that suicide is multifaceted and rarely the result of any single cause (Apter, 2010).

One of the major challenges for research in this field is the need to define the role of personality and trait-like dimensions in predisposing to suicidal behavior. The aim of this chapter is to review the past and current literature on the long-known link between aggression, impulsivity, and suicide.

Suicide and suicidal behavior

Suicide is an act of intentionally terminating one's own life (Nock *et al.*, 2008). A suicide attempt is defined as such when the following characteristics are present: (a) self-initiated, potentially injurious behavior; (b) intent to die; and (c) a nonfatal outcome (Van Orden *et al.*, 2010; Witte *et al.*, 2008). Suicide may be preceded by suicidal thoughts, threats, gestures, non-suicidal self-injuries, and suicide attempts of various degrees of lethality, all of which are generally lumped together under the rubric of 'suicidality'. There is also some value in separating out medically serious suicide attempts (MSSA) from the non-medically serious suicide attempt (NMSSA) (Beautrais, 2001, 2003), as the study of this subgroup can best shed light on actual suicide attempters (Marzano *et al.*, 2009; Levi-Belz *et al.*, 2013).

Aggression and impulsivity: a single or two distinct constructs?

There are a growing number of studies on impulsivity and aggression. Yet a consensus definition of the constructs aggression and impulsivity remains elusive and is beset by a lack of conceptual clarity (for review, see Gvion and Apter, 2011). This is largely due to the confusion between terms such as 'aggression', 'aggressiveness', 'impulsivity' and 'impulsive-aggression'.

In the psychological and psychiatric literature **aggression** is defined as any behavior intended to harm another person who is motivated to avoid being harmed (Baron and Richardson, 1994). Terms such as aggression and violence are used to describe destructive behavior, angry feelings, hostile fantasies and indirect attacks on objects (Gothelf *et al.*, 1997).

Although the literature uses terms such as aggression, violence, irritability, and anger interchangeably, it is important to specify differences and over-laps. Trait anger is the tendency to feel anger more intensely, more often and for a longer period of time than others (Deffenbacher *et al.*, 1996). The definition of trait irritability includes being angrier, in general and taking offense at the slightest provocation as well as the propensity to be offensive in the use of aggressive behavior (Bettencourt *et al.*, 2006), trait irritability and violence are conceptually related (Glasser, 1985) to trait aggressiveness (Caprara and Renzi, 1981) and the construct of trait anger overlaps with trait aggressiveness (Buss and Perry, 1992). There is also a difference between two forms of aggression: reactive and proactive aggression. Reactive aggression (RA) is an aggressive response to a perceived threat or provocation, and as such it is emotionally charged, poorly controlled, and impulsive, whereas proactive aggression (PA) is defined as an unemotional, highly controlled, and premeditated behavior that anticipates a reward (Kemps *et al.*, 2005; Conner *et al.*, 2009).

Impulsivity is an ill-defined concept encompassing a broad range of behaviors that reflect impaired self-regulation (Evenden, 1999; Whiteside and Lynam, 2001). Cyders and colleagues (2007) distinguish five facets of impulsivity: sensation seeking, lack of deliberation, lack of persistence, positive urgency, and negative urgency (the latter two meaning the tendency to act rashly in response to positive and negative affective states, respectively). Patton and colleagues (2005) define impulsivity in terms of attentional, motor, and non-planning impulsiveness and look at impulsivity as a stable trait that can be evaluated using personality questionnaires. Others assess behavioral impulsivity using measures such as the Immediate Memory Task (IMT) (Keilp *et al.*, 2005), or consider it as a state that can be assessed by taking individuals' subjective accounts of state impulsivity (Michaelis *et al.*, 2003). A recent meta-analysis found a significant but rather small association between different measures across studies (Cyders and Coskunpinar, 2011).

Given its robust relations to aggressive and delinquent behaviors, early appearance in development, and overlap with domains of general personality, increasing attention is being paid to impulsivity as a predictor of aggressive behaviors (Krueger *et al.*, 1996). Some authors suggested that overlap between aggression and impulsivity is robust and universal and that they should be considered together, as a single phenotype (Mann and Currier, 2009), others, however, believe they represent two distinct latent dimensions (Critchfield *et al.*, 2004). Be that as it may, the association among impulsivity, aggression, and suicidality is well documented both in research and in clinical practice across diagnoses (for review, see Gvion and Apter, 2011). Some recent studies have suggested aggressive impulsive behavior as the underlying link between a family history of suicide and new attempts by probands especially in youth (Brent and Melhem, 2008; Chachamovich *et al.*, 2009).

One of the problems that arise when trying to decide which is most relevant to suicidal behavior is the lack of clarity of the definitions: there are studies that use the terms aggression and hostility synonymously (Michaelis *et al.*, 2004). Others use composites of constructs, namely impulsivity, hostility, and aggression and terming them inter-changeably, as impulsive aggression (McGirr *et al.*, 2008, 2009). Problems also arise from the fact that aggressive acts may be impulsive or premeditated, and impulsivity is a trait encompassing spontaneous, poorly planned, and situationally inappropriate behaviors, without necessarily including aggression (McGirr *et al.*, 2008). It is also important to distinguish between trait impulsivity and state impulsivity (Baca-Garcia *et al.*, 2005). From a suicidology perspective, they are all facets of the same underlying predisposition, none a necessary and sufficient cause of the other, never precluding the other, but each a manifestation of a predisposition to suicide subsumed under the impulsive aggressive suicide diathesis (McGirr *et al.*, 2007; Brent and Mann, 2005).

Aggression-impulsivity psychopathology and suicidal behavior

Anger, aggression, and impulsivity are associated with suicide attempts. Although current models suggest that aggression and impulsivity may contribute to a summary factor predictive of suicidal behavior in patients with various types of psychiatric diagnoses (Mann and Currier, 2009), many studies examined the influence of each construct independently from the other.

Impulsivity, psychopathology and suicidal behavior

Numerous studies that have examined different aspects of suicidality in different clinical populations have concluded that those with higher impulsivity levels tend to be more likely to engage in suicidal acts (Forcano *et al.*, 2009; Gut-Fay *et al.*, 2001; Yen and Siegler, 2003). Gut-Fay and and colleagues (2001) for example, found that schizophrenic patients with co-morbid substance abuse produced higher trait impulsivity scores and reported a higher number of suicide attempts when compared to those without a history of substance abuse. Similarly Swann and colleagues (2005) evaluated bipolar patients with and without a definite history of attempted suicide using the Barratt Impulsiveness Scale and a behavioral laboratory performance measure. They found that a history of medically severe suicide attempts was associated with impulsive responses on an immediate memory task. In another study Dumais *et al.* (2005a) noted an association of suicide with high levels of impulsivity and aggression, in addition to alcohol and drug dependence, and cluster B personality disorders. Finally, Maser and colleagues (2002) compared the personality characteristics of three groups of patients with affective disorders who were followed naturalistically for 14 years. Impulsivity was common to both suicide attempters and completers, and together with assertiveness was the best predictor of completed suicide beyond 12 months.

Impulsive and suicidal behaviors are among the most characteristic features of cluster B diagnosis (Gunderson, 2001; Paris, 2002). Zouk and colleagues (2006) investigated suicide completers with very extreme phenotypes, defined as a score above the 70th and below the 30th percentile on the Barret Impulsivity Scale (BIS). Compared to less impulsive suicide completers, the highly impulsive subjects were more likely to have a cluster B diagnosis, exhibited higher measures of aggressive behavior, and as well as a life-time and six-month prevalence of alcohol and drug dependence.

Suicide attempts in alcoholics have also been linked to behavioral disinhibition, impulsivity, and aggression (Mezzich *et al.*, 1997). For example, Wojnar and colleagues (2009) studied patients with alcohol dependence. A stop-signal procedure was used as a behavioral measure of impulsivity. Forty-three percent of the subjects reported life-time suicide attempts, of which 62 percent were impulsive. The only significant factor that distinguished patients with impulsive suicide attempts from patients with a non-impulsive suicide attempts and non-suicidal patients was a higher level of behavioral impulsivity. Similar results were obtained by Pompili and colleagues (2009) who compared a psychiatric group with substance dependence and another without. The substance dependent group had a tendency towards more impulsive aggressive personality and a history of suicidal thoughts and behaviors. The statistical significance of these finding was, however, low.

Studies of young populations consider the presence of impulsive behaviors and maladaptive personality traits as possible factors that play a role in the risk of suicide (Renaud *et al.*, 2008). In a recent study Ghanem *et al.* (2013) found that youth attempters had higher total scores and subscales of impulsivity than controls.

It is not known whether impulsivity increases the risk of suicide independently of aggressive traits (Baud, 2005) or if it is related to the medical severity of suicide attempts. Some authors reported evidence of higher levels of impulsivity in individuals who died by suicide than those who did not (Swann *et al.*, 2005; Dumais *et al.*, 2005b) whereas others found that although people who attempt

suicide tend to be more impulsive than people who do not, the actual act of completed suicide is often not made impulsively (Anestis *et al.*, 2007). Simon *et al.*
(2001) reported that only 24 percent of survivors of near-lethal suicide attempts
had thought about their attempt for less than 5 minutes. Those who made their
attempt within 5 minutes of deciding to do so were less likely to have considered
another method of suicide. They also had a greater likelihood of discovery and a
lower expectation of death. Baca-Garcia and colleagues (2001, 2005) claimed
that impulsivity is a characteristic of non-lethal suicide attempts or suicide gestures whereas planned suicide involves a more subjective element drawn from the
desired outcome and the perceived lethality of the act of self-harm. Baca-Garcia
and colleagues (2005) assessed attempt impulsivity (i.e., state) and attempter
(i.e., trait) impulsivity in an inpatient population. They found that impulsivity of
the attempter was not a good predictor of impulsivity of the attempt (i.e., attempting suicide without prior planning) and that non-impulsive attempts (i.e., those
that involved prior planning) were more lethal compared to impulsive attempts.
These findings highlight the importance of planning and preparation for suicide
in determining lethality. An additional study (Wyder and De Leo, 2007) surveyed
a community sample regarding past suicidal behavior. Only one quarter of these
described a pattern consistent with an impulsive attempt. Finally Witte and
colleagues (2008) compared adolescents who had planned a suicide attempt but
did not actually attempt; adolescents who did not plan a suicide but attempted;
and those who both planned and attempted suicide. They found that individuals
who planned suicide without attempting were significantly less impulsive than
those who attempted without planning and those who planned and attempted.
Furthermore, participants who attempted without planning were less impulsive
than those who both planned and attempted.

Other authors emphasized the mediatory role of the intent to die at the time
of the suicide attempt. Hawton (1986) observed that less than 50 percent
of subjects with a history of suicide attempts really wanted to die; he defined
their attempts as little-planned impulsive acts. Motives reported in impulsive
suicides ranged from escaping from an intolerable situation to manipulation
(Carballo *et al.*, 2006; Oquendo *et al.*, 2000).

When evaluating impulsivity within suicidality, research has focused on direct,
proximate, and indirect causal factors. For example, Mann and colleagues (1999)
propose a stress-vulnerability model of suicidality. Their model suggests that it is
not just stressors (e.g., job loss, end of a romantic relationship) that can lead an
individual to undertake a suicidal act. They postulate that, additionally, vulnerability towards experiencing more suicidal ideation and to acting in a more
impulsive manner needs to be present which then increases the likelihood of
individuals being more inclined to act on suicidal ideation. Furthermore,
impulsivity can increase risk for other suicide-related factors such as alcohol or
drug use, and thereby indirectly contribute to the risk of a suicide attempt
(Mann *et al.*, 1999).

Joiner (2007) proposed the interpersonal psychological theory of attempted
and completed suicide which claims that in order to die by suicide an individual

must have both the desire and the capability. The desire to die by suicide stems from a thwarted sense of belongingness and the feeling of being a burden on others. However, the capability to engage in suicidal behavior is separate from the desire to engage in suicidal behavior. The capability to die by suicide is acquired through a process of habituation that allows the individual to overcome the pain and fear associated with suicidal behavior. Pre-existing factors sometimes accelerate the process. Thus, according to Joiner (2007), impulsivity is only distally related to suicide: impulsive individuals may be more likely to have experiences that are painful or provocative which, in turn, confer an increased risk of suicidal behavior via habituation. Along the same lines, Witte *et al.* (2008) proposed that certain behaviors may promote the individual's capability of committing lethal suicide, such as prostitution, drug use, self-mutilation, and violence. With practice and repetition, the fear- and pain-inducing aspects of such provocative behaviors are reduced, and they become rewarding.

Aggression, psychopathology and suicidal behavior

The correlation between aggression and suicidality has been studied across psychiatric samples, and non-psychiatric populations. Popular conceptualizations of suicide among schizophrenic patients have posited that many suicides of schizophrenic patients involve the use of violent methods to commit suicide thus implying a correlation between aggression and suicidality. Although some studies did find that patients suffering from schizophrenia usually attempt suicide with a potentially lethal method (Fenton *et al.*, 1997), this was not confirmed by other studies. Symonds and colleagues (2006) compared suicidal intent, violence of method, and motive in patients suffering from schizophrenia and adjustment reactions with self-harm. The schizophrenic group did not significantly use more violent methods. The use of a violent method was also not significantly associated with the presence of positive symptoms in schizophrenia. Along the same lines Mitrev and Massaldjieva (2004) found no significant relation between current aggressive behavior and current suicide risk, as well as between lifetime aggression and lifetime suicide behavior in male inpatients with schizophrenia and other psychotic disorders. Finally, in a study by McGirr and colleagues (2006), it was found that impulsive-aggressive behaviors did not play a role in schizophrenic and chronic psychotic suicide.

Depression is also associated with suicide risk; several studies found a correlation between suicide attempters suffering from depression and high levels of impulsive and aggressive behaviors (Pendse *et al.*, 1999), especially when comorbid with Borderline Personality Disorder or substance use disorders (Cheng *et al.*, 1997). It remains unclear whether the association between impulsive and aggressive behaviors and the risk of suicide is at least partly explained by Axis I disorders that are commonly associated with suicide, such as major depressive disorders. In an attempt to clarify that question, Dumais and colleagues (2005a) compared a large sample of male suicide completers who died during an episode of major depression to living depressed males. They found that impulsive aggressive personality disorders and alcohol abuse were two independent predictors of suicide in major depression.

Bipolar disorder is also associated with suicidal behavior. Aggression but not impulsivity appears to be a factor in this group. Oquendo and colleagues (2000), and Michaelis and colleagues (2004) report that hostility was elevated in bipolar suicide attempters relative to non-attempters.

In clinical practice, impulsiveness and hostility may function as suicide attempt risk indicators because they indicate the likelihood of Borderline Personality Disorder (BPD), which itself carries a heightened risk for suicidal behavior. Therefore many studies investigated the association between suicide attempts and violence among individuals with personality disorders, especially BPD (Zalsman *et al.*, 2006). One of the studies (McGirr *et al.*, 2007) found that individuals with BPD who died by suicide differed from those typically encountered in acute psychiatric settings. They suggest that the lethality of BPD suicide attempts results from an interaction between impulsivity and the violent-aggressive features associated with cluster B comorbidity. Similar results were obtained by Brodsky and colleagues (2006) who found that attempters with comorbid BPD and major depressive disorder (MDD) had a higher number of lifetime suicide attempts, and had higher levels of lifetime aggression, hostility and impulsivity, compared with attempters with major depression only.

There is also a robust association of aggression and suicidal behavior in hospitalized adolescents. Two types of suicidal behavior were found: one characterized by depressive symptoms and another characterized by impulsivity (Apter *et al.*, 1988, 1995). This model of two types of suicidal behavior was affirmed in a later study on younger male subjects (mean age 9.81) (Greening *et al.*, 2008). The association of aggression with suicidal behavior was also found in non-patient adolescents. Conner and colleagues (2004) gathered data from a community sample of 625 adolescent and young adult males. Impulsivity and irritability were associated strongly with suicidal ideation after accounting for alcohol dependence and other aggression-related constructs including psychopathy. Vermeiren and colleagues (2003) conducted a school-based study, using self-report measures. They observed that suicidal and violent adolescents shared characteristics related to internalizing problems, aggression, and risk-taking behavior.

In an attempt to study the relationship between aggression and suicide completion, different approaches have been taken. One of them compared medically serious suicide attempters (MSSAs) to healthy controls. Trait aggression was significantly higher in the MSSA group (Doihara *et al.*, 2008), however, that study did not include a non-medically serious suicide attempters (NMSSAs) control group. In another study personality-disordered individuals, particularly those who are more impulsive and aggressive and who have a co-morbid depressive disorder were found to have a higher risk for more frequent and more medically severe suicidal behavior in comparison to individuals with Major Depressive

Disorder (MDD) or Bipolar Depression (BD) alone (Black *et al.*, 1988; McGlashan, 1987). Contrary to that, in a recent study our group compared MSSA to NMSSA and to psychiatric non-suicidal controls. We found that aggression and impulsivity distinguished suicide attempters from non-attempters. However, they did not distinguish the MSSA group from the NMSSA group and thus did not predict the lethality of the suicide attempt (Gvion *et al.*, 2014).

Gender is a factor that is closely related to suicide attempts and to the lethality of the attempt. It has been found across different studies, that actual suicide is more prevalent among men, whereas nonfatal suicidal behaviors are more prevalent among women (Kessler *et al.*, 2005). Aggression or one of its facets (e.g., anger, violence) might be related to the difference found between female and masculine suicidal behavior and completion.

Summary

Aggression-impulsivity are risk factors for suicide attempts. The association between aggression, impulsivity, and suicidal behavior is well documented and is based on decades of research and clinical practice. In analyzing the reciprocal relationship between aggressiveness impulsivity and suicide behavior it is important to make a distinction between acts (or observable behaviors, e.g. an aggression) and traits or predispositions (e.g. impulsivity or aggressiveness), which are non-observable, inferred constructs. It is also important to better define the various suicidal behaviors. Looking at aggression and impulsivity in near lethal attempters may be very different from examining these associations in suicide attempt repeaters who frequently are present at emergency rooms.

Nevertheless the literature is confusing and contradictory and not easy to organize in a coherent manner. This is probably due to the difficulty in defining and separating out these concepts and the fact that there is much overlap between them. Thus, some of the data collected to date on the role of aggression and impulsivity in suicide and suicide lethality needs to be reconsidered in light of differences among the studies in definitions used, methods employed, and the selected population. The future probably lies in looking at some basic under-lying biological phenotypes such as those described in the work of Mann and Currier (2009) or some of the sociological problem behavior theories of Jessor (1991). Since aggression and impulsivity are so ubiquitous in suicidal behaviors and so obvious a target for intervention, this area of enquiry must be pursued despite all the inherent difficulties involved in such an endeavor.

References

Anestis, M. D., Selby, E. A., and Joiner, T. E. (2007). The role of urgency in maladaptive behaviors. *Behavior Research and Therapy*, 45(12), 3018–3029.

Apter, A. (2010). Clinical aspects of suicidal behavior relevant to genetics. *European Psychiatry*, 25(5), 257–259.

Apter, A., Bleich, A., Plutchik, R., Mendelsohn, S., and Tyano, S. (1988). Suicidal behavior, depression, and conduct disorder in hospitalized adolescents. *Journal of the American Academy of Child and Adolescence Psychiatry*, 27(6), 696–699.

Apter, A., Gothhelf, D., Orbach, I., Weisman, R., Ratzoni, G., Har Even, D., and Tyano, S. (1995). Correlation of suicide and violent behavior in different diagnostic categories in hospitalized adolescent patients. *Journal of the American Academy of Child and Adolescence Psychiatry*, 34(7), 912–918.

Baca-Garcia, E., Diaz-Sastre, C., Basurte, E., Prieto, R., Ceverino, A., Saiz-Ruiz, J., and de Leon, J. (2001). A prospective study of the paradoxical relationship between impulsivity and lethality of suicide attempts. *The Journal of Clinical Psychiatry*, 62(7), 560–564.

Baca-Garcia, E., Diaz-Satre, C., Garcia-Resa, E., Blasco, H., Braquehais Conesa, D., Oquendo, M.A., *et al.* (2005). Suicide attempts and impulsivity. *European Archives of Psychiatry and Clinical Neuroscience*, 255(2), 152–156.

Baron, R. A., and Richardson, D. (1994). *Human Aggression*. New York, NY: Plenum Press.

Baud, P. (2005). Personality traits as intermediary phenotypes in suicidal behavior: Genetic issues. *American Journal of Medical Genetics*, 133C(1), 34–42.

Beautrais, A. L. (2001). Suicide and serious suicide attempts: Two populations or one? *Psychological Medicine*, 31(5), 837–845.

Beautrais, A. L. (2003). Suicide and serious suicide attempts in youth: A multiple-group comparison study. *The American Journal of Psychiatry*, 160(6), 1093–1099.

Bettencourt, B. A., Talley, A., Benjamin, A. J., and Valentine, J. (2006). Personality and aggressive behavior under provoking and neutral conditions: A meta-analytic review. *Psychological Bulletin*, 132(5), 751–777.

Black, D. W., Bell, S., Hulbert, J., and Nasrallah, A. (1988). The importance of Axis II in patients with major depression. *Journal of Affective Disorders*, 14(2), 115–122.

Brent, D. A., and Mann, J. J. (2005). Family genetic studies, suicide, and suicidal behavior. *American Journal of Medical Genetics*, 133C(1), 13–24.

Brent, D. A., and Melhem, N. (2008). Familial transmission of suicidal behavior. *The Psychiatric Clinics of North America*, 31(2), 157–177.

Brodsky, B. S., Groves, S. A., Oquendo, M. A., Mann, J. J., and Stanley, B. (2006). Interpersonal precipitants and suicide attempts in borderline personality disorder. *Suicide and Life-Threatening Behavior*, 36(3), 313–322.

Buss, A. H., and Perry, M. (1992). The Aggression Questionnaire. *Journal of Personality and Social Psychology*, 63(3), 452–459.

Caprara, G. V. and Renzi, P. (1981). The frustration-aggression hypothesis vs. irritability. *Recherches de Psychologue Sociale*, 3, 75–80.

Carballo, J. J., Oquendo, M. A., Giner, L., Zatsman, G., Roche, A. M., and Sher, L. (2006). Impulsive-aggressive traits and suicidal adolescents and young adults with alcoholism. *International Journal of Adolescent Medical Health*, 18(1), 15–19.

Cavanagh, J. T., Carson, A., Sharpe, M., and Lawrie, S. M. (2003). Psychological autopsy studies of suicide: A systematic review. *Psychological Medicine*, 33(3), 395–405.

Chachamovich, E., Stefanello, S., Botega, N., and Turecki, G. (2009). Which are the recent clinical findings regarding the association between depression and suicide? *Revista Brasileira de Psiquiatria*, 31(Suppl.1), S18–S25.

Cheng, A. T., Mann, A. H., and Chan, K. A. (1997). Personality disorder and suicide: A case control study. *British Journal of Psychiatry*, 170, 441–446.

Conner, K. R., Meldrum, S., Wieczorek, W. F., Duberstein, P. R., and Welte, J. W. (2004). The association of irritability and impulsivity with suicidal ideation among 15- to 20-year-old males. *Suicide and Life-Threatening Behavior*, 34(4), 363–373.

Conner, K. R., Swogger, M. T., and Houston, R. J. (2009). A test of reactive aggression-suicidal behavior hypotheses: Is there a case for proactive aggression? *Journal of Abnormal Psychology*, 118(1), 235–240.

Critchfield, K. L., Levy, K. N., and Clarkin, J. F. (2004). The relationship between impulsivity, aggression, and impulsive-aggression in borderline personality disorder: An empirical analysis of self-report measures. *Journal of Personality Disorders*, 18(6), 555–570.

Cyders, M., and Coskunpinar, A. (2011). Measurement of constructs using self-report and behavioral lab tasks: Is there overlap in nomothetic span and construct representation for impulsivity? *Clinical Psychological Review*, 31(6), 965–982.

Cyders, M. A., Smith, G. T., Spillane, N. S., Fischer, S., Annus, A. M., and Peterson, C. (2007). Integration of impulsivity and positive mood to predict risky behaviour: Development and validation of a measure of positive urgency. *Psychological Assessment*, 19(1), 107–118.

Deffenbacher, J. L., Oetting, E. R., Thwaites, G. A., Lynch, R. S., Baker, D. A., Stark, R. S., *et al.* (1996). State-trait anger theory and the utility of the Trait Anger Scale. *Journal of Counseling Psychology*, 43(2), 131–148.

Doihara, C., Kawanishi, C., Yamada, T., Sato, R., Hasegawa, H., Furuno, T., *et al.* (2008). Trait aggression in suicide attempters: A pilot study. *Psychiatry and Clinic Neurosciences*, 62(3), 352–354.

Dumais, A., Lesage, A. D., Alda, M., Rouleau, G., Dumont, M., Chawky, N., *et al.* (2005a). Risk factors for suicide completion in major depression: A case-control study of impulsive and aggressive behaviors in men. *The Journal of Psychiatry*, 162(11), 2116–2124.

Dumais, A., Lesage, A. D., Lalovi, A., Séguin, M., Tousignant, M., Chawky, N., and Turecki, G. (2005b). Is violent method of suicide a behavioral marker of lifetime aggression? *The American Journal of Psychiatry*, 162(7), 1375–1378.

Evenden, J. (1999). Impulsivity: A discussion of clinical and experimental findings. *Journal of Psychopharmacology*, 13(2), 180–192.

Fenton, W. S., McGlashan, T. H., Victor, B. J., and Blyler, C. R. (1997). Symptoms, subtype, and suicidality in patients with schizophrenia spectrum disorders. *The American Journal of Psychiatry*, 154(2), 199–204.

Forcano, L., Fernández-Aranda, F., Alvarez-Moya, E., Bulik, C., Granero, R., Gratacòs, M., *et al.* (2009). Suicide attempts in bulimia nervosa: Personality and psychopathological correlates. *European Psychiatry*, 24(2), 91–97.

Ghanem, M., Gamaluddin, H., Mansour, M., Samiee, A. A., Shaker, N. M., and El Rafei, H. (2013). Role of impulsivity and other personality dimensions in attempted suicide with self-poisoning among children and adolescents. *Archives of Suicide Research*, 17(3), 262–274.

Glasser, M. (1985). Aspects of Violence, paper given to the Applied Section of the British Psychoanalytical Society.

Gothelf, D., Apter, A., and van Praag, H. (1997). Measurement of aggression in psychiatric patients. *Psychiatry Research*, 71(2), 83–95.

Greening, L., Stoppelbein, l., Fite, P., Dhossche, D., Erath, S., Brown, J., *et al.* (2008). Pathways to suicidal behaviors in childhood. *Suicide and Life-Threatening Behavior*, 38(1), 35–45.

Gunderson, J. G. (2001). *Borderline Personality Disorder: A Clinical Guide*. Washington, DC: American Psychiatric Publishing.

Gut-Fay and, A., Dervaux, A., Olie, J., Loo, H., Poirier, M., and Krebs, M. (2001). Substance abuse and suicidality in schizophrenia: A common risk factor linked to impulsivity. *Psychiatry Research*, 102(1), 65–72.

Gvion, Y., and Apter, A. (2011). Aggression, impulsivity and suicide behavior: A review of the literature. *Archives of Suicide Research*, 15(2), 93–112.

Gvion, Y., and Apter, A. (2012). Suicide and suicidal behavior. *Public Health Review*, 34(2), 1–20.

Gvion, Y., Horesh, N., Levi-Belz, Y., Fischel, T., Trves, I., Weise, M., *et al.* (2014). Aggression-impulsivity, mental pain, and communication difficulties in medically serious and medically non-serious suicide attempters. *Comprehensive Psychiatry*, 55(1), 40–50.

Hawton, K. (1986). *Suicide and Attempted Suicide Among Children and Adolescents.* Newbury Park, CA: Sage Publications.

Hawton, K., and van Heeringen, K. (2009). Suicide. *Lancet*, 373(9672), 1372–1381.

Jessor, R. (1991). Risk behavior in adolescence: A psychosocial framework for understanding and action. *Journal of Adolescent Health*, 12(8), 597–605.

Joiner, T. E. (2007). *Why People Die by Suicide*. Cambridge, MA: Harvard University Press.

Keilp, J. G., Sackeim, H. A., and Mann, J. J. (2005). Correlates of trait impulsiveness in performance measures and neuropsychological tests. *Psychiatry Research*, 135(3), 191–201.

Kemps, M., Matthys, W., de Vries, H., and van Engeland, H. (2005). Reactive and proactive aggression in children: A review of theory, findings and the relevance for child and adolescent psychiatry. *European Child and Adolescent Psychiatry*, 14(1), 11–19.

Kessler, R. C., Berglund, P., Borges, G., Nock, M. K., and Wang, P. S. (2005). Trends in suicide ideation, plans, gestures, and attempts in the United States, 1990–1992 to 2001–2003. *The Journal of American Medical Association*, 293(20), 2487–2495.

Krueger, R. F., Caspi, A., Moffitt, T. E., White J., and Stouthamer-Loeber, M. (1996). Delay of gratification, psychopathology, and personality: Is low self-control specific to externalizing problems? *Journal of Personality*, 64(1), 107–129.

Levi-Belz, Y., Gvion, Y., Horesh, N., and Apter, A. (2013). Attachment patterns in medically serious suicide attempts: The mediating role of self-disclosure and loneliness. *Suicide and Life-Threatening Behavior*, 43(5), 511–522.

Mann, J. J., and Currier, D. (2009). Biological predictors of suicidal behavior in mood disorders. In D. Wasserman and C. Wasserman (Eds), *Oxford Textbook of*

Suicide Prevention: A Global Perspective (pp. 335–341). Oxford: Oxford University Press.

Mann, J. J., Waternaux, C., Haas, G. L., and Malone, K. M. (1999). Toward a clinical model of suicidal behavior in psychiatric patients. *American Journal of Psychiatry*, 156(2), 181–189.

Marzano, L., Rivlin, A., Fazel, S., and Hawton, K. (2009). Interviewing survivors of near-lethal self-harm: A novel approach for investigating suicide amongst prisoners. *Journal of Forensic and Legal Medicine*, 16(3), 152–155.

Maser, J. D., Akiskal, H. S., Schettler, P., Scheftner, W., Mueller, T., Endicott, J., *et al.* (2002). Can temperament identify affectively ill patients who engage in lethal or near lethal suicide behavior? A 14-year prospective study. *Suicide and Life-Threatening Behavior*, 32(1), 10–32.

McGirr, A., Alda, M., Seguin, M., Cabot, S., Lesage, A., and Turecki, G. (2009). Familial aggregation of suicide explained by cluster B traits: A three-group family study of suicide controlling for major depressive disorder. *The American Journal of Psychiatry*, 166(10), 1124–1134.

McGirr, A., Paris, J., Lesage, A., Renaud, J., and Turecki, G. (2007). Risk factors for suicide completion in borderline personality disorder: A case-control study of cluster B comorbidity and impulsive aggression. *Journal of Clinical Psychiatry*, 68(5), 721–729.

McGirr, A., Renaud, J., Bureau, A., Seguin, M., Lesage, A., and Turecki G. (2008). Impulsive-aggressive behaviors and completed suicide across the life cycle: A predisposition for younger age of suicide. *Psychological Medicine*, 38(3), 407–417.

McGirr, A., Tousignant, M., Routhier, D., Pouliot, L., Chawky, N., Margolese, H. C., and Turecki, G. (2006). Risk factors for completed suicide in schizophrenia and other chronic psychotic disorders: A case-control study. *Schizophrenia Research*, 84(1), 132–143.

McGlashan, T. H. (1987). Borderline personality disorder and unipolar affective disorder. *The Journal of Nervous and Mental Disease*, 175(8), 467–473.

Mezzich, A. C., Giancola, P. R., Tarter, R. E., Lu, S., Parks, S. M., and Barrett, C. M. (1997). Violence, suicidality, and alcohol/drug use involvement in adolescent females with psychoactive substance use disorder and controls. *Alcoholism, Clinical and Experimental Research*, 21(7), 1300–1307.

Michaelis, B. H., Goldberg, J. F., Davis, G. P., Singer, T. M., Garno, J. L., and Wenze, S. J. (2004). Dimensions of impulsivity and aggression associated with suicide attempts among bipolar patients: A preliminary study. *Suicide and Life-Threatening Behavior*, 34(2), 172–176.

Michaelis, B. H., Goldberg, J. F., Singer, T. M., Garno, J. L., Ernst, C. L., and Davis, G. P. (2003). Characteristics of first suicide attempts in single versus multiple suicide attempters with bipolar disorder. *Comprehensive Psychiatry*, 44(1), 15–20.

Mitrev, I. N., and Massaldjieva, R. I. (2004). Suicidal behaviour and aggression in psychiatric inpatients. *Folia Med (Plovdiv)*, 46(4), 22–26.

Nock, M. K., Borges, G., Bromet, E. J., Alonso, J., Angermeyer, M., Beautrais, A., *et al.* (2008). Cross-national prevalence and risk factors for suicidal ideation, plans and attempts. *British Journal of Psychiatry*, 192(2), 98–105.

Oqendo, M. A., Waternaux, C., Brodsky, B., Parsons, B., Haas, G. L., Malone, K. M., and Mann, J. J. (2000). Suicidal behavior in bipolar mood disorder:

Clinical characteristics of attempters and non attempters. *Journal of Affective Disorders*, 59(2), 107–117.

Paris, J. (2002). Chronic suicidality among patients with borderline personality disorder. *Psychiatric Services*, 53(6), 738–742.

Patton, J. H., Stanford, M.. S., and Barratt, E. S., (2005). Factor structure of the Barratt Impulsivity Scale. *Journal of Clinical Psychology*, 51(6), 768–774.

Pendse, B., Westrin, A., and Engstrom, G. (1999). Temperament traits in seasonal affective disorder, suicide attempters with non-seasonal major depression and healthy controls. *Journal of Affective Disorder*, 54(1), 55–65.

Pompili, M., Immamorati, M., Lester, D., Akiskal, H. S., Rihmer, Z., del Casale, A., *et al.* (2009). Substance abuse, temperament and suicide risk: Evidence from a case-control study. *Journal of Addictive Diseases*, 28(1), 13–20.

Renaud, J., Berlim, M. T., McGirr, A., Tousignant, M., and Turecki, G. (2008). Current psychiatric morbidity, aggression/impulsivity, and personality dimensions in child and adolescent suicide: A case-control study. *Journal of Affective Disorders*, 105(1–3), 221–228.

Simon, O. R., Swann, A. C., Powell, K, E., Potter, L. B., Kresnow. M. J., and O'Carroll, P. W. (2001). Characteristics of impulsive suicide attempts and attempters. *Suicide and Life-Threatening Behavior*, 32(1 Suppl.), 49–59.

Simon, R. I. (2008). Suicide. In R. E. Hales, S. C. Yudofsky, and G. O. Gabbard (Eds), *The American Psychiatric Publishing Textbook of Psychiatry*, 5th edition (p. 1644). Washington, DC: American Psychiatric Publishing Inc.

Swann, A. C., Dougherty, D. M., Pazzaglia, P. J., Pham, M., Steinberg, J. L., and Moeller, F. G. (2005). Increased impulsivity associated with severity of suicide attempt history in patients with bipolar disorder. *The American Journal of Psychiatry*, 162(9), 1680–1688.

Symond, C. S., Taylor, S., Tippins, V., and Turkington, D. (2006). Violent self-harm in schizophrenia. *Suicide and Life-Threatening Behavior*, 36(1), 44–49.

Van Orden, K., Witte, T. K., Cukrowicz, K. C., Braithwaite, S. R., Selby, E. A., and Joiner, T. E., Jr. (2010). The Interpersonal theory of suicide. *Psychological Review*, 117(2), 575–600.

Vermeiren, R., Schwab-Stone, M., Ruchkin, V., King, R., Heeringen, V., and Deboutte, D. (2003). Suicidal behavior and violence in male adolescents: A school-based study. *Journal of the American Academy of Child and Adolescent Psychiatry*, 42(1), 41–48.

Whiteside, S. P. and Lynam, D. R. (2001). The Five Factor Model and impulsivity: Using a structural model of personality to understand impulsivity. *Personality and Individual Differences*, 30(4), 669–689.

Witte, T. K., Merrill, K. A., Stellrecht, N. E., Bernert, R. A., Hollar, D. L., Schatschneider, C., and Joiner T. E. Jr. (2008). Impulsive youth suicide attempters are not necessarily all that impulsive. *Journal of Affective Disorders*, 107(1–3), 107–116.

Wojnar, M., Ilgen, M.A., Czyz, E., Strobbe, S., Klimkiewicz, A., and Jakubczyk, A. (2009). Impulsive and non-impulsive suicide attempts in patients treated for alcohol dependence. *Journal of Affective Disorders*, 115(1–2), 131–139.

Wyder, M., and De Leo, D. (2007). Behind impulsive suicide attempts: Indications from a community study. *Journal of Affective Disorders*, 104(1–3), 167–173.

Yen, S. and Siegler, I. C. (2003). Self-blame, social introversion and male suicides: Prospective data from a longitudinal study. *Archives of Suicide Research*, 7(1), 17–27.

Zalsman, G., Braun, M., Arendt, M., Grunebaum, M. F., Sher, L., Burke, A. K., *et al.* (2006). A comparison of medical lethality of suicide attempts in bipolar and major depressive disorders. *Bipolar Disorder*, 8(5 pt2), 558–565.

Zouk, H., Tousignant, M., Seguin, M., Lesage, A., and Turecki G. (2006). Characterization of impulsivity in suicide completers: Clinical, behavioral and psychosocial dimensions. *Journal of Affective Disorders*, 92(2–3), 195–204.

6 Psycho-social stress and suicidal behaviour

Vsevolod A. Rozanov

The role of stress (stressful life events) in the suicidal process is well established. At the individual level actual stress interacts with genetic predispositions, personality features and protective factors producing positive or negative outcomes (Wasserman, 2001). At the population level effects of stress are mostly modulated by social factors which form the 'framework'. For the human being the majority of changes that need adaptation or produce frustrations and threats belong to the social sphere. In modern industrialized societies with a high work load, rapid changes in society, competitiveness, social inequalities and frequent readjustment to new conditions, stress causes a variety of health problems which are mostly psychosomatic by nature or involve mental health (Lundberg, 2006). These effects are understood within the concept of psycho-social determinants of health, i.e. factors that mediate the effect of social structure on individual and population health outcomes and are conditioned by contexts in which these factors exist or evolve (Martikainen *et al.*, 2002).

The analysis of this concept presented by the above-mentioned authors suggests a distinction between the macro-, meso- and micro-levels as a socio-logical framework. It considers 'psycho-social' as a meso-level concept, which is modified by macro-social factors. Macro-level in turn includes a set of characteristics which relate to ownership and control of land and businesses, legal and welfare structures, as well as distribution of income and other resources between groups and individuals. Meso-level is understood as a more local set of parameters, such as social networks and level of support provided by them, work/activity control, effort/reward balance at work, security, autonomy, home control and work/family conflicts. The central idea of a psycho-social explanation of health outcomes is that social processes at macro- and meso-levels lead to perceptions and psychological processes at the individual (micro-) level. These psychological factors can influence health through direct psychobiological processes or through modified behaviours and lifestyles. So, psycho-social stress should be understood less at the individual level and more at the community level as a response to deprivation, social injustice, inequalities or related events and feelings. Rapid changes in social structures need to be taken into consideration such as revolutions, countries' disintegration, etc. This model is presented on Figure 6.1.

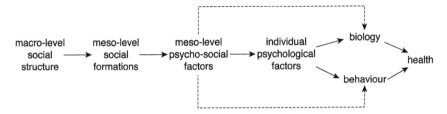

Figure 6.1 Schematic representation of psycho-social pathways to health or disease (from Martikainen *et al.* (2002), by permission).

Rapid changes in society that modify macro-level factors, usually referred to as transition periods are of the greatest interest to us within this chapter. Recently these processes were widely represented in the post-Soviet space and in the countries of the former Soviet bloc. There are many publications which explore the public health consequences of such transition. One of the first, Wolfgang Rutz pointed out the dramatic lowering of life expectancy and excessive mortality from external causes in the former USSR countries in 1993–2001, explaining this by the advent of the severe stress that has overtaken hundreds of millions of its inhabitants (Rutz, 2006). Among the factors that accompany rapid societal changes (macro-level disruption) Rutz discusses growing mental ill health, depression and aggression, alcoholism and addiction, violence and suicidality, risk-taking behaviours and destructive lifestyles, the rise of cardio- and cerebrovascular diseases as well as accidents, both in traffic and in workplaces. These negative manifestations have deep roots in psychological mechanisms which include the loss of dignity and identity, loss of status, helplessness, loss of control and capacity to be in charge of one's own life, the anomie and loss of values, impairment of social connectedness, as well as the lack of existential cohesion and meaning in life (Rutz, 2006). These psychological perceptions and frustrations are accompanied by biological mechanisms involving stress hormones with their diverse effects that provoke various diseases, possibly tackling genetic mechanisms (Schneiderman *et al.*, 2005; McEven, 2012; Rozanov, 2012a).

In concordance with these views, Kopp and Rethelyi (2004), looking at the transforming societies, have pointed out that chronic stress is the main cause of the morbidity and mortality crisis, and draw attention to such global psychological models as depression and learned helplessness that form the basis for negative health and behaviour outcomes. In turn, Ginter and Simko (2010) stressed that the main causes of mortality in the post-totalitarian Europe are the cardiovascular diseases and external causes. They also stressed the role of unhealthy life styles and alcohol consumption.

Actually the idea that psycho-social stress is a factor of great influence that impairs health has been around for many years (Guntem, 1977). It was pointed out that consumption of alcohol, alcoholism, psychosomatic syndromes, as well as consumption of drugs and tobacco and mental ill health together with criminality can serve as important indicators of chronic psycho-social stress. On the other hand, it was noticed that when measuring the impact of societal stress it is difficult to differentiate between stressors, indicators of stress and indicators of coping behaviours (Guntem, 1977). Further it was stated that the population statistics of myocardial infarction and cerebral stroke may be referred to as clear indicators of the level of psycho-social stress in society (Denisova *et al.*, 2005; Egido *et al.*, 2012). Nevertheless, suicide was not very clearly identified among this set of psycho-social stress indicators, possibly due to the complexity of this phenomenon and its dependence on many other factors, all of which is very difficult to untangle.

We are going to demonstrate that changes and variations in suicide rates observed in different countries undergoing rapid socio-economic transitions can be understood to a great extent as the result of the changing level of psycho-social stress. We believe that the concept of psycho-social stress provides additional possibilities for understanding variations in suicide, sometimes clearer than Durkheim's sociological theory that explores the integration and regulation of society as the main internal factors and which are very difficult to measure. To support this, we analyze changes in suicide mortality in the 15 new independent states that appeared on the world map after the USSR collapsed on the eve of the year 1992. Suicide rates changes over a certain historical period (from 1980 to 2010) will be compared with other and stress-related diseases' mortality rates. The information source is the European Health for All Database (EHAD) provided by the WHO web-site. For most 'post-Soviet' countries the above-mentioned database contains data starting from the 1980s, when they were still Soviet republics, up to 2011–2012. Here we are going to discuss psycho-social stress effects while previously we explored these data mainly from the point of view of the role of alcohol consumption (Rozanov, 2012b).

It is well known that for the last 30 years the most prominent fluctuations in suicide rates were observed in the post-Soviet era. These dramatic fluctuations that contrast with the stable situation in European Union countries (see Figure 6.2A) have been analyzed by researchers repeatedly (Mäkinen, 2000; Rutz, 2006; Varnik and Mokhovikov, 2009; Varnik *et al.*, 2010; Kõlves *et al.*, 2013). All authors agree on the role of stress in the observed fluctuations. Discussion centres on such factors as 'community syndrome of excessive morbidity and premature mortality', 'economic distress', and the 'general pathogenic social stress' which accompanies political changes and social disorganization on the peak of processes of disintegration and further transition to a different macro-level social structure. It was noticed by all authors that the developments in suicide have been very different in various Eastern European countries, and that the same causes cannot apply to all of them though high stress on the societal level has been involved. From this point of view it is interesting to compare changes in suicide mortality with other stress-related mortality indices – all external causes, cardiovascular and cerebrovascular mortality (Figure 6.2B). It is clear that these indices had the same temporal pattern as suicides which are also in full accordance with the concept of psycho-social stress.

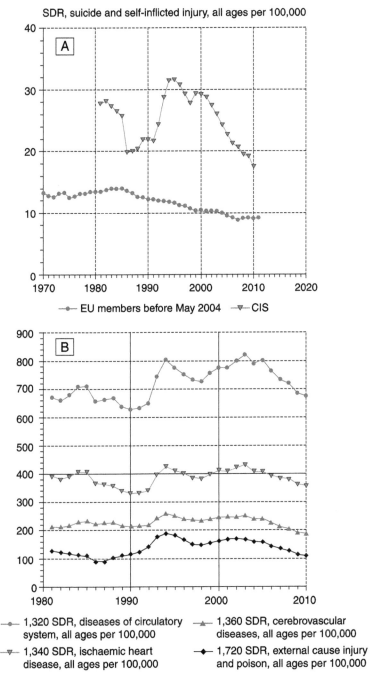

Figure 6.2 (A) Suicide rates in the EU and the 12 former USSR countries and (B) stress-related mortality in the post-Soviet space, for 100,000 of population.

Source: European Health for All Database (WHO).

As can be seen in Figure 6.2A the average suicide rate fluctuations very well reflect the social and economic processes and transformations taking place in the country in the given historical period. Thus, with the beginning of 'perestroika' (the democratization and openness initiative which started in 1985), the level of suicides decreased, reached a quite acceptable level (20 per 100,000) and stayed at that figure up to 1991. It is important to notice that this period was full of social optimism, a feeling of positive change, a turn towards more open discussions, transparency, justice, freedom and contacts with the foreign countries, which of course meant a lowering of psycho-social stress. However, economic problems had been accumulating and very soon the situation changed completely. The collapse of the USSR (the very end of 1991) provoked a sharp increase in the number of suicides (60 per cent increase compared to 1985–1986 data), which remained very high till 1995. These fluctuations were connected with the economic problems in society, especially the 'shock therapy' during privatization, as well as such adverse factors as loss of identity, internal migration and several armed conflicts which took place in the post-Soviet era during the painful period of 1991–1997. Suicide rates started to decrease after 1995, but only after the economy had started to stabilize. Still this short decrease was followed with a new sharp increase which coincided with the economic crisis and default in the Russian Federation in 1998. This rise was short-term and after it suicide indexes started going down all over the post-Soviet territory up to the present moment, as can be seen from Figure 6.2A.

This stress involved all the population in the whole country, but as we will see further the reaction to it with regard to suicide rates was very diverse in different parts of the former empire. This is the main subject of our discussion, and we are going to support the idea that existing attitudes to suicide, restrictions or permissions regarding certain forms of self-destructive behaviour and possible 'canalization' of psycho-social stress are the main mechanisms that create variations in suicide rates in different cultures under similar stressful conditions. To prove this, we are using an approach in which countries are classified by the level of suicides and the changes of different indicators under stress are compared within the groups that are formed on the basis of the similarity of suicide rates. Our conclusions are based on qualitative and visual perception of graphs depicting the time changes in mortality indices in the different countries that emerged after the fall of the USSR.

One can see variations of suicide rates between republics which were once united in one country in Figure 6.3. As can be noted from the data provided, the figures might be eight times different (for example, during the Soviet times, the suicide rate in Lithuania reached 32 per 100,000 and in Armenia the rate was 4 per 100,000). The most remarkable issue is that in Figure 6.3 it is possible to see two distinct groups of republics inside the USSR and further when they became independent. The first group unites high suicide rate (HSR) countries. In this group there are all the Baltic republics (Latvia, Lithuania and Estonia), all the Slavic republics (Russia, Ukraine and Belarus) and Kazakhstan. The second distinct group unites low suicide rate (LSR) countries. Here we can see all the

Caucasus republics (Georgia, Armenia, Azerbaijan), and three Middle East republics (Tadzhikistan, Turkmenistan, Uzbekistan). Also, a medium suicide rate group can be identified in Figure 6.3 which is represented by Moldova and Kirgizstan, which is not so distinct.

It is obvious that HSR and LSR countries are clustered geographically and united by certain common features from the point of view of economic development and cultural peculiarities. High rate countries are united by their northern location, dependence of their economies on industrial development and world economic tendencies, a high urbanization level, and multinational population. In other words, these are 'modernist' type countries that are integrated into the global economic and social processes. In such countries many of the culturally specific features gradually decrease, giving way to more global tendencies. The majority of the populations in the particular set of countries that belong to the HSR group profess Christianity, except Kazakhstan where half of the inhabitants are Muslims.

The LSR countries are diverse in their religions (Georgians and Armenians are Christians while Middle Asia peoples are Muslims), but all of them have lower levels of economic development, they are mostly peripheral agricultural economies, with profound ethno-cultural specificity, almost mono-ethnic with very traditional meso-social systems (families, communities, villages, etc.). All these countries are located in southern peripheral regions (Caucasus and the Middle East). They are historically destined to resist global tendencies, trying to preserve their own mentality, culture, way of life and the specific social and manufacture structure.

However, the existence of the 'medium suicide rate group' is less understandable – it is rather complicated to explain what Moldova and Kirgizstan have in common other than the suicide rate. To avoid this ambiguity, we will further consider only those groups of countries that clearly differ from each other. We are aware of the fact that this is a limitation of our analysis, however, at this stage we believe it is necessary to present the most logical part of it.

It is necessary to say that for more than 70 years of the existence of the USSR, all countries (the former republics) were united politically, economically and ideologically within one union; but as can be seen from Figure 6.3, they have kept profound differences in suicidal behaviour. Such stability is not a surprise. When speaking about aggregate suicide rates, all the countries in the world are known to have their national level which keeps respective countries at more or less the same ranking position in the general list, even though certain variations are possible (Makinen and Wasserman, 1997). Besides, a stable gradient of increasing suicide activity can be observed when moving from West to East and from South to North along the Eurasian continent (Cantor, 2000; Bertolote and Fleischman, 2009). This may be also observed inside large countries and it can also be seen in modern Russia and Ukraine. Historical national levels of stability and geographical gradients of suicide rates are important markers of the existence of some strong factors which determine this stability in contrast to other causes of death.

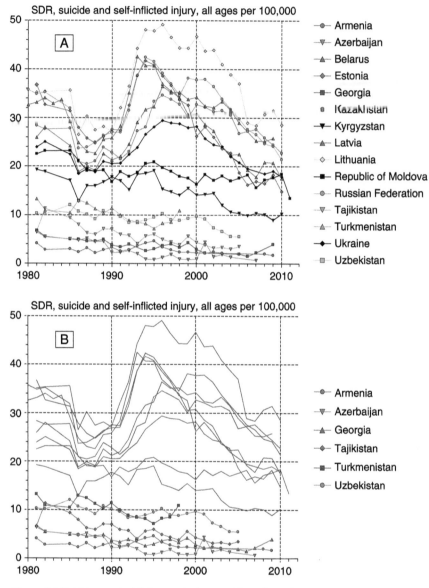

Figure 6.3 Suicide rates in 15 former Soviet republics, all genders, all ages. General overview (A); highlighted low suicide rates group (B); and high suicide rates group (C).

Source: European Health for All Database (WHO).

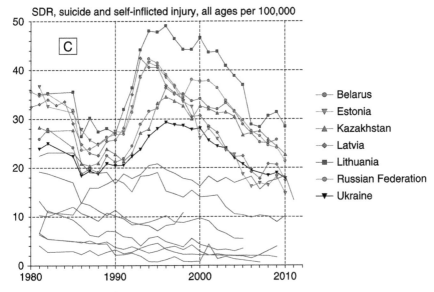

Figure 6.3 (Continued)

This may be due to different complex reasons, but mostly may be understood as 'cultural resistance' (Makinen and Wasserman, 1997).

Deeper analysis of Figure 6.3 gives a lot of interesting observations. First, sharp fluctuations in suicide rates for the last 30 years were typical only for the HSR countries. In LSR countries (Caucasus and the Middle East republics) all of the occurring changes of psycho-social stress that have influenced suicidal behaviour in the Slavic and Baltic ethnicities had no effect, judging from their suicide rates. Thus, at first glance we can suppose that there are countries that are contrastingly different from each other in terms of 'high suicide rate and sharp reaction to the psycho-social stress' and 'low-suicide rate and blunted reaction to psycho-social stress'. On the other hand this conclusion is based only on suicide rates as indicators. However, reactions to psycho-social stress are not only confined to suicide rate, but are represented by mortality from other stress-related diseases, homicides, traffic accidents and other causes, as was mentioned by Rutz (2006) and other authors. This is very well confirmed by Figure 6.2B which shows, that a temporal pattern of mortality due to these reasons was actually the same as changes in suicide rate. It means that stress was actually displayed, and furthermore detailed data will confirm it. On the other hand it was suicide particularly that varied so much in the differing cultural and geographical clusters.

Another important fact becomes obvious when gender differences in suicide rates are represented. The data provided by Figure 6.4 show that social and economic problems of the period of transition impacted the female population much less compared to the male population (Figure 6.4A–A1). Actually almost all excessive suicide mortality in the period from 1989 to 1997 was due to suicide

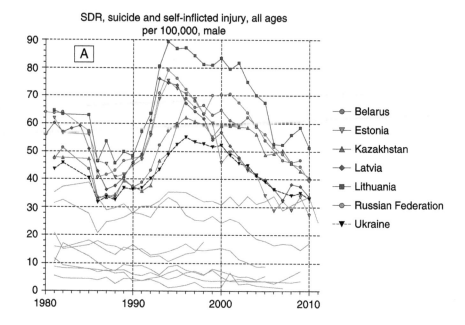

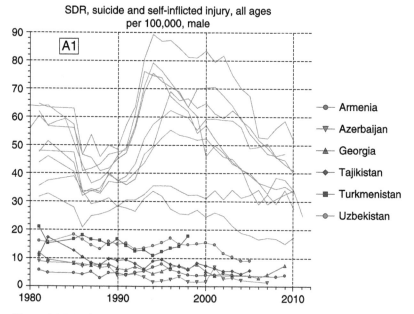

Figure 6.4 Suicide rates in former USSR republics, gender aspect (A–A1: suicide among men in HSR and LSR countries; B–B1: suicides among women in HSR and LSR countries in positions that best reflect changes).

Source: European Health for All Database (WHO).

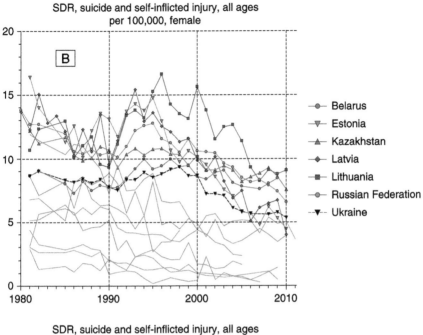

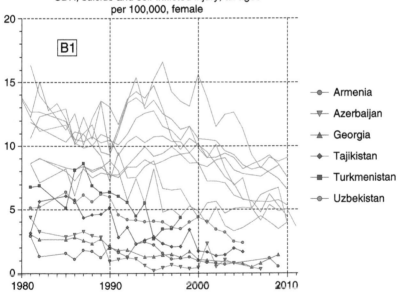

Figure 6.4 (Continued)

in males from HSR countries. The pattern of change of male suicides in the LSR countries was different – there was no marked rise in rates at the respective period of time. As a result, differences in suicide rates between HSR and LSR countries increased. At the peak of the rise (1995) in HSR countries rates in males varied from 52.54 per 100,000 (Ukraine) to 86.82 (Lithuania) with the mean 68.78, while in LSR countries variation was from 1.65 (Azerbaijan) to 15.31 (Uzbekistan) with the mean for this group 8.43 per 100,000. Thus the estimated ratio between HSL and LSR countries for male suicides reached 8.16. Moreover, in HSR countries suicide rates in males have peaked on average to 75 per cent in the period from 1986 to 1995.

Presentation of suicide rates in females (Figure 6.4B–B1) reveals that women in HSR countries also have higher rates than in LSR countries though the differences are not so marked as among males. According to EHAD, in women corresponding indices in the LSR group varied from 0.19 (Azerbaijan) to 4.07 (Uzbekistan) with the mean 2.21 in LSR countries and from 8.54 (Ukraine) to 15.28 (Lithuania) with the mean 12.02 per 100,000. So, the estimated average HSR/LSR ratio in female suicides reached 5.43. In HSR countries women also showed the rise in the period from 1986 to 1995 on average to 23 per cent.

From these figures and calculations as well as from the diagrams it is clear that excessive mortality shortly after the fall of the USSR almost all befell males in HSR countries (Figure 6.4A–A1). Among men and women from LSR countries there was no substantial reaction to the occurring social and economic perturbations, and since the time of being part of the USSR up to the present moment there has been a gradual decrease in suicide rates (Figure 6.4, A–A1, B–B1). These smooth positive changes are in contrast with pronounced peaks in suicide rates among men in the Baltic and Slavic states. There is a temptation to conclude that Caucasus and the Middle East republics did not suffer so much due to disintegration of the union, but we are going to show that this may be a wrong conclusion.

Substantial differences in suicides in post-Soviet countries can be explained from several points of view, but the economic factor is the first to be noted. It goes without saying, that Russia, Ukraine, Belarus, Kazakhstan and the Baltic countries underwent huge losses as a result of economic difficulties, general market disintegration, rapid mass privatization, impoverishment of huge contingents, sky-rocketing social inequality, etc. No doubt it impacted people's lives severely at a certain period of history. There is no doubt that these stressful changes involved all former republics, including the peripheral regions. The Caucasian and Middle East countries suffered even more due to their peripheral location and specialization regarding industrial development. In this respect we consider it useful to look at other indicators of psycho-social stress – mortality rates from the disease traditionally related to stress, specifically, ischaemic heart disease. These data are provided in Figure 6.5, where the countries are again clustered according to their suicide rates.

It is clear that when looking at ischaemic heart disease mortality, differences between HSR and LSR countries practically disappear. If we take the chosen 'reference' countries from contrasting clusters (Armenia and Lithuania), male mortality rate according to EHAD from these pathological states in Lithuania is comparable with the male mortality rate in Armenia (534 per 100,000 vs. 532 per 100,000 in 1995). Mortality rate among females is even higher in Armenia (347 and 318 per 100,000 respectively). Moreover these data clearly indicate that the mortality rate among men and women from such types of stress-related diseases does not differ very much, though in females it is marginally lower than in males. A similar picture can be observed when mortality rates from a wider range of diseases of the circulatory system and cerebrovascular diseases are analyzed (not presented here in the diagrams, but clear from the database). This is very well supported by recent studies that prove the role of psycho-social stress as a risk factor for cerebrovascular diseases (Egido *et al.*, 2012). Differences between two groups of countries are also not very marked if we take such indicators of psycho-social stress such as traffic accidents and traumatic injuries. We are not able to present corresponding diagrams here due to limited space.

We believe that these data can be interpreted as a shining example of the fact that psycho-social stress hit all post-Soviet countries at approximately the same level. It becomes apparent when cardio-vascular pathologies mortality rates and especially circulatory system diseases are considered. These pathological states are known as diseases with a strong psychosomatic component and with stress-dependent pathogenesis. From this an important deduction can be drawn regarding mortality rates from suicides that differentiate the countries so much. These differences are induced by psycho-social stress that touched, as we state, all countries to a more or less similar degree, but were strongly modulated by culturally conditioned levels of attitudes, traditional restrictions or permissions for such an act as suicide in the particular society, culture or ethos. This resulted in a marked rise in suicides in HSR countries and a blunted rise in LSR countries. In other words, the problem of historically established differences in suicide rates is actually the problem of cultural tolerance towards such types of self-destructive acts as suicide. This coincides with the opinion of other authors who put culture, religion, norms and traditions forward as factors that most strongly influence national suicide rates (Cantor, 2000; Cheng and Chau-Shoun, 2000; Wasserman, 2009).

If we take this point of view, the HSR and LSR clusters can be seen a result of how stress was 'finding its way', but less a result of the differences in stress itself. Both northern and southern nations, males and females when facing crucial points in their history were being forced to go through the collapse of the country that had provided security, relative economic stability, independence from critical phenomena in a more global economic context, suffered considerable difficulties, socio-economic and existential problems. The differences in suicidal behaviour are called forth by certain life roles, behaviour patterns, and ethno-cultural norms and traditions typical to this or that particular ethnicity as they have been formed historically.

Some evidence to prove our reasoning is also found in gender differences in suicidal behaviour in HSR and LSR countries. It is well established that males

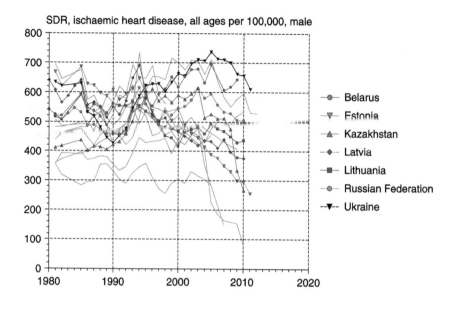

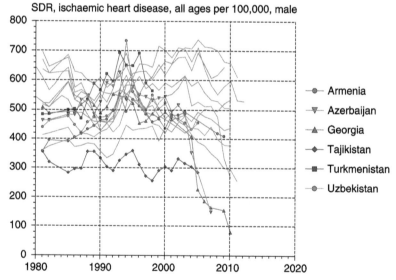

Figure 6.5 Mortality rates from cardio-vascular diseases among men and women in HSR and LSR countries.

Source: European Health for All Database (WHO).

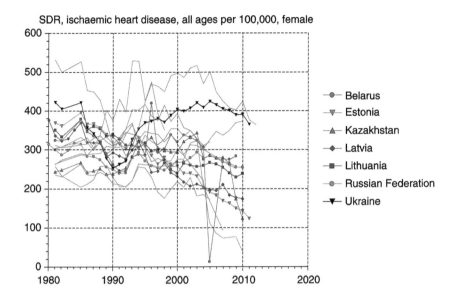

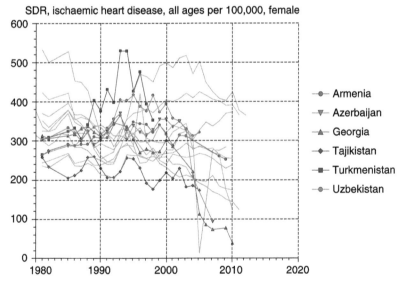

Figure 6.5 (Continued)

complete suicides much more frequently than females, and consequently suicide is often considered as a 'male phenomenon' (Rutz and Rihmer, 2009). Nevertheless it is a subject of great cultural influence how suicide is viewed among males and females (Beautrais, 2006; Canetto, 2009). In this respect, the considerable predominance of male suicides in the Slavic and Baltic countries (5–6 times higher) can be regarded as the consequence of cultural 'permissions'. Not only suicide is seen as 'allowed', it is actually sometimes encouraged as a positive male behavioural pattern (the way 'to solve all problems', 'save face', 'go away with dignity' and so on). Suicides among men and women in LSR countries may be examined from the same point of view. Here male suicides are less dominating (just 2–3 times higher than in females). At the same time, we should keep in mind that these countries' culture does not support any type of suicide. Apparently, this has an impact mostly on the male population and as a result we can see lower indexes and a lower male–female ratio in LSR countries.

With regards to the role of psycho-social stress, correlations between suicide rates and alcohol consumption in the given environment should be also viewed. The role of alcohol in suicides at the national level in the former USSR has been discussed in suicidology many times. Analyzing the situation, Värnik and Wasserman (1992), and later Wasserman *et al.* (1994) have pointed out that significant decline in suicide rates in the republics of the former USSR in 1984–1988 was observed shortly after the introduction of the anti-alcohol policy. Logically restrictions of alcohol sale and lowering of the consumption at the national level were supposed to be factors in suicide prevention (Wasserman and Värnik, 1998) and possibly it really saved many lives. On the other hand it may explain the lowering of suicides and other external causes' mortality while the synchronous lowering of cardiovascular and cerebrovascular mortality (Figure 6.2) is not so easy to understand following this reasoning. Besides, the problem of alcohol is very complicated. Official data in the USSR were far from reality due to the availability of home-made alcohol, the amount of which, according to different sources, made up 25–40 per cent of the official figures (Feldbrugge, 1989), so the efforts of the government maybe were not very effective. Very soon after the USSR collapsed alcohol consumption as well as alcohol-related mortality went up especially in the HSR countries (Nemtsov, 2003; Pridemore, 2006). In other words, we may see a concurrent pattern of changes, which is most likely associated with psycho-social stress. As societal optimism grows, the consumption of alcohol goes down, and vice versa. This process is accompanied with the effect of 'mutual reinforcement' of the oscillations in alcohol consumption and suicide rate. Alcohol can play a compensatory role in depression and suicide tendencies (Liu *et al.*, 1998; Thomas, Randall and Carrigan, 2003), especially for younger people, though it can have a negative impact in terms of suicide planning for older people and in a long-term perspective (Blow *et al.*, 2004; Sher, 2006). The relationship between alcohol and suicidality is also strongly determined by a culture that functions as a moderator between stress, suicidality and alcohol consumption. While in one given country with traditional style of drinking there is a strong correlation between alcohol consumption and suicide, when several countries are taken into consideration, such factors like wet or dry drinking cultures have a greater influence (Ramstedt, 2001) and correlations between suicides and alcohol are not found while the impact of economic factors remains remarkable (Kõlves *et al.*, 2013).

It must be also taken into consideration that the collapse of the USSR had certain peculiarities; it was not only the case of economic difficulties. Dismantling of the socialist system, often fair but having now lost its social attractiveness, and transition to the capitalist way of life, alluring with its welfare, intensified the polarization of society, which in itself became an additional source of stress. This was also the result of the harsh and rapid large-scale privatization (King, Hamm and Stuckler, 2009). These processes were accompanied by economic hardship, unemployment, population impoverishment, decline in health-care resources and weakening of government control over the alcohol and drugs market. From this point of view, the collapse of the USSR was a rather unique 'natural experiment' where the population effects of psycho-social stress could be clearly registered and studied and the fact that there is a long-lasting interest in the health and suicide consequences of this geopolitical event confirms it.

Summing up, we can state that the approach used in this chapter (dividing all post-Soviet countries into two groups based on historically determined suicide levels) allows the promotion of the role of psycho-social stress as a factor of increased suicide mortality during the period of transition from one social-economic system to another. We consider that here we can see the classical influence of macro-level factors on the meso-level, which is moderated by the micro-level (personality) according to Martikainen *et al.* (2002) with the central role of psycho-social stress. It is necessary to notice here that stress in Russian culture refers not only to a personal perception but is generally understood as a societal process (Petila and Rytkonen, 2008). This possibly reflects one more dimension of perception of stress in society – the conceptual tool in interpreting social processes and popular discourse widely used in contemporary life.

On the other hand we must consider the complicated and ambiguous character of the concomitant phenomena, the interconnection between stress and alcohol consumption, the heterogeneity in mortality rate fluctuations caused by national features during the switch to a market economy, mixed populations and migration processes (King *et al.*, 2009; Kõlves *et al.*, 2013). Our analysis is qualitative, not quantitative. Sometimes it reveals reflections of the insider, not only scientific interest. Nevertheless it indicates that the interpretation of data on the reactivity of suicide rates in different countries to serious psycho-social stress at a certain historical period is explained with ethno-cultural peculiarities. National traditions, the significance of cultural norms, the ability to preserve one's own identity and values under the pressure of global tendencies seem to be important factors that determine variations in suicidal behaviour and its historical dynamics.

References

Beautrais, A. L. (2006). Women and suicidal behavior. *Crisis: The Journal of Crisis Intervention and Suicide Prevention*, 27(4), 153–156.

Bertolote, J. M. and Fleischman, A. (2009). A global perspective on the magnitude of suicide mortality. In D. Wasserman and C. Wasserman (Eds), *Oxford Textbook on Suicidology and Suicide Prevention* (pp. 91–98). New York: Oxford University Press.

Blow, F. C., Brockmann, L. M., and Barry, K. L. (2004). Role of alcohol in late-life suicide. *Alcoholism: Clinical and Experimental Research*, 28(5 Suppl), 48S–56S.

Canetto, S. S. (2009). Prevention of suicidal behavior in females. In D. Wasserman and C. Wasserman (Eds), *Oxford Textbook on Suicidology and Suicide Prevention* (pp. 241–247). New York: Oxford University Press.

Cantor, C. H. (2000). Suicide in the Western world. In K. Hawton and K. van Heeringen (Eds), *The International Book of Suicide and Attempted Suicide* (pp. 9–28). Chichester: John Wiley and Sons.

Cheng, A. T. A. and Chau-Shoun, L. (2000). Suicide in Asia and Far East. In K. Hawton and K. van Heeringen (Eds), *The International Book of Suicide and Attempted Suicide* (pp. 29–48). Chichester: John Wiley and Sons.

Denisova, T. P., Shkoda, A. S., Malinova, L. I., and Astaf'eva, N. G. (2005). Social stress as a risk factor for ischemic heart disease. *Terapevticheskii Arkhiv*, 77(3), 52–55.

Egido, J. A, Castillo, O., Roig, B., Sanz, I., Herrero, M. R., Garay, M. T., *et al.* (2012). Is psycho-physical stress a risk factor for stroke? *Journal of Neurology, Neurosurgery and Psychiatry*, 83(11), 1104–1110.

Feldbrugge, F. J. M. (1989). The Soviet second economy in a political and legal perspective. In E. L. Feige (Ed.), *The Underground Economies. Tax Evasion and Information Distortion* (pp. 297–338). Cambridge: Cambridge University Press.

Ginter, E. and Simko V. (2010). Health of Europeans twenty years after the fall of the Berlin wall. *Bratislavske Lekarske Listy*, 111(7), 398–403.

Guntem, G. (1977). The long-term Apendorf study: Paradigm for the study of long-acting psychosocial stressors. *Schweizer Archiv für Neurologie und Psychiatrie*, 121(1), 97–113.

King, L., Hamm, P., and Stuckler, D. (2009). Rapid large-scale privatization and death rates in ex-communist countries: An analysis of stress-related and health system mechanisms. *International Journal of Health Services*, 39(3), 461–489.

Kõlves, K., Milner, A., and Värnik, P. (2013). Suicide rates and socioeconomic factors in Eastern European countries after the collapse of the Soviet Union: Trends between 1990 and 2008. *Sociology of Health and Illness*, 35(6), 956–970.

Kopp, M. S. and Rethelyi, J. (2004). Where psychology meets physiology: Chronic stress and premature mortality – the Central-Eastern European health paradox. *Brain Research Bulletin*, 62(5), 351–367.

Liu, Y., Rao, K., and Fei, J. (1998). Economic transition and health transition: Comparing China and Russia. *Health Policy*, 44(2), 103–122.

Lundberg, U. (2006). Stress, subjective and objective health. *International Journal of Social Welfare*, 15(suppl. 1), S41–S48.

Mäkinen, I. H. (2000). Eastern European transition and suicide mortality. *Social Science and Medicine*, 51(9), 1405–1420.

Mäkinen, I. H. and Wasserman, D. (1997). Suicide prevention and cultural resistance: Stability in European countries' suicide ranking, 1970–1988. *Italian Journal of Suicidology*, 7(2), 73–85.

Martikainen, P., Bartley, M., and Lahelma, E. (2002). Psychosocial determinants of health in social epidemiology. *International Journal of Epidemiology*, 31(6), 1091–1093.

McEven, B. S. (2012). Brain on stress: How the social environment gets under the skin. *Proceedings of the National Academy of Sciences of the United States of America*, 109(2), 17180–17185.

Nemtsov, A. (2003). Suicides and alcohol consumption in Russia, 1965–1999. *Drug and Alcohol Dependence*, 71(2), 161–168.

Petila, I. and Rytkonen, M. (2008). Coping with stress and by stress: Russian men and women talking about transition, stress and health. *Social Sciences and Medicine*, 66(2), 327–338.

Pridemore, W. A. (2006). Heavy drinking and suicide in Russia. *Social Forces*, 85(1), 413–440.

Ramstedt, M. (2001). Alcohol and suicide in 14 European countries. *Addiction*, 96(Suppl.1), S59–75.

Rozanov, V. A. (2012a). Epigenetics: Stress and behavior. *Neurophysiology*, 44(4), 332–350.

Rozanov, V. A. (2012b). Suicide, psycho-social stress and alcohol consumption in the countries of the former USSR. *Suicidology (Suitsidologiya)*, 4, 28–39.

Rutz, W. (2006). Social psychiatry and public mental health: present situation and future objectives. Time for rethinking and renaissance? *Acta Psychiatrica Scandinavica*, 113(Suppl 429), 95–100.

Rutz, W. and Rihmer, Z. (2009). Suicide in men. Suicide prevention for the male person. In D. Wasserman and C. Wasserman (Eds), *Oxford Textbook on Suicidology and Suicide Prevention* (pp 249–255). New York: Oxford University Press.

Schneiderman, N., Ironson, G., and Siegel, S. D. (2005). Stress and health: Psychological, behavioral, and biological determinants. *Annual Review of Clinical Psychology*, 1, 607–628.

Sher, L. (2006). The relationship between the frequency of alcohol use and suicide rates in young people. *International Journal of Adolescents' Medicine and Health*, 18(1), 81–85.

Thomas, S. E., Randall, C. L., and Carrigan, M. H. (2003). Drinking to cope in socially anxious individuals: A controlled study. *Alcoholism: Clinical and Experimental Research*, 27(12), 1937–1943.

Varnik, A. and Mokhovikov, A. (2009). Suicide during transition in the former Soviet republics. In D. Wasserman and C. Wasserman (Eds), *Oxford Textbook on Suicidology and Suicide Prevention* (pp. 191–197). New York: Oxford University Press.

Varnik, A., Sisask, M., and Varnik, P. (2010). *Baltic Suicide Paradox*. Tallinn: TLU Press.

Värnik, A. and Wasserman, D. (1992). Suicides in the former Soviet republics. *Acta Psychiatrica Scandinavica*, 86(1), 76–78.

Wasserman, C. (2009). Suicide: Considering religion and culture. In D. Wasserman and C. Wasserman (Eds), *Oxford Textbook on Suicidology and Suicide Prevention* (pp. 3–5). New York: Oxford University Press.

Wasserman, D. (2001). *Suicide: An Unnecessary Death*. London: Martin Dunitz.

Wasserman, D., and Varnik, A. (1998). Suicide-preventive effect of perestroika in the former USSR: The role of alcohol restriction. *Acta Psychiatrica Scandinavica, Supplementum*, 394, 1–4.

Wasserman, D., Varnik, A., and Eklund, G. (1994). Male suicides and alcohol consumption in the former USSR. *Acta Psychiatrica Scandinavica*, 89(5), 306–313.

7 From social adversity to psychological pain

A pathway to suicide

Philippe Courtet and Emilie Olié

The World Health Organization (WHO) estimates about 1.5 million deaths by suicide per year worldwide by 2020. Emile Durkheim (Durkheim, 1897) viewed suicide as a social fact. According to his theory the variations in suicidal rate on a macro-level could also be explained by society-scale phenomena rather than individual's feelings and motivations. Nowadays, suicidal acts may be best understood within a stress-vulnerability model, where it is assumed that only vulnerable patients, when submitted to environmental stressors, will kill themselves. We will discuss how social adversity and psychological pain interact in this model and help in a better understanding of suicidal process at individual level.

Social crisis

If suicide is a major health problem in occidental countries, it is not yet the case in developing countries. On the one hand, it cannot be excluded that it is due to the lack of epidemiological data. On the other hand, it could suggest that economic expansion may be associated with increased suicidal risk because it exposes more people to crisis and bankruptcy. Moreover, according to Durkheim's theory (Durkheim, 1897), economic development would lead to the destruction of the social protections afforded by traditional communities and the increase of individualism that would favour suicide. In addition, both prosperity phases and financial crises would influence suicidal rates because they disturb the normal course of economic life. If prosperity phases increase suicidal rates, European suicide rates would have increased between 1945 and 1975. But the reverse was observed: stagnation in the suicide rate during economic expansion and increase in young people parallel to the increase in unemployment. Epidemiological data show that the richer a country is (reflected by the gross domestic product), the higher the level of suicide. However, in occidental countries, wealth and suicide vary inversely: the poorest outlying urban areas are the most affected by suicide (Baudelot and Establet, 2013). A recent series of publications in high-ranking scientific journals have examined the impact of the current economic recession on suicide rates in European populations. Stuckler, Basu, Suhrcke, Coutts, and McKee (2009) have reported a significant increase in suicide mortality at ages younger than 65 years in relation to the increase in unemployment in 26 European countries between 1970 and 2007; unemployment being a strong indicator of the socio-economic situation of a country. Moreover, social labour market protections interacted with the effect of unemployment on suicide rates. Every US$10 per person increased investment in active labour market programmes induced a significant reduction of the effect of unemployment on suicides. Thus, in the twenty-first century, three major points have to be highlighted to underline a possible relationship between economic crisis and suicide:

- the suicide rate of employees is becoming more similar to the suicide rate of workers while working conditions are getting worse;
- an increase of suicide rate for young working men has been observed since 1970, i.e. the beginning of the oil crisis;
- suicides occur in the workplace, sometimes serial suicides in (inter)national companies (i.e. France Telecom).

High risk populations

Since the early study of Durkheim (1897) that demonstrated the relationship between suicide and social factors, many authors have repeatedly shown that social and economic factors are associated with spatial and temporal variation in suicide occurrence (Rezaeian *et al.*, 2005). Theories of suicidal behaviour suggest that the desire to die can arise from the disruption of interpersonal relationships. A theory of Joiner *et al.* (2005) attributes suicide to an individual's acquired capability to enact self-harm, perceived burdensomeness, and thwarted belongingness. Perceived burdensomeness is a mental state characterized by the belief that others would 'be better off if I were gone'.

Isolated elderly

Among this population, identified socio-environmental correlates include: population density (Hempstead, 2006; Middleton *et al.*, 2006), proportion of elderly people (Aihara and Iki, 2003), and single person households (Hempstead, 2006). Single person households are considered a measure of anomie ('personal feeling of lack of social norms') and this has been used to construct Congdon's Social Fragmentation Index, but only using people younger than 65 years of age (Whitley *et al.*, 1999). Living alone can induce the feeling of being at odds with social norms feeling. Rurup *et al.* (2011) have reported that having a low social network and feeling alone were associated with the occurrence of suicidal ideation. The elderly are more prone to be isolated. Purcell *et al.* (2012) have demonstrated a significant main effect of family connectedness on suicide ideation in depressed adults over 50 years old. It may suggest that having a stronger connection to family members decreased the likelihood of reporting suicide ideation. In addition, in a study of 26 European countries, Yur'yev *et al.* (2010) found a negative association between the social representation of people over 70 years old and suicide. Perception of the elderly as having higher status, recognition of their economic contribution and higher moral standards, and friendly feelings towards and admiration of them were inversely correlated with suicide mortality. Suicide rates were lower in countries where the elderly live with their families more often.

Prisoners

The global prison population in 2008 was estimated at 9.8 million with a median rate of imprisonment of 145 prisoners per 100,000 persons, most of whom are aged between 18 and 44 years (Walmsley, 2009). If the excess mortality from suicide in prison is a fact that nobody can ignore (Fazel *et al.*, 2011), the existence of a persistent increase of suicidal risk even after release is more confidential. The risk of suicide has increased eight-fold for men, and 36 times for women compared to the general population (Pratt *et al.*, 2006). Familial disruption, poor attainment, social disadvantage, substance abuse, isolation, unemployment, and psychiatric morbidity are each associated with suicide. But the fact remains that as a society we are failing a group of particularly vulnerable individuals, whose interdependent social and health problems fall too easily between compartmentalized community services. Suicides in released prisoners reflect not only shortcomings in agencies involved, but ultimately society's attitudes to rehabilitation and re-integration.

Psychosocial stress

At the individual level, the transition to the suicidal act is usually precipitated by psychosocial stress. Nearly all suicide victims have experienced at least one or more adverse life event within one year of death (concentrated in last few months). Interpersonal conflict brought the greatest risk of suicidal act, followed by relationship breakdown, forensic events, unemployment, job problems, financial problems, bereavement, and domestic violence. Some of the risk associated with interpersonal events, forensic events, unemployment, and loss events is independent of mental disorder (Foster, 2011). All these factors are related to social features and threaten the social status of the individual. Indeed, such events decrease the potential for social investment defined as the ratio between the social value of an individual to others and their social burden on others (Allen and Badcock, 2003). When this ratio reaches a point where social value and social burden are approaching equivalence, the individual is in danger of social exclusion and becomes hypersensitive to signals of rejection.

Social bounds are essential for the survival of humans. Thus, when threatened with exclusion, individuals either adapt their behaviours in order to increase the degree of social acceptability promoting a return to baseline or may adopt aggressive behaviour including antisocial or self-injurious behaviours (Williams, 2007). This is in line with Durkheim's altruistic suicide, which takes place when a subject identifies with a social group for whom he or she is willing to sacrifice his/her own life.

Suicidal vulnerability

Forty years of clinical as well as scientific research have produced evidence that environmental factors alone may not explain the suicidal act. The proposed understanding of the clinical model of suicidal behaviour is a model of stress vulnerability. It is now accepted that only individuals harbouring suicidal vulnerability, when subjected to stressors, commit the act (Mann, 2003). Suicidal vulnerability has been demonstrated to be underlain by stable traits enduring all through life related to genetic, biological, cognitive abnormalities as well as clinical characteristics:

- personal and familial history of suicide, impulsive aggressive personality traits, hopelessness and neuroticism;
- serotonergic system and hypothalamo-pituitary axis dysfunction;
- dysfunctional emotional and cognitive processing such as deficits in problem solving, altered decision-making relying on dysfunctional prefrontal regions;
- role of genetic and epigenetic factors.

Social exclusion

Early traumatic life events are strongly associated with suicidal vulnerability. Retrospective cohort and longitudinal studies have shown that childhood exposure to a harmful environment, such as sexual abuse, emotional neglect, disturbed relationship with parents or parental mental illness, have a devastating effect and dramatically increase the risk of suicidal behaviour (Agerbo *et al.*, 2002). According to the theory of attachment (Bowlby, 1977), the perception of being rejected or neglected in childhood would, in adulthood, lead to rejection sensitivity and the perception of feeling unwanted in general – and hence contribute to suicidal risk (Ehnvall *et al.*, 2008). In addition, alterations in decision-making (Jollant *et al.*, 2007), a putative suicidal endophenotype involved in the ability of the individual to make choices in daily life (Courtet *et al.*, 2011), are correlated to the occurrence of problematic affective relationships (Jollant *et al.*, 2007). When exploring decision-making capacities of patients with a past history of suicidal act, it appears that they tend to keep on choosing options with high immediate rewards but disadvantageous long-term outcomes, whereas patients (without any past suicidal history) and healthy controls learn to avoid these options and turn towards choices with low immediate gains but long-term benefits (Jollant *et al.*, 2005). Interestingly, this pattern of responses is similar in ostracized animals, which have an impaired inhibition against eating non-nutritive foods and avoidance of less tasty, nutritive foods (Baumeister *et al.*, 2006). Using functional MRI, prefrontal regions associated with suicidal vulnerability (Jollant *et al.*, 2008, 2010; van Heeringen *et al.*, 2011) have also been involved in studying response to rejection-related stimuli. Indeed, compared to controls, suicide attempters had increased activity in the right anterior cingulate cortex in response to mildly happy versus neutral faces and increased activity in the right orbitofrontal cortex in response to angry versus neutral faces (Jollant *et al.*, 2008). These results may indicate that suicide attempters could be less prone to detect positive social cues and more sensitive to signals of rejection. To study exclusion, a paradigm based on a virtual ball-tossing game (Cyberball Game) was developed: while playing, subjects are either included or excluded by other players. In response to exclusion, healthy controls showed hyperactivation of the dorsal anterior cingulate and the right ventral prefrontal cortices (Eisenberger *et al.*, 2003). Moreover, Bolling *et al.* (2011) have found greater functional connectivity of the anterior cingulate cortex to regions of the default mode network during social exclusion. These results show that exclusion is salient for humans and relies on regions involved in both emotion regulation and executive functions. Interestingly, emotional support through supportive messages may attenuate social distress associated with exclusion. Functional MRI showed that participants who experienced greater attenuation of social pain exhibited lower ventral anterior cingulate cortex and higher left lateral prefrontal cortex activation (Onoda *et al.*, 2009). It may suggest that emotional support enhances cognitive inhibition through lateral prefrontal cortex, which regulates emotional distress relying on the cingulate cortex.

Social and psychological pains

Being excluded or rejected signals a threat for which reflexive detection in the form of pain and distress is adaptive for survival (Williams, 2007). Social pain is defined as the unpleasant experience associated with potential or actual damage to one's sense of social connection or social value (owing to social rejection, exclusion, negative social evaluation or loss) (Eisenberger, 2012; Eisenberger and Lieberman, 2004). Indeed, for Shneidman (1993) psychological pain or 'psychache' is 'the introspective experience of negative emotions such as dread, despair, fear, grief, shame, guilt, frustrated love, loneliness and loss' and relies on the frustration of psychological needs. Thus we assume that social pain should be considered as a subtype of psychological pain emerging from the threat of affiliation. Unbearable pain, particularly psychological pain, is a frequent theme of suicide notes. Suicidal acts should be considered as the expression of an attempt to escape from this psychological suffering. Using visual analogic scales, our group has recently reported that depressed patients with a recent or past history of suicide attempt expressed significantly higher levels of psychological pain than depressed patients without any history of suicide attempt (Olié *et al.*, 2009). The intensity of psychological pain has been associated with suicidal ideation independent of depression (Lester, 2000; Mee *et al.*, 2011; Olié *et al.*, 2009). High psychological pain is associated with a history of suicide attempt (Flamenbaum, 2007, 2009; Holden *at al.*, 2001; Mills *et al.*, 2005), suicide planning (Mee *et al.*, 2011), and suicidal intention (Flamenbaum, 2007). However, the association between psychological pain and suicide attempts has not always been replicated (Lester, 2000; Pompili *et al.*, 2008). Psychological pain was found to predict suicide attempts, but not suicidal ideation in the general population (Flamenbaum, 2009; Troister, 2009). On the contrary, in a cross-sectional study, psychological pain was predictive of suicidal ideation in suicide attempters (Flynn and Holden, 2007). In a two-year follow-up study, the authors also reported that psychological pain contributed to the statistical prediction of suicidal ideation, independent of depression and hopelessness (Troister and Holden, 2012). Similarly to social pain and suicidal vulnerability, psychological pain relies mainly on the prefrontal cortex, associated with suicidal behaviour (review in Jollant *et al.*, 2011; van Heeringen *et al.*, 2011). Increased cerebral blood flow in the right dorsolateral prefrontal cortex, the right inferior frontal gyrus, the left inferior temporal gyrus and the right occipital cortex was reported in depressed patients with high levels of psychological pain in comparison to those with low levels of pain (van Heeringen *et al.*, 2010).

People may seek death through suicide as a means of relief from a painful internal state (Orbach *et al.*, 2003). Clinical experience suggests that suicidal ideation can function as a coping mechanism, in that some people are able to tolerate high levels of pain and/or disability by telling themselves that if their distress becomes unbearable, they at least have the option of ending their distress through suicide. In other words, suicidal behaviour becomes a problem-solving behaviour in order to 'stop the painful flow of consciousness' (Shneidman, 1993). Indeed, the role of painful defeat or entrapment in suicidal process was highlighted by the *cry of pain mode* (O'Connor *et al.*, 2008; Panagioti *et al.*, 2012) and motivations to escape from painful self-awareness were mentioned in the *escape theory* of suicide (Baumeister, 1990).

Therapeutic perspectives

Promoting social bounds

Interestingly, the quality of social support is a protective factor for suicide. Contacting people by telephone one month after being discharged from an emergency department for deliberate self-poisoning may help reduce the number of re-attempted suicides over one year (Vaiva *et al.*, 2006) independent of the effect of the identification of subjects at suicidal risk and the implementation of a crisis intervention. Religion is another protective factor against suicide (Dervic *et al.*, 2004). Beyond the protective nature of a religious affiliation through the moral opposite of suicide objection, we could assume that religion promotes social links and favours affiliative needs.

As social exclusion may play a role in the suicidal process, future research focused on prosocial pathways through oxytocin/vasopressin system is justified. Examination of animal research provided evidence that the oxytocin system is involved in response to social separation. The intranasal administration of oxytocin reduces aversion to angry faces, a signal of rejection and salient emotion to study suicidal vulnerability (Evans *et al.*, 2010). Lower levels of oxytocin in cerebrospinal fluid have been reported in suicide attempters in comparison to both patients without a history of suicide attempt and healthy controls (Jokinen *et al.*, 2012).

Relieving pain

There is increasing evidence that physical and psychological/social pains not only overlap in colloquial language, but also at the clinical and neuroanatomical levels: both states may involve suffering and activate the 'pain matrix' (experiencing social distress activates the insular, cingulate, and secondary somatosensory cortices) (Courtet *et al.*, 2011; Eisenberger, 2012; Kross *et al.*, 2011). Interestingly, in a population-based study, we recently reported that people with a past history of suicide attempts were more prone to consume prescribed opioid drugs than subjects having a lifetime history of depression without a suicidal act and healthy controls (Olié *et al.*, 2013). Despite the fact that pain was not measured during the follow-up period, we hypothesize that subjects with a history of suicide attempt have an increased pain perception, assessed by an increased consumption of opioid analgesics. Because people carrying suicidal vulnerability may perceive high levels of psychological pain, it may lead practitioners to prescribe analgesic drugs for undifferentiated states of physical or psychological pain. The implication of endogenous opioid systems in suicide needs further investigations. μ-opioid receptors have long been implicated in the modulation of responses to emotional stressors, in the quality of parental attachment (Moles *et al.*, 2004; Copeland *et al.*, 2011). If psychological pain is the core of the suicidal act, relieving it efficiently is thus needed to prevent suicide.

A single infusion of ketamine, a well-known analgesic drug, leads to a rapid resolution of suicidal ideation in patients with treatment-resistant major depressive disorder (DiazGranados *et al.*, 2010). However, the reduction of suicidal thoughts remains to be attributed to either the antidepressant or analgesic effect. One on-going study is now investigating the specific anti-suicidal ideation effect of intravenous ketamine in depressed inpatients (www.clinicaltrial.gov). Further studies are needed to test the efficacy of analgesics on psychological pain and suicidal risk.

Conclusion

Suicidal mortality is evitable and should be prevented. To succeed, a double approach is needed: to promote social protections by the community and to develop pharmacological targets for vulnerable people. On the one hand psychosocial stresses leading to social pain are environmental factors precipitating the suicidal act. On the other hand, it is suggested that suicidal vulnerability is associated with an increased perception of psychological pain. Psychological pain seems to be a common construct for understanding suicide and social exclusion should be closely considered in the suicidal process. Assessment of such pain may have important implications in intervention research, considering that psychological pain could be a therapeutic target

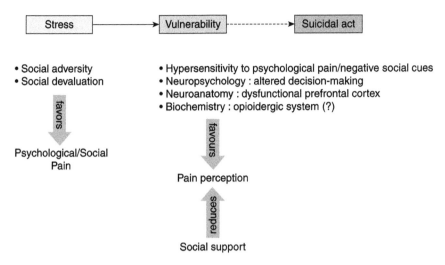

Figure 7.1 Stress-vulnerability model including social/psychological pain (proposed by the authors).

on its own. New avenues for improving the understanding of physiopathology and treatment of suicidal behaviours will be discussed in the light of psychological/social pain (Figure 7.1).

References

Aihara, H., and Iki, M. (2003). An ecological study of the relations between the recent high suicide rates and economic and demographic factors in Japan. *Journal of Epidemiology*, 13(1), 56–61.

Agerbo, E., Nordentoft, M., and Mortensen, P. B. (2002). Familial, psychiatric, and socioeconomic risk factors for suicide in young people: nested case-control study. *British Medical Journal*, 325, 74.

Allen, N. B., and Badcock, P. B. (2003). The social risk hypothesis of depressed mood: evolutionary, psychosocial, and neurobiological perspectives. *Psychological Bulletin*, 129(6), 887–913.

Baudelot, C., and Establet, R. (2013). Suicide et crises économiques. In Philippe Courtet (Ed.), *Suicide et environnement social* (pp. 13–19). Paris: Dunod Publisher.

Baumeister, R. F. (1990). Suicide as escape from self. *Psychological Review*, 97(1), 90–113.

Baumeister, R. F., Gailliot, M., DeWall, C. N., and Oaten, M. (2006). Self-regulation and personality: How interventions increase regulatory success, and how depletion moderates the effects of traits on behavior. *Journal of Personality*, 74(6), 1773–1801.

Bolling, D. Z., Pitskel, N. B., Deen, B., Crowley, M. J., Mayes, L. C., and Pelphrey, K. A. (2011). Development of neural systems for processing social exclusion from childhood to adolescence. *Developmental Science*, 14(6), 1431–1444.

Bowlby, J. (1977). The making and breaking of affectional bonds. I. Aetiology and psychopathology in the light of attachment theory. An expanded version of the Fiftieth Maudsley Lecture, delivered before the Royal College of Psychiatrists, 19 November 1976. *British Journal of Psychiatry*, 130, 201–210.

Copeland, W. E., Sun, H., Costello, E. J., Angold, A., Heilig, M. A., and Barr, C. S. (2011). Child mu-opioid receptor gene variant influences parent–child relations. *Neuropsychopharmacology*, 36(6), 1165–1170.

Courtet, P., Gottesman, I. I., Jollant, F., and Gould, T. D. (2011). The neuroscience of suicidal behaviors: What can we expect from endophenotype strategies? *Translational Psychiatry*, 1(5), e7.

Dervic, K., Oquendo, M. A., Grunebaum, M. F., Ellis, S., Burke, A. K., and Mann, J. J. (2004). Religious affiliation and suicide attempt. *American Journal of Psychiatry*, 161(12), 2303–2308.

DiazGranados, N., Ibrahim, L. A., Brutsche, N. E., Ameli, R., Henter, I. D., Luckenbaugh, D. A., et al. (2010). Rapid resolution of suicidal ideation after a single infusion of an N-methyl-D-aspartate antagonist in patients with treatment-resistant major depressive disorder. *Journal of Clinical Psychiatry*, 71(12), 1605–1611.

Durkheim, E. (1897). *Le suicide: étude de sociologie*, Paris: Quadrige/PUF.

Ehnvall, A., Parker, G., Hadzi-Pavlovic, D., and Malhi, G. (2008). Perception of rejecting and neglectful parenting in childhood relates to lifetime suicide attempts for females – but not for males. *Acta Psychiatrica Scandinvica*, 117(1), 50–56.

Eisenberger, N. I. (2012). The pain of social disconnection: Examining the shared neural underpinnings of physical and social pain. *Nature Review Neurosciences*, 13(6), 421–434

Eisenberger, N. I., and Lieberman, M. D. (2004). Why rejection hurts: A common neural alarm system for physical and social pain. *Trends in Cognitive Sciences*, 8(7), 294–300.

Eisenberger, N. I., Lieberman, M. D., and Williams, K. D. (2003). Does rejection hurt? An FMRI study of social exclusion. *Science*, 302(5643), 290–292.

Evans, S., Shergill, S. S., and Averbeck, B. B. (2010). Oxytocin decreases aversion to angry faces in an associative learning task. *Neuropsychopharmacology*, 35(13), 2502–2509.

Fazel, S., Grann, M., Kling, B., and Hawton, K. (2011). Prison suicide in 12 countries: An ecological study of 861 suicides during 2003–2007. *Social Psychiatry and Psychiatric Epidemiology*, 46(3), 191–195.

Flamenbaum, R. (2007). Psychache as a mediator in the relationship between perfectionism and suicidality. *Journal of Counseling Psychology*, 54(1), 51–61.

Flamenbaum, R. (2009). Testing Shneidman's theory of suicide: psychache as a prospective predictor of suicidality and comparison wih hopelessness. Doctoral thesis, Queen's University, Kingston.

Flynn, J. J., and Holden, R. R. (2007). Predictors of suicidality in a sample of suicide attempters. *Canadian Psychology*, 48(2a), 317.

Foster, T. (2011). Adverse life events proximal to adult suicide: A synthesis of findings from psychological autopsy studies. *Archive of Suicide Research*, 15(1), 1–15.

Hempstead, K. (2006). The geography of self-injury: Spatial patterns in attempted and completed suicide. *Social Science and Medicine*, 62(12), 3186–3196.

Holden, R. R., Mehta, K., Cunningham, E., and McLeod, L. D. (2001). Development and preliminary validation of a scale of psychache. *Canadian Journal of Behavioural Science*, 33(4), 224–232.

Joiner, T. E., Jr., Brown, J. S., and Wingate, L. R. (2005). The psychology and neurobiology of suicidal behavior. *Annual Review of Psychology*, 56, 287–314.

Jokinen, J., Chatzittofis, A., Hellstrom, C., Nordstrom, P., Uvnas-Moberg, K., and Asberg, M. (2012). Low CSF oxytocin reflects high intent in suicide attempters. *Psychoneuroendocrinology*, 37(4), 482–490.

Jollant, F., Bellivier, F., Leboyer, M., Astruc, B., Torres, S., Verdier, R., *et al.* (2005). Impaired decision making in suicide attempters. *American Journal of Psychiatry*, 162(2), 304–310.

Jollant, F., Guillaume, S., Jaussent, I., Castelnau, D., Malafosse, A., and Courtet, P. (2007). Impaired decision-making in suicide attempters may increase the risk of problems in affective relationships. *Journal of Affective Disorders*, 99(1–3), 59–62.

Jollant, F., Lawrence, N. S., Giampietro, V., Brammer, M. J., Fullana, M. A., Drapier, D., *et al.* (2008). Orbitofrontal cortex response to angry faces in men with histories of suicide attempts. *American Journal of Psychiatry*, 165(6), 740–748.

Jollant, F., Lawrence, N. L., Olié, E., Guillaume, S., and Courtet, P. (2011). The suicidal mind and brain: A review of neuropsychological and neuroimaging studies. *World Journal of Biological Psychiatry*, 12(5), 319–339.

Jollant, F., Lawrence, N. S., Olié, E., O'Daly, O., Malafosse, A., Courtet, P., and Phillips, M. L. (2010). Decreased activation of lateral orbitofrontal cortex during risky choices under uncertainty is associated with disadvantageous decision-making and suicidal behavior. *Neuroimage*, 51(3), 1275–1281.

Kross, E., Berman, M. G., Mischel, W., Smith, E. E., and Wager, T. D. (2011). Social rejection shares somatosensory representations with physical pain. *Proceedings of the National Academy of Sciences*, 108(15), 6270–6275.

Lester, D. (2000). Psychache, depression, and personality. *Psychological Reports*, 87(3), 940.

Mann, J. J. (2003). Neurobiology of suicidal behaviour. *Nature Review Neurosciences*, 4(10), 819–828.

Mee, S., Bunney, B. G., Bunney, W. E., Hetrick, W., Potkin, S. G., and Reist, C. (2011). Assessment of psychological pain in major depressive episodes. *Journal of Psychiatric Research*, 45(11), 1504–1510.

Middleton, N., Sterne, J. A., and Gunnell, D. (2006). The geography of despair among 15-44-year-old men in England and Wales: Putting suicide on the map. *Journal of Epidemiological Community Health*, 60(12), 1040–1047.

Mills, J. F., Green, K., and Reddon, J. R. (2005). An evaluation of the Psychache Scale on an offender population. *Suicide and Life-Threatening Behavior*, 35(5), 570–580.

Moles, A., Kieffer, B. L., and D'Amato, F. R. (2004). Deficit in attachment behavior in mice lacking the mu-opioid receptor gene. *Science*, 304(5679), 1983–1986.

O'Connor, R. C., Fraser, L., Whyte, M. C., Machale, S., and Masterton, G. (2008). A comparison of specific positive future expectancies and global hopelessness as predictors of suicidal ideation in a prospective study of repeat self-harmers. *Journal of Affective Disorders*, 110(3), 207–214.

Olié, E., Courtet, P., Poulain, V., Guillaume, S., Ritchie, K., and Artero, S. (2013). History of suicidal behaviour and analgesic use in community-dwelling elderly. *Psychotherapy and Psychosomatics*, 82(5), 341–343.

Olié, E., Guillaume, S., Jaussent, I., Courtet, P., and Jollant, F. (2009). Higher psychological pain during a major depressive episode may be a factor of vulnerability to suicidal ideation and act. *Journal of Affective Disorders*, 120(1–3), 226–230.

Onoda, K., Okamoto, Y., Nakashima, K., Nittono, H., Ura, M., and Yamawaki, S. (2009). Decreased ventral anterior cingulate cortex activity is associated with reduced social pain during emotional support. *Social Neurosciences*, 4(5), 443–454.

Orbach, I., Mikulincer, M., Sirota, P., and Gilboa-Schechtman, E. (2003). Mental pain: A multidimensional operationalization and definition. *Suicide and Life-Threatening Behavior*, 33(3), 219–230.

Panagioti, M., Gooding, P. A., and Tarrier, N. (2012). Hopelessness, defeat, and entrapment in posttraumatic stress disorder: Their association with suicidal behavior and severity of depression. *The Journal of Nervous and Mental Disease*, 200(8), 676–683.

Pompili, M., Lester, D., Leenaars, A. A., Tatarelli, R., and Girardi, P. (2008). Psychache and suicide: A preliminary investigation. *Suicide and Life-Threatening Behavior*, 38(1), 116–121.

Pratt, D., Piper, M., Appleby, L., Webb, R., and Shaw, J. (2006). Suicide in recently released prisoners: A population-based cohort study. *Lancet*, 368(9530), 119–123.

Purcell, B., Heisel, M. J., Speice, J., Franus, N., Conwell, Y., and Duberstein, P. R. (2012). Family connectedness moderates the association between living alone and suicide ideation in a clinical sample of adults 50 years and older. *American Journal of Geriatric Psychiatry*, 20(8), 717–723.

Rezaeian, M., Dunn, G., St Leger, S., and Appleby, L. (2005). The ecological association between suicide rates and indices of deprivation in English local authorities. *Social Psychiatry and Psychiatric Epidemiology*, 40(10), 785–791.

Rurup, M. L., Deeg, D. J., Poppelaars, J. L., Kerkhof, A. J., and Onwuteaka-Philipsen, B. D. (2011). Wishes to die in older people: A quantitative study of prevalence and associated factors. *Crisis*, 32(4), 194–203.

Shneidman, E. S. (1993). Suicide as psychache. *Journal of Nervous and Mental Diseases*, 181(3), 145–147.

Stuckler, D., Basu, S., Suhrcke, M., Coutts, A., and McKee, M. (2009). The public health effect of economic crises and alternative policy responses in Europe: An empirical analysis. *Lancet*, 374(9686), 315–323.

Troister, T. (2009). A prospective study of psychache and its relationship to suicidality. (Master of Science), Queen's University, Kingston.

Troister, T., and Holden, R. R. (2012). A two-year prospective study of psychache and its relationship to suicidality among high-risk undergraduates. *Journal of Clinical Psychology*, 68(9), 1019–1027.

Vaiva, G., Ducrocq, F., Meyer, P., Mathieu, D., Philippe, A., .et al. (2006). Effect of telephone contact on further suicide attempts in patients discharged from an emergency department: Randomised controlled study. *British Medical Journal*, 332(7552), 1241–1245.

van Heeringen, C., Bijttebier, S., and Godfrin, K. (2011). Suicidal brains: A review of functional and structural brain studies in association with suicidal behaviour. *Neuroscience and Biobehavioral Reviews*, 35(3), 688–698.

van Heeringen, K., Van den Abbeele, D., Vervaet, M., Soenen, L., and Audenaert, K. (2010). The functional neuroanatomy of mental pain in depression. *Psychiatry Research*, 181(2), 141–144.

Walmsley, R. (2009). *World Prison Population List,* Eighth Edition. King's College, London: International Centre for Prison Studies. Retrieved from www.kcl.ac.uk/depsta/law/news/news_details.php?id=203.

Whitley, E., Gunnell, D., Dorling, D., and Smith, G. D. (1999). Ecological study of social fragmentation, poverty, and suicide. *British Journal of Medicine*, 319(7216), 1034–1037.

Williams, K. D. (2007). Ostracism. *Annual Review of Psychology*, 58, 425–452.

Yur'yev, A., Leppik, L., Tooding, L. M., Sisask, M., Varnik, P., Wu, J., and Varnik, A. (2010). Social inclusion affects elderly suicide mortality. *Internal Psychogeriatry*, 22(8), 1337–1343.

8 Clustering and contagion of suicidal behaviour

Ella Arensman and Carmel McAuliffe

Internationally, there is growing public and professional interest in clustering and contagion in suicidal behaviour. There are indications of increasing clustering and contagion effects in suicidal behaviour associated with the rise of modern communication systems (Larkin and Beautrais, 2012; Robertson *et al.*, 2012). Yet, the research in this area and information on effective response procedures and prevention strategies are limited (Haw *et al.*, 2013; Larkin and Beautrais, 2012). Even in recent times, Boyce (2011) referred to the lack of research as 'Suicide clusters: the undiscovered country'. The methodological approaches in assessing clustering and contagion of suicidal behaviour are wide-ranging and internationally, there is a lack of consistency regarding the definition of clustering and contagion and regarding the statistical techniques assessing spatio-temporal aspects (Haw *et al.*, 2013; Larkin and Beautrais, 2012; Mesoudi, 2009).

Defining suicide clusters and contagion

Internationally, there is a lack of consistency in defining suicide clusters, which is partly due to limited data and absence of controlled studies. Most studies so far included narrative reports of potential suicide clusters without appropriate statistical verification.

A frequently used definition to indicate time-space clustering (point cluster) is

> a temporary increase in the frequency of suicides within a small community or institution, relative to both the baseline suicide rate before and after the point cluster and the suicide rate in neighbouring area.
>
> (Gould, Wallenstein, and Kleinman, 1990;
> Haw *et al.*, 2013; Joiner, 1999; Mesoudi, 2009)

Larkin and Beautrais (2012) went a step further and introduced an operational definition:

> A suicide cluster is a series of three or more closely grouped deaths within three months that can be linked by space or social relationships. In the

absence of transparent social connectedness, evidence of space and time linkages are required to define a candidate cluster. In the presence of a strong demonstrated social connection, only temporal significance is required.

A concept introduced in recent times is the so-called echo clusters, which refers to 'the occurrence of subsequent, but temporally distinct clusters of suicide, which take place in the same location after an initial suicide' (Hanssens, 2010; Larkin and Beautrais, 2012).

Another type of suicide clusters is being referred to as mass clusters, and is commonly defined as 'a temporary increase in the total frequency of suicides within an entire population relative to the period immediately before and after the cluster, with no spatial clustering'. Mass clusters are typically associated with high-profile celebrity suicides that are publicized and disseminated in the mass media (Haw *et al.*, 2013; Hegerl *et al.*, 2013; Ladwig *et al.*, 2012; Mesoudi, 2009; Stack, 2000).

Based on a recent review, contagion is a concept derived from the study of infectious diseases and increasingly applied to cluster suicides. The underlying assumption is that 'suicidal behaviour may facilitate the occurrence of subsequent suicidal behaviour, either directly (via contact or friendship with the index suicide) or indirectly (via the media)' (Haw *et al.*, 2013). Those who are part of an at-risk population and have geographical and psychosocial proximity to a suicide are particularly vulnerable (Haw *et al.*, 2013).

Methodological issues

Research has tended to focus either on descriptive reports, or on the statistical verification of point and mass clusters. However, while both approaches have their merits when taken in isolation, it is their combination that offers the best opportunity to further our understanding of the mechanisms of suicide clustering (Arensman *et al.*, 2013). Thus, in examining suicide clustering, it is important to both verify the statistical significance of emerging clusters across space and time, and also to examine the level of contagion (interrelatedness) of cases that occur within clusters.

In recent years, research has moved beyond the exploratory stage and started to systematically examine clustering patterns, using geospatial analysis, such as SaTScan (Kulldorff, 1997). SaTScan has previously been used mainly to examine clustering patterns in infectious diseases, and this technique offers an innovative means of furthering our understanding of space-time (point) suicide clusters (Bando *et al.*, 2012; Cheung *et al.*, 2012; Larkin and Beautrais, 2012). The use of scan statistics allows us to statistically verify suicide clusters across both space and time. The method tests whether the number of cases within any spatial/ temporal window exceeds the number expected by random process. Detection of these types of clusters offers the potential to explore the factors underlying clustering and will facilitate the implementation of intervention and post-intervention strategies.

Epidemiological aspects of suicide clustering

Taking into account that the perception of clustering itself can be a risk factor for suicide, suicide clusters therefore differ from many other event clusters (Rezaeian, 2012). Most studies have reported on suicide clustering in adolescents and young adults, and indicate that clusters account for 2–15 per cent of all teen suicides (Insel and Gould, 2008). However, recent research has also identified clustering of suicides among adults and older people, in particular, men (Arensman *et al.*, 2013; Chotai, 2005; Larkin and Beautrais, 2012). Generally, males are over-represented among suicide clusters (Haw *et al.*, 2013; Qi *et al.*, 2012), but recent studies show that females may represent up to 24 per cent of those involved in a cluster (Jones *et al.*, 2013). Recent studies investigating spatial and time-space suicide clustering, found that suicide clustering was associated with lower socio-economic status (Exeter and Boyle, 2007; Qi *et al.*, 2012) and areas representing a higher proportion of indigenous population (Hanssens, 2010; Qi *et al.*, 2012). Larkin and Beautrais (2012) investigated the prevalence of echo clusters in New Zealand between 1990 and 2007. They identified nine distinct regions in which echo clustering had occurred. The average time between initial suicide clusters and echo clusters was 7.6 years with a range from 1.2 to 16.9 years.

In addition to geographical clusters, there is growing evidence showing time-space suicide clusters among specific populations and settings, such as psychiatric inpatients, adolescents and young adults in community settings (Haw *et al.*, 2013), schools (Poijula *et al.*, 2001), and universities (MacKenzie, 2013). In a recent study by Hawton *et al.* (2013), evidence was found for time-space clustering of self-harm in prisons in England and Wales, in particular among women and which was significantly associated with subsequent suicide.

The role of the media

There is evidence that suicide clustering and contagion are more prominent when media coverage is extensive and when suicides are glamorized and reported upon in detail (Niederkrotenthaler *et al.*, 2012; Pirkis *et al.*, 2006), with a stronger impact on suicides that are similar to the respective model in terms of age group, gender and suicide method (Niederkrotenthaler *et al.*, 2009). In this regard, Ladwig and colleagues (2012) found an 81 per cent increase in railway suicides during a period of six weeks after the death of a well-known German football goal-keeper who jumped in front of a train. Hegerl *et al.* (2012) looked at the long-term effects, and identified an 18.8 per cent increase in railway suicides during the two years after this event compared to the two years before. Regarding the impact of the media, the authors concluded that media reports followed the media guidelines to some extent, but it remains uncertain as to what the extent of the increase in railway suicides might have been if the media had followed the guidelines more thoroughly (Ladwig *et al.*, 2012). Media reports covering details of less well-known people, but elaborating on specific details of suicide methods, such as carbon monoxide poisoning by burning barbecue charcoal and inhaling hydrogen sulphide gas were also associated with significant increases in subsequent suicides and attempted suicides involving the same method (Hagihara *et al.*, 2013; Liu *et al.*, 2007). A study on the impact of newspaper reporting of hydrogen sulphide suicide on imitative suicide attempts in Japan identified an immediate effect of media reports on subsequent suicide attempts. The time lag between exposure to newspaper reports of suicide and suicide attempts was one or three days, and the magnitude of the impact of front page articles was greater than that of suicide articles in general (Hagihara *et al.*, 2013). A study by Jones *et al.* (2013) found that following statistical verification, the size of a suicide cluster among young people in the Bridgend area of South Wales, was smaller and shorter in duration than reported in the media. However, most deaths in the suicide cluster occured after the media had started reporting on initial cases of suicide.

There is growing evidence supporting the negative impact of new media on suicide contagion and clustering. Information on specific suicide methods on websites is associated with significant increases in suicides involving these methods and suicide pacts among two or more people (Hitosugi, 2006; JijiPress, 2008; Lee *et al.*, 2005; Rajagopal, 2004). A systematic review by Daine *et al.* (2013) showed that internet use may exert both positive and negative effects on young people at risk of self-harm or suicide. In terms of positive effects, young people, who self-harm or are suicidal, commonly use the internet for seeking support and coping with difficulties. However, there is also evidence indicating that the internet exerts a negative influence by normalising self-harm and potentially discouraging disclosure or professional help-seeking (Daine *et al.*, 2013).

Robertson *et al.* (2012) identified an association between suicide contagion and clustering, and social networking and SMS text messaging. The cluster involved eight young people aged 15–18 years in a city in New Zealand, and which occurred over a six-month period. The young people attended different schools and were living in different communities within the city, and most of them were linked by social networking sites, including sites created in memory of earlier suicide cases, text messaging and physical proximity. Seven of the eight suicide cases were male, and mental health and relationship problems were present in most of the cases. The study indicates that electronic communications increased the risk of suicide contagion, and this also facilitated the rapid spread of information and rumour throughout the community (Robertson *et al.*, 2012).

Risk factors associated with suicide clustering and contagion

In this section we try to address two separate but interrelated questions: First, what are the characteristic risk factors among individuals involved in a cluster? And, second, what makes an individual vulnerable to contagion?

The research evidence from narrative and statistical studies investigating point clusters consistently focuses to adolescents and young adults as being most at risk of suicide clustering (Bechtold, 1988; Davies and Wilkes, 1993; Gould *et al.*, 1990; Grigg, 1988; Johansson *et al.*, 2006; Poijula *et al.*, 2001; Tower, 1989;

Ward and Fox, 1977; Wilkie *et al.*, 1998; Wissow *et al.*, 2001). While suicide clustering is understood to be between two and four times more common among young people aged 15–24 years than among other age groups (Gould *et al.*, 1990), it is nonetheless a rare phenomenon even among the young. In a study investigating possible suicide clusters in Wales between 2000 and 2009 (Jones *et al.*, 2013), a temporo-spatial analysis only detected clustering when it was restricted to the sub-group of deaths that occurred among 15–34-year-olds. However, less than 1 per cent of possible suicide deaths among young people in Wales during this time were identified as being cluster-related. Larkin and Beautrais (2012) reported from their study investigating geospatial and temporal distribution of suicides occurring in Canterbury province in New Zealand between 1991 and 2008 that 1.1 per cent of teenage suicides over that time were cluster-related. While cluster suicides were significantly younger than singleton suicides (median age 29 and 37 years respectively), only one of the nine clusters they identified was composed exclusively of young people aged 20 years or younger. All eight remaining clusters included at least one individual aged 35 years or older. They argue that adult participation in cluster suicides is a neglected area. Chotai (2005) compared suicide cluster cases with singleton cases in northern Sweden and found that middle-aged and older males were most at risk, although the author points out the low number of teenage suicides in the overall sample. A report on suicides ascertained in the Cork region in Ireland between August 2010 and June 2012 identified two point clusters using geospatial techniques. The first cluster included 12 men and one woman with a median age of 47 years and an inter-quartile range (IQR) of 37.5 to 54 years. The second cluster comprised three men and four women with a median age of 39 years and IQR between 32 and 50 years (Arensman *et al.*, 2013).

Suicide cluster deaths occur more frequently among males (Bechtold, 1988; Chotai, 2005; Davies and Wilkes, 1993; Grigg, 1988; Ward and Fox, 1977; Wissow *et al.*, 2001). In one review of point clusters among adolescents (Insel and Gould, 2008) females were identified as being at greater risk of attempted suicide while males were at greater risk of completed suicide, consistent with findings from studies of non-cluster suicidal behavior.

Individuals who die in suicide clusters tend to have high risk profiles (Haw *et al.*, 2013). Cluster victims are repeatedly described in the research literature as *vulnerable* individuals (Davies and Wilkes, 1993; Larkin and Beautrais, 2012; Ward and Fox, 1977). For example, Larkin and Beautrais report from their study of nine clusters that almost one-quarter (23.3 per cent) of all cluster cases combined had a lifetime history of inpatient psychiatric admission, and almost half (46.5 per cent) had a history of outpatient psychiatric care. One-fifth (20.9 per cent) had a diagnosis of alcohol abuse or dependence with almost one in four having a pattern of problem alcohol use in the year prior to death. Drug problems in the year prior to death were reported for 14 per cent of cases. Almost half (42 per cent) had a lifetime history of suicide attempt, and one in five (18.6 per cent) had made at least one suicide attempt in the year prior to death. More than half (51 per cent) had a lifetime history of threatening suicide and 40 per cent were known to have made a suicide threat in the year prior to death. One in three cluster decedents (34.9 per cent) had attempted suicide in the month prior to their death.

Despite this high prevalence of risk factors identified in descriptive studies of suicide clusters, for example, drug and alcohol abuse, employment problems and past history of self-harm, are common risk factors for suicide in general and not unique to clustering (Haw *et al.*, 2013). A fairly consistent trend in the limited literature available is the lack of differences between cluster and singleton suicides. Larkin and Beautrais (2012) found that cluster compared to singleton suicides were similar on demographic characteristics including gender, marital status, ethnicity, education and employment status. They found no differences between singleton, cluster or index suicides on psychosocial or psychiatric characteristics including occurrence of stressful life events, presence of a suicide note, physical health problems at the time of death, recent visit to a GP, history of inpatient or outpatient psychiatric treatment, lifetime diagnosis of a psychiatric illness, alcohol or drug use in the year prior to death, lifetime or past year history of self-harm or suicide threat, or having a friend relative or partner who had died by suicide. They did find, however, that clusters of suicides were more likely to include people involved in suicide pacts (9.3 per cent vs. 0.9 per cent, $p < 0.05$). Compared to other cases in a cluster, index cases were more likely to have financial problems at the time of their death (11.6 per cent vs. 33.3 per cent, $p < 0.05$).

A lack of methodologically sound studies has hampered our identification of specific risk profiles among cluster suicides. In their review, Haw and colleagues (2013) were only able to identify two case-control studies comparing suicide cluster cases with singleton suicides (Chotai, 2005) or living controls (Davidson *et al.*, 1989). In both studies, other methodological limitations arose. For example, in the study by Chotai (2005) only a limited range of possible risk factors was examined (gender, age, marital status, area of residence, season of birth and method of suicide); while in the study by Davidson and colleagues, 14 teenagers in two suicide clusters were compared with living controls (three living controls for each suicide). Therefore, variables that characterized the suicides could not be assumed to characterize cluster suicides specifically, as non-cluster suicides were not included as a control group. In the study by Larkin and Beautrais (2012), cluster suicides ($n = 43$) were compared with all non-cluster suicides ($n = 216$) occurring in the region over the same time period. Although the cluster cases were significantly younger than the singleton cases (median age 29 years compared with 37 years respectively), they were not matched by age and gender. Despite their younger age, cluster cases had similar lifetime rates of diagnosed psychiatric illness, inpatient psychiatric treatment and outpatient psychiatric treatment; and similar proportions had a friend, relative or partner who had died by suicide. Cluster cases had even higher rates of lifetime suicide attempts and past year suicide attempts, although this was not significant. It is possible that some of the differences between cluster and singleton suicides were not detected as a result of inadequate power.

Responding to suicide clusters and contagion

Early identification of emerging suicide clusters and contagion is crucial in order to facilitate a strategic and co-ordinated response. It would be required to have timely access to detailed information on the cases of suicide involved in order to determine risk factors and interrelatedness among the suicide cases (Arensman *et al.*, 2013). In a number of countries, such as the US, Australia, New Zealand, England and Wales, and Ireland, guidelines to respond to emerging suicide clusters, have been developed and implemented. However, evaluations have not yet been published.

A co-ordinated response involving relevant public health, health and bereavement support services should be established in order to respond to the needs of people affected, such as next of kin, friends, colleagues and people affected in the community or setting (e.g. school, psychiatric ward) and to prevent further suicidal behaviour (Askland *et al.*, 2003; LIFE, 2012; Robertson *et al.*, 2012). Due to multiple losses in a short space of time, family members and friends may experience complicated grief, which requires involving expertise in the area of suicide bereavement support (Spiwak *et al.*, 2012). Another key element of a response plan is involving the media in order to ensure adherence to media guidelines for suicide reporting and appropriate and balanced media reports. Monitoring of social networking sites by suicide prevention agencies enables access to conversations which may be related to possible subsequent suicides (Robertson *et al.*, 2012). In order to enhance responding to a suicide cluster and to the needs of those who are affected and of the professionals involved, the need for training should be explored and addressed, and crisis responses should be linked to a long-term programme of suicide risk reduction and community recovery (LIFE, 2012).

References

Arensman, E., Wall, M. A., McAuliffe, C., Corcoran, P., Williamson, M. E., McCarthy, M. J., *et al.* (2013). *Second Report of the Suicide Support and Information System.* Cork: NSRF.

Askland, K. D., Sonnenfeld, N., and Crosby, A. (2003). A public health response to a cluster of suicidal behaviors: Clinical psychiatry, prevention, and community health. *Journal of Psychiatric Practice*, 9(3), 219–227.

Bando, D., Moreira, R., Pereira, J., and Barrozo, L. (2012). Spatial clusters of suicide in the municipality of São Paulo 1996–2005: An ecological study. *BMC Psychiatry*, 12(124), 1–8.

Bechtold, D. W. (1988). Cluster suicide in American Indian adolescents. *American Indian and Alaska Native Mental Health Research*, 1(3), 26–35.

Boyce, N. (2011). Suicide clusters: The undiscovered country. *The Lancet*, 378(9801), 1452.

Cheung, Y. T. D., Spittal, M. J., Pirkis, J., and Yip, P. S. F. (2012). Spatial analysis of suicide mortality in Australia: Investigation of metropolitan-rural-remote differentials of suicide risk across states/territories. *Social Science and Medicine*, 75(8), 1460–1468.

Chotai, J. (2005). Suicide aggregation in relation to socio-demographic variables and the suicide method in a general population: Assortative susceptibility. *Nordic Journal of Psychiatry*, 59(5), 325–330.

Daine, K., Hawton, K., Singaravelu, V., Stewart, A., Simkin, S., and Montgomery, P. (2013). The power of the web: A systematic review of studies of the influence of the internet on self-harm and suicide in young people. *PloS One*, 8(10), e77555.

Davidson, L. E., Rosenberg, M. L., Mercy, J. A., Franklin, J., and Simmons, J. T. (1989). An epidemiologic study of risk factors in two teenage suicide clusters. *JAMA: the Journal of the American Medical Association*, 262(19), 2687–2692.

Davies, D., and Wilkes, T. C. (1993). Cluster suicide in rural western Canada. *The Canadian Journal of Psychiatry*, 38(7), 515–519.

Exeter, D. J., and Boyle, P. J. (2007). Does young adult suicide cluster geographically in Scotland? *Journal of Epidemiology and Community Health*, 61(8), 731–736.

Gould, M. S., Wallenstein, S., and Kleinman, M. (1990). Time-space clustering of teenage suicide. *American Journal of Epidemiology*, 131(1), 71–78.

Grigg, J. R. (1988). Imitative suicides in an active duty military population. *Military Medicine*, 153(2), 71–78.

Hagihara, A., Abe, T., Omagari, M., Motoi, M., and Nabeshima, Y. (2014). The impact of newspaper reporting of hydrogen sulfide suicide on imitative suicide attempts in Japan. *Social Psychiatry and Psychiatric Epidemiology*, 49(2), 221–229.

Hanssens, L. (2010). 'Echo Clusters' – Are they a unique phenomenon of indigenous attempted and completed suicide? *Aboriginal and Islander Health Worker Journal*, 34(1), 17–26.

Haw, C., Hawton, K., Niedzwiedz, C., and Platt, S. (2013). Suicide clusters: A review of risk factors and mechanisms. *Suicide and Life-Threatening Behavior*, 43(1), 97–108.

Hawton, K., Linsell, L., Adeniji, T., Sariaslan, A., and Fazel, S. (2013). Self-harm in prisons in England and Wales: An epidemiological study of prevalence, risk factors, clustering, and subsequent suicide. *The Lancet, Early Online Publication*, 16 December 2013. doi:10.1016/S0140-6736(13)62118-2

Hegerl, U., Koburger, N., Rummel-Kluge, C., Gravert, C., Walden, M., and Mergl, R. (2013). One followed by many? – Long-term effects of a celebrity suicide on the number of suicidal acts on the German railway net. *Journal of Affective Disorders*, 146(1), 39–44.

Hitosugi, M. (2006). Group suicide due to charcoal burning with administration of melatonin. *Japanese Journal of Toxicology*, 19(1), 55–56.

Insel, B. J. and Gould, M. S. (2008). Impact of modeling on adolescent suicidal behavior. *Psychiatric Clinics of North America*, 31(2), 293–316.

JijiPress. (2008). The number of suicides by hydrogen sulfide between January and November, 2008 exceeds 1,000, Online press article cited in Hagihara *et al.*, 2013.

Johansson, L., Lindqvist, P., and Eriksson, A. (2006). Teenage suicide cluster formation and contagion: Implications for primary care. *BMC Family Practice*, 7(32), 1–5.

Joiner, T. E. (1999). The clustering and contagion of suicide. *Current Directions in Psychological Science*, 8(3), 89–92.

Jones, P., Gunnell, D., Platt, S., Scourfield, J., Lloyd, K., Huxley, P., *et al.* (2013). Identifying probable suicide clusters in Wales using national mortality data. *PloS One*, 8(8), 1–9.

Kulldorff, M. (1997). A spatial scan statistic. *Communications in Statistics-Theory and Methods*, 26(6), 1481–1496.

Ladwig, K. H., Kunrath, S., Lukaschek, K., and Baumert, J. (2012). The railway suicide death of a famous German football player: Impact on the subsequent frequency of railway suicide acts in Germany. *Journal of Affective Disorders*, 136(1), 194–198.

Larkin, G., and Beautrais, A. (2012). *Geospatial Mapping of Suicide Clusters*. Auckland: Te Pou o Te Whakaaro Nui.

Lee, D. T., Chan, K. P., and Yip, P. S. (2005). Charcoal burning is also popular for suicide pacts made on the internet. *BMJ: British Medical Journal*, 330(7491), 602–603.

LIFE. (2012). *Developing a Community Plan for Preventing and Responding to Suicide Clusters*. Melbourne: Centre for Health Policy, Programs and Economics, Melbourne School of Population Health, The University of Melbourne.

Liu, K. Y., Beautrais, A., Caine, E., Chan, K., Chao, A., Conwell, Y., (2007). Charcoal burning suicides in Hong Kong and urban Taiwan: An illustration of the impact of a novel suicide method on overall regional rates. *Journal of Epidemiology and Community Health*, 61(3), 248–253.

MacKenzie, D. W. (2013). Applying the Anderson-Darling test to suicide clusters. *Crisis*, 34(6), 434–437.

Mesoudi, A. (2009). The cultural dynamics of copycat suicide. *PLoS One*, 4(9), e7252.

Niederkrotenthaler, T., Fu, K.W., Yip, P. S., Fong, D. Y., Stack, S., Cheng, Q., and Pirkis, J. (2012). Changes in suicide rates following media reports on celebrity suicide: A meta-analysis. *Journal of Epidemiology and Community Health*, 66(11), 1037–1042.

Niederkrotenthaler, T., Till, B., Kapusta, N. D., Voracek, M., Dervic, K., and Sonneck, G. (2009). Copycat effects after media reports on suicide: A population-based ecologic study. *Social Science and Medicine*, 69(7), 1085–1090.

Pirkis, J. E., Burgess, P. M., Francis, C., Blood, R. W., and Jolley, D. J. (2006). The relationship between media reporting of suicide and actual suicide in Australia. *Social Science and Medicine*, 62(11), 2874–2886.

Poijula, S., Wahlberg, K. E., and Dyregrov, A. (2001). Adolescent suicide and suicide contagion in three secondary schools. *International Journal of Emergency Mental Health*, 3(3), 163–168.

Qi, X., Hu, W., Page, A., and Tong, S. (2012). Spatial clusters of suicide in Australia. *BMC Psychiatry*, 12(86), 1–11.

Rajagopal, S. (2004). Suicide pacts and the internet: Complete strangers may make cyberspace pacts. *BMJ: British Medical Journal*, 329(7478), 1298–1299.

Rezaeian, M. (2012). Suicide clusters: Introducing a novel type of categorization. *Violence and Victims*, 27(1), 125–132.

Robertson, L., Skegg, K., Poore, M., Williams, S., and Taylor, B. (2012). An adolescent suicide cluster and the possible role of electronic communication technology. *Crisis: The Journal of Crisis Intervention and Suicide Prevention*, 33(4), 239–245.

Spiwak, R., Sareen, J., Elias, B., Martens, P., Munro, G., and Bolton, J. (2012). Complicated grief in Aboriginal populations. *Dialogues in Clinical Neuroscience*, 14(2), 204–209.

Stack, S. (2000). Media impacts on suicide: A quantitative review of 293 findings. *Social Science Quarterly*, 81(4), 957–971.

Tower, M. (1989). A suicide epidemic in an American Indian community. *American Indian and Alaska Native Mental Health Research*, 3(1), 34–44.

Ward, J. A., and Fox, J. (1977). A suicide epidemic on an Indian reserve. *The Canadian Psychiatric Association Journal/La Revue de l'Association des psychiatres du Canada*, 22(8), 423–426.

Wilkie, C., Macdonald, S., and Hildahl, K. (1998). Community case study: Suicide cluster in a small Manitoba community. *Canadian Journal of Psychiatry*, 43(8), 823–828.

Wissow, L. S., Walkup, J., Barlow, A., Reid, R., and Kane, S. (2001). Cluster and regional influences on suicide in a Southwestern American Indian tribe. *Social Science and Medicine*, 53(9), 1115–1124.

Part II

Varied research evidence and assessment perspectives

9 Suicidal ideation and behavior among sexual minority youth

Correlates, vulnerabilities, and protective factors

*Samantha Pflum, Kaitlin Venema,
Joseph Tomlins, Peter Goldblum
and Bruce Bongar*

Compared to their heterosexual peers, sexual minority youth continue to experience significant health disparities. These youth report differentially higher rates of anxiety, depression, suicidality, low self-esteem, and substance use (D'Augelli et al., 2002; Friedman et al., 2006; Poteat et al., 2009; Rivers and Noret, 2008). Since 2001, the United States Surgeon General has identified sexual minority youth as a 'vulnerable population' (Surgeon General, 2001). As a result of environmental stressors such as peer bullying, family rejection, and community-based victimization, sexual minority youth may be at particularly high risk for suicide. Suicidal ideation, attempts, and completions are among the most concerning disparities for this population (Poteat et al., 2011).

Rates of suicidal ideation and attempts vary based on sampling approaches, definitions of constructs, geographical location, help-seeking, and other factors. However, several decades of research have consistently demonstrated that lesbian, gay, bisexual, and queer/questioning youth report higher levels of suicidal ideation and attempts than heterosexual youth (Cochran and Mays, 2013; Goodenow et al., 2006; Mustanski et al., 2010; Russell and Joyner, 2001; Russell and Toomey, 2012). Among sexual minorities, the odds of attempting suicide are approximately two to seven times higher than the odds of suicide attempt among heterosexuals (King et al., 2008; Haas et al., 2010). A Rhode Island-based study demonstrated that 10 percent of sexual minority adolescents, as compared to just over 3 percent of heterosexual teens, reported suicide attempts severe enough to warrant medical attention (Jiang et al., 2010). The 2001 Massachusetts Youth Risk Behavior Survey reported a similar pattern, with 20 percent of LGB youth requiring medical attention after a suicide attempt, as compared to 4.7 percent of heterosexual youth (Massachusetts Department of Education, 2002). As a group, LGB youth experience greater levels of suicidal ideation and behavior than their heterosexual peers (Suicide Prevention Resource Center [SPRC], 2008). Sexual orientation itself does not lead to suicidality among LGB youth; rather, environmental reactions to non-heterosexual orientations increase suicide risk in this population (Savin-Williams and Ream, 2003).

Suicide deaths among LGB youth

Cross-sectional research suggests that sexual minority youth are 'far more likely' to commit suicide than their heterosexual peers (Hershberger and D'Augelli, 1995; Plöderl *et al.*, 2013). However, completed suicides among this population have not been thoroughly documented or examined empirically. Less is known about completed suicides due to lack of data on sexual minority individuals in probability studies, as well as the difficulty in determining sexual orientation postmortem (Cochran and Mays, 2013). Sexual orientation is rarely assessed in psychological autopsy studies, which involve the reconstruction of suicidal deaths through interviews with survivors (Copeland, 1993). Youth may not be 'out' to loved ones or may be unsure of their sexual identity, further confounding the accurate measurement of suicide completions among LGB youth. Additionally, studies of completed suicides among heterosexuals and sexual minorities have been flawed by the use of non-representative samples, such as incarcerated individuals and psychiatric patients (McDaniel *et al.*, 2001). When information on sexual orientation is collected, data on completed suicides tends to drastically exaggerate or minimize the rate of completed suicides among sexual minorities (SPRC, 2008).

Although definitive data on suicide rates for LGB youth are lacking, extant research indicates that the most reliable predictors of suicide risk among both heterosexuals and sexual minorities are suicidal ideation and prior suicide attempts (SPRC, 2008). Based on the higher rate of suicide attempts among LGB youth and the seriousness of their suicide attempts, it is likely that LGB youth experience higher rates of suicide deaths than their heterosexual peers (SPRC, 2008). Some research indicates that sexual minority youth have more risk factors and fewer protective factors than their heterosexual peers, placing them at higher risk for suicidal behavior and completions (SPRC, 2008). LGB youth who are homeless, living in foster care, and/or involved in the juvenile justice system are at even higher risk for suicide attempts and completions than their LGB peers who do not endorse these risk factors (SPRC, 2008).

The etiology of increased suicide risk among LGB youth

Sexual minority stress

The minority stress model (Meyer, 2003) helps to elucidate some of the connections between sexual minority identity and suicidality. In most industrialized societies, individuals identifying as lesbian, gay, or bisexual are part of a stigmatized and devalued cultural group. This disadvantaged social position leads to the experience of minority stress (Meyer, 2003). For LGB individuals, 'stigma, prejudice, and discrimination create a hostile and stressful social environment that causes mental health problems' (Meyer, 2003, p. 674). These widespread experiences of stigma negatively impact self-perception and increase the expectation of social rejection (Hatzenbuehler, 2009; Meyer, 2003).

Eventually, the elevated level of social adversity contributes to higher psychiatric morbidity (Hatzenbuehler, 2009; Meyer, 2003).

Sexual minorities consistently report more everyday experiences of discrimination; perceptions of discrimination are closely linked to mental health morbidity among lesbian, gay, and bisexual individuals (Almeida *et al.*, 2009; Cochran and Mays, 2007; Herek, 2009; Mays and Cochran, 2001). Moreover, stress associated with the awareness, discovery, and disclosure of one's LGB identity is a unique risk factor for sexual minority youth. LGB youth are at greater risk for suicide attempts if they 'come out' to others at an earlier age (Remafedi *et al.*, 1991). Particularly for youth, stigma-based experiences that appear 'minor' can build up over time, resulting in serious mental health consequences (Meyer *et al.*, 2011). Micro-aggressions, brief ignominies that communicate derogation towards LGB individuals, can lead to or exacerbate mental health issues (Nadal, 2008; Sue *et al.*, 2007). These can take the form of heterosexist terminology, use of derogatory terms, and the assumption of a universal heterosexual experience (Nadal, 2008). As a result of continued exposure to stressful events – however small – sexual minorities may experience more adverse mental health outcomes than their heterosexual peers (Meyer, 2003).

The psychological mediation framework

Based on findings from the minority stress framework, psychiatric epidemiology, and general psychological processes related to morbidity, Hatzenbuehler (2009) put forth a psychological mediation framework to elucidate the etiology of mental health disparities among sexual minorities. This framework posits that, through experiences of stigma-induced stress, sexual minorities become more vulnerable to psychological processes that contribute to psychopathology in heterosexual individuals (Hatzenbuehler, 2009). Relative to heterosexuals, the experience of stigma-related stress causes increases in emotional dysregulation, social difficulties, and cognitive processes influencing risk for psychopathology (Hatzenbuehler, 2009). By taking both unique and general stressors into account, this framework provides a more advanced understanding of influences upon mental health disparities in the LGB population.

Correlates of suicidality among sexual minority youth

Ecological systems theory (Bronfenbrenner, 1979) can be used as a framework to explore the components of elevated risk, correlates of suicidality, and relevant protective factors for LGB youth. Correlates of suicidality can be found at many ecological levels ranging from the immediate microsystem (e.g., family, peers, school) to the macrosystem (e.g., general societal and cultural norms) (Bronfenbrenner, 1979). Among LGB youth, suicide attempters have been found to experience higher levels of both general stress and stress related to their sexual minority identities (Savin-Williams and Ream, 2003). Such stressors can be localized in various socio-ecological levels, such as individual vulnerability to mental health problems, conflict with rejecting family members, and intolerant social environments.

Depression: prevalence and etiology

Compared to their heterosexual counterparts, sexual minority youth are at increased risk for both internalizing and externalizing symptoms (Hatzenbuehler, 2009). Major depressive disorder is the most commonly experienced mental health condition among sexual minorities, including both youth and adults (Cochran and Mays, 2013). Approximately 20 percent of sexual minorities experience significant depressive symptoms on an annual basis, and sexual minorities are twice as likely than heterosexuals to suffer from depression (Cochran and Mays, 2013; Hatzenbuehler *et al.*, 2010). Given its close association with suicidality, depression will be the focus of this section.

Interpersonal theories of depression posit that stressors, particularly those related to stigma, alter interpersonal relationships and render individuals more vulnerable to psychopathology (Hatzenbuehler, 2009). For sexual minorities, stigma-related stress may lead to isolation, internalized homophobia, and as a consequence, diminished social support (Hatzenbuehler, 2009; Link *et al.*, 1997). Concerns about rejection and negative evaluation may cause sexual minorities to avoid close relationships for fear of others discovering their stigmatized identities (Pachankis, 2008). Although this avoidance enables the temporary escape from rejection, identity concealment may lead to greater loneliness, isolation, and social anxiety (Pachankis, 2008).

Social isolation has been linked to greater psychological distress, particularly symptoms of depression and anxiety (Hatzenbuehler, 2009). Additionally, the chronicity of stressors faced by sexual minorities often engenders hopelessness, a construct that is associated with both depression and suicidality (Russell and Joyner, 2001). Chronic exposure to discrimination, rejection, and interpersonal victimization can lead to negative self-schemas and internalized homophobia, in which negative societal views of homosexuality are turned against the self. Cross-sectional research has demonstrated that LGB individuals have lower self-esteem than heterosexual individuals, a construct that has been linked to stigma-related stressors (Plöderl and Fartacek, 2005). In turn, negative self-esteem is predictive of suicidality (Savin-Williams and Ream, 2003).

Peer victimization

Victimization based on known or suspected sexual minority identity is the most common form of bias-related violence (Pilkington and D'Augelli, 1995; Herek, 1989). Negative outcomes of such victimization include disruptions of the coming out process, increased internalized homophobia, decreases in self-esteem and self-worth, heightened fears for personal safety, and exacerbations of mental health symptoms (Pilkington and D'Augelli, 1995). As a result of societal stressors and prejudices, sexual minority youth are particularly vulnerable to mental health problems, a vulnerability that can be exacerbated by victimization (Hershberger and D'Augelli, 1995).

For sexual minority youth, there is a strong correlation between discrimination, victimization, and increased self-harm, suicidal ideation, and suicide attempts (Goldblum *et al.*, 2012; Hershberger and D'Augelli, 1995; Poteat *et al.*, 2011). Compared to victimization that is not bias-based, victimization based on sexual minority status (homophobic victimization) is associated with significantly higher levels of both suicidal ideation and attempts (Russell *et al.*, 2012). Although these results have been based primarily on cross-sectional studies, recent longitudinal findings offer prospective evidence of this relationship. Among diverse sexual minority youth, early reports of victimization predicted future suicidal ideation and deliberate self-harm (Liu and Mustanski, 2012). After suicide attempt history, victimization based on sexual minority status was the strongest predictor of self-harm (Liu and Mustanski, 2012).

School climate and overall school safety are strongly connected to the experience of peer victimization among LGB youth. The Gay, Lesbian, and Straight Education Network (GLSEN) revealed that 84.9 percent of LGB students in elementary, middle, and high schools heard homophobic remarks from peers, teachers, and school staff (Kosciw *et al.*, 2012). Additionally, 63.5 percent of sexual minority students felt unsafe and unwelcome at school, and 81.9 percent were verbally harassed because of their sexual orientation (Kosciw *et al.*, 2012).

Homophobic victimization has been shown to predict suicidality, depression, substance use, and school problems among sexual minority youth (Birkett *et al.*, 2009; Poteat *et al.*, 2011). Students who experienced high levels of victimization based on sexual orientation endorsed higher levels of depression and lower levels of self-esteem (Kosciw *et al.*, 2012). Even in the absence of direct homophobic victimization, youth may experience increased anxiety, depression, and isolation in schools with pervasive use of anti-gay language (Birkett *et al.*, 2009). Feeling unsafe and unwelcome in school is associated with heightened levels of suicidal ideation and suicide attempts (Poteat *et al.*, 2011); such experiences may also be connected to a sense of thwarted belongingness, a primary component of the interpersonal theory of suicide (Joiner, 2010). Serious suicide attempts requiring medical attention are more common among sexual minority youth attending schools perceived as safe for most youth (Goodenow *et al.*, 2006). Thus, overall ratings of school safety may not be representative of the experiences of LGB youth. While heterosexual students thrive in such schools, LGB students may suffer significantly.

Family relationships

For sexual minority youth, families may not be sources of solace from external prejudice and victimization. Many fear coming out to their families, noting that the prospect of such disclosure is 'extremely troubling' (Hershberger and D'Augelli, 1995, p. 65). LGB youth report rejection, harassment, and abuse from immediate family members, and are more likely to experience long-term parental maltreatment (Corliss *et al.*, 2001; Pilkington and D'Augelli, 1995). LGB children may be more likely to experience maltreatment by their parents in families with multiple siblings (Balsam *et al.*, 2005). Ryan and colleagues (2009) demonstrated that LGB young adults who noted higher levels of family rejection during adolescence were 8.4 times more likely to report having attempted suicide, 5.9 times more likely to report high levels of depression, 3.4 times more likely to report illegal drug use, and 3.4 times more likely to report having engaged in unprotected sexual activity (compared to peers from families with low or moderate levels of rejection). LGB youth from families with low or moderate levels of rejection were found to be at significantly lower risk for these negative mental health outcomes (Ryan *et al.*, 2009). Such findings have important implications for understanding the etiology of psychiatric symptoms, particularly suicidality, among sexual minorities. Although such research has not definitively established causality, it has indicated a strong and significant link between parental rejection and negative mental health outcomes in LGB youth (Ryan *et al.*, 2009).

Protective factors

In examining health disparities between sexual minority and heterosexual youth, it is apparent that some of these disparities may be due to lower levels of protective factors among sexual minority youth (Saewyc, 2011). When present, these factors can help to mitigate risk and to support positive development for LGB youth (Saewyc, 2011). As members of a stigmatized group, sexual minority youth can develop a variety of coping strategies and support systems to minimize the negative psychological consequences of societal bias.

Family support

A supportive home environment can be crucial for decreasing suicide risk among sexual minority youth. For LGB adolescents, family acceptance and support are associated with positive health outcomes in young adulthood, including self-esteem, social support, and general health (Hershberger and D'Augelli, 1995; Poteat *et al.*, 2011; Ryan *et al.*, 2010). Family support helps to protect against negative health outcomes, including depression, substance abuse, suicidal ideation, and suicide attempts (Poteat *et al.*, 2011; Ryan *et al.*, 2010; SPRC, 2008). Such support may be capable of attenuating the effects of sexual orientation-based victimization (Poteat *et al.*, 2011). In regards to the long-term effects of homophobic bullying, adults who recalled having positive friendships and strong family or community relationships during adolescence reported greater resilience and positive mental health outcomes later in life (Rivers, 2011). Parents are capable of promoting the overall health of sexual minority youth by providing both general support and sexual orientation-specific support (such as affirming their child's LGB identity) (Poteat *et al.*, 2011). Specific suggestions for parental promotion of health can be found in the Recommendations section of this chapter.

School-based protective factors

School-based support can promote positive mental health outcomes for LGB youth. Feelings of safety and connectedness at school are associated with lower levels of suicide attempts (Saewyc, 2011). Several studies have explored the role of Gay-Straight Alliances (GSAs) in relation to mental health outcomes among LGB youth. Findings indicate that sexual minority youth attending schools with GSAs report more positive health and academic outcomes than youth in schools without GSAs, including lower rates of suicide attempts (Birkett *et al.*, 2009; Goodenow *et al.*, 2006; Poteat *et al.*, 2013; Saewyc, 2011).

GSAs may function to reduce suicidality by decreasing the victimization that has been linked to suicidal ideation and attempts (Goodenow *et al.*, 2006). Schools that promote student diversity, have LGBT-inclusive curricula, and have anti-bullying policies that specify the protection of sexual minorities have been shown to reduce high-risk behaviors among sexual minority students (Goodenow *et al.*, 2006). Inclusive anti-bullying policies have a strong negative association with suicide attempts, even when victimization and social support are taken into account (Goodenow *et al.*, 2006).

Health professionals

Health professionals also play a role in supporting the acceptance of sexual minority youth within families (Ryan *et al.*, 2010). The Family Acceptance Project (FAP) is a San Francisco-based research and intervention program designed to assess and improve parental support for sexual minority children (Ryan *et al.*, 2010). Mental health and medical providers can help families identify supportive behaviors that can protect against risk and promote healthy psychological development. Such behaviors include talking with children about their LGBT identity, advocating for youth when they are mistreated due to their sexual minority identity, and connecting an LGBT child to an LGBT adult role model (Ryan *et al.*, 2010). As family acceptance is associated with reduced odds of suicidal ideation and attempts, it can be crucial for health professionals to facilitate positive family reactions to a youth's 'coming out' process (Ryan *et al.*, 2010). Educating families of sexual minority youth about the serious negative health impact of family rejection (including depression, suicidality, and substance use) can mitigate risk and help improve health outcomes in LGB youth (Ryan *et al.*, 2010).

For LGB students who are bullied at school or are rejected by their parents, psychologists, counselors, and nurses often serve as first responders. Rates of suicidality among LGB youth have been shown to decrease in schools that offer supportive nonacademic counseling (Goodenow *et al.*, 2006). Mental health and medical professionals can provide a safe space for students to disclose their concerns, but must first signal to youth that they are open to diversity in sexual orientation and relationships. After 'passing the test', professionals may experience increased disclosure of information related to being LGB and increased willingness to discuss concerns related to sexual minority status (Weiss, 1994). Without education and training on LGB-specific issues, health professionals may not have the competencies required to address difficulties that are unique to sexual minorities (American Psychological Association, 2012).

Recommendations

Based on the information on suicidal ideation and behavior among LGB youth presented in this chapter, we provide a number of recommendations intended to maximize protective factors among LGB youth.

For mental health and medical professionals

- Seek further training on sexual minority-specific issues in order to facilitate continued professional development. Specific guidelines for working with this population can be derived from the American Psychological Association's *Guidelines for Psychological Practice with Lesbian, Gay, and Bisexual Clients* (2012).
- When LGB youth present with symptoms of depression and/or suicidality, conduct a thorough assessment of risk and protective factors. A lack of protective factors has been linked to suicidality, making it essential to capitalize on young clients' existing strengths and healthy coping skills.
- Identify local LGB support programs and online resources to educate parents about how to support their LGB children.
- Build a network of referrals that specialize in providing clinical, educational, and support services for LGB youth.
- Speak with LGB adolescents about family reactions to their sexual identity. For families who have trouble accepting their child's sexual identity, refer to LGB community support programs and for supportive counseling.
- Advise parents that negative reactions to their child's LGB identity negatively influences their child's mental health. More information on this research can be found through the Family Acceptance Project (www.familyproject.sfsu.edu).

For teachers and school administrators

- Implement and support policies and procedures to prevent harassment due to LGB identity. Ensure that sexual orientation and gender identity are explicitly included in nondiscrimination and anti-bullying policies.
- Provide education about LGB issues to students, administrators, staff, and teachers to increase safety in schools. Encourage the implementation of LGB-inclusive curricula.
- Support the establishment and maintenance of a Gay-Straight Alliance (GSA) to facilitate social support and decrease bullying and suicidality among LGB students. Encourage teachers and school staff to place LGBTQ-affirmative stickers (e.g., Human Rights Campaign, Trevor Project) on their doors to signal openness and safety.

- Regularly monitor classrooms, hallways, and cafeterias for the presence of anti-gay comments. Seek support from your local chapter of GLSEN (www.glsen.org) if you witness homophobic victimization.

For parents and families

- Be attuned to signs that a child may be experiencing symptoms of depression and/or thoughts of suicide (hopelessness, withdrawal, school failure, talking about 'not wanting to be here', etc). Seek support from a mental health professional if any of these signs are noted.
- A supportive home environment is crucial for attenuating suicidality among LGB youth. Express affection, validation, and support related to all aspects of your child's identity, particularly their sexual minority identity.
- Advocate for your child whenever he or she faces peer victimization. Engage with organizations that support families of LGB youth, such as Parents and Friends of Lesbians and Gays (PFLAG). If it is difficult to accept your child's LGB identity, consider seeking support from an organization such as the Family Acceptance Project (www.familyproject.sfsu.edu).

Conclusion and future directions

Contemporary research underscores the importance of understanding the diverse experiences of LGB youth. Family relationships, peer victimization, and mental health concerns are risk factors that are particularly salient for this population. Fostering safe and supportive environments for LGB youth, both in school and at home, is essential to decreasing suicidal ideation and behavior. The development of Gay-Straight Alliances, implementation of LGB-inclusive school criteria, and facilitation of parental openness to sexual minority identities can minimize risk and bolster protective factors. LGB suicide prevention should target families, peers, and schools, and should incorporate health professionals in prevention efforts.

More research is needed to identify rates of completed suicide among LGB youth, a development that will aid in the promotion of specific protective factors and prevention efforts for this population (McDaniel *et al.*, 2001). Future research, particularly large-scale epidemiological studies, would benefit from the inclusion of diverse sexual orientation and gender identity variables (SPRC, 2008). Incorporating questions related to discrimination, peer victimization, and mental health problems can also improve understanding of the factors associated with suicidality among LGB youth. The recommendations and suggestions for future research included in this chapter aim to reduce mental health disparities between LGB and heterosexual youth. Importantly, such recommendations intend to promote the health, safety, and validation of LGB youth as valuable, emboldened members of our communities.

References

Almeida, J., Johnson, R. M., Corliss, H. L., Molnar, B. E., and Azrael, D. (2009). Emotional distress among LGBT youth: The influence of perceived discrimination based on sexual orientation. *Journal of Youth and Adolescence*, 38(7), 1001–1014.

American Psychological Association (2012). Guidelines for psychological practice with lesbian, gay, and bisexual clients. *American Psychologist*, 67(1), 10–42.

Balsam, K. F., Rothblum, E. D., and Beauchaine, T. P. (2005). Victimization over the life span: A comparison of lesbian, gay, bisexual, and heterosexual siblings. *Journal of Consulting and Clinical Psychology*, 73(3), 477–487.

Birkett, M., Espelage, D. L., and Koenig, B. (2009). LGB and questioning students in schools: The moderating effects of homophobic bullying and school climate on negative outcomes. *Journal of Youth and Adolescence*, 38(7), 989–1000.

Bronfenbrenner, U. (1979). *The Ecology of Human Development.* Cambridge, MA: Harvard University Press.

Cochran, S. D. and Mays, V. M. (2007). Physical health complaints among lesbians, gay men, and bisexual and homosexually experienced heterosexual individuals: Results from the California Quality of Life Survey. *American Journal of Public Health*, 97(11), 2048–2055.

Cochran, S. D. and Mays, V. M. (2013). Sexual orientation and mental health. In J. C. Patterson and A. R. D'Augelli (Eds), *Handbook of Sexual Orientation and Mental Health* (pp. 204–222). New York: Oxford University Press.

Copeland A. (1993). Suicide among AIDS patients. *Medicine, Science and the Law*, 33(1), 21–28.

Corliss, H., Cochran, S. D., and Mays, V. M. (2001). Experiences of parental maltreatment during childhood in a United States population-based survey of adults: Does sexual orientation make a difference? *Child Abuse and Neglect*, 26(11), 1165–1178.

D'Augelli, A. R., Pilkington, N. W., and Hershberger, S. L. (2002). Incidence and mental health impact of sexual orientation victimization of lesbian, gay, and bisexual youths in high school. *School Psychology Quarterly*, 17(2), 148–167.

Friedman, M. S., Koeske, G. F., Silvestre, A. J., Korr, W. S., and Sites, E. W. (2006). The impact of gender-role nonconforming behavior, bullying, and social support on suicidality among gay male youth. *Journal of Adolescent Health*, 38(5), 621–623.

Goldblum, P., Testa, R. J., Pflum, S., Hendricks, M. L., Bradford, J., and Bongar, B. (2012). The relationship between gender-based victimization and suicide attempts in transgender people. *Professional Psychology: Research and Practice*, 43(5), 468–475.

Goodenow, C., Szalacha, L., and Westheimer, K. (2006). School support groups, other school factors, and the safety of sexual minority adolescents. *Psychology in the Schools*, 43(5), 573–589.

Haas, A. P., Eliason, M., Mays, V. M., Mathy, R. M., Cochran, S. D., D'Augelli, A. R., *et al.* (2010). Suicide and suicide risk in lesbian, gay, bisexual, and transgender populations: Review and recommendations. *Journal of Homosexuality*, 58(1), 10–51.

Hatzenbuehler, M. L. (2009). How does stigma 'get under the skin?': A psychological mediation framework. *Psychological Bulletin*, 135(5), 707–730.

Hatzenbuehler, M. L., Hilt, L. M., and Nolen-Hoeksema, S. (2010). Gender, sexual orientation, and vulnerability to depression. In J. C. Chrisler and D. R. McCreary (Eds), *Handbook of Gender Research in Psychology* (pp. 133–151). New York: Springer.

Herek, G. M. (1989). Hate crimes against lesbians and gay men: Issues for research and social policy. *American Psychologist*, 44(6), 948–955.

Herek, G. M. (2009). Hate crimes and stigma-related experiences among sexual minority adults in the United States: Prevalence estimates from a national probability sample. *Journal of Interpersonal Violence*, 24(1), 54–74.

Hershberger, S. L. and D'Augelli, A. R. (1995). The impact of victimization on the mental health and suicidality of lesbian, gay, and bisexual youths. *Developmental Psychology*, 31(1), 65–74.

Jiang, Y., Perry, D. K., and Hesser, J. E. (2010). Adolescent suicide and health risk behaviors: Rhode Island's 2007 Youth Risk Behavior Survey. *American Journal of Preventive Medicine*, 38(5), 551–555.

Joiner, T. (2010). *Myths about Suicide*. Boston, MA: Harvard University.

King, M., Semlyen, J., Tai, S. S., Killaspy, H., Osborn, D., Popelyuk, D., and Nazareth, I. (2008). A systematic review of mental disorder, suicide, and deliberate self harm in lesbian, gay and bisexual people. *BMC Psychiatry*, 8(70), 1–33.

Kosciw, J. G., Greytak, E. A., Bartkiewicz, M. J., Boesen, M. J., and Palmer, N. A. (2012). *The 2011 National School Climate Survey: The Experiences of Lesbian, Gay, Bisexual and Transgender Youth in Our Nation's Schools*. New York: GLSEN.

Link, B. G., Struening, E. L., Rahav, M., Phelan, J. C., and Nuttbrock, L. (1997). On stigma and its consequences: Evidence from a longitudinal study of men with dual diagnosis of mental illness and substance abuse. *Journal of Health and Social Behavior*, 38(2), 177–190.

Liu, R. T. and Mustanski, B. (2012). Suicidal ideation and self-harm in lesbian, gay, bisexual, and transgender youth. *American Journal of Preventive Medicine*, 42(3), 221–228.

Massachusetts Department of Education (2002). *2001 Massachusetts Youth Risk Behavior Survey Results*. Retrieved from www.lgbtdata.com/uploads/1/0/8/8/10884149/ds007_yrbs_ma_report_2001.pdf.

Mays, V. M. and Cochran, S. D. (2001). Mental health correlates of perceived discrimination among lesbian, gay, and bisexual adults in the United States. *American Journal of Public Health*, 91(11), 1869–1876.

McDaniel, J. S., Purcell, D., and D'Augelli, A. R. (2001). The relationship between sexual orientation and risk for suicide: Research findings and future directions for research and prevention. *Suicide and Life-Threatening Behavior*, 31(1), 84–105.

Meyer, I. H. (2003). Prejudice, social stress, and mental health in lesbian, gay, and bisexual populations: Conceptual issues and research evidence. *Psychological Bulletin*, 129(5), 674–697.

Meyer, I. H., Ouellette, S. C., Haile, R., and McFarlane, T. A. (2011). 'We'd Be Free': Narratives of life without homophobia, racism, or sexism. *Sexuality Research and Social Policy*, 8(3), 204–214.

Mustanski, B. S., Garofalo, R., and Emerson, E. M. (2010). Mental health disorders, psychological distress, and suicidality in a diverse sample of lesbian, gay, bisexual, and transgender youths. *American Journal of Public Health*, 100(12), 2426–2432.

Nadal, K. L. (2008). Preventing racial, ethnic, gender, sexual minority, disability, and religious microaggressions: Recommendations for promoting positive mental health. *Prevention in Counseling Psychology: Theory, Research, Practice, and Training*, 2(1), 22–27.

Pachankis, J. E. (2008). The psychological implications of concealing a stigma: A cognitive-affective-behavioral model. *Psychological Bulletin*, 133(2), 328–345.

Pilkington, N. W. and D'Augelli, A. R. (1995). Victimization of lesbian, gay, and bisexual youth in community settings. *Journal of Community Psychology*, 23(1), 34–56.

Plöderl, M., and Fartacek, R. (2005). Suicidality and associated risk factors among lesbian, gay, and bisexual compared to heterosexual Austrian adults. *Suicide and Life-Threatening Behavior*, 35(6), 661–670.

Plöderl, M., Wagenmakers, E. J., Tremblay, P., Ramsay, R., Kralovec, K., Fartacek, C., and Fartacek, R. (2013). Suicide risk and sexual orientation: A critical review. *Archives of Sexual Behavior*, 42(5), 715–727.

Poteat, V. P., Aragon, S. R., Espelage, D. L., and Koenig, B. W. (2009). Psychosocial concerns of sexual minority youth: Complexity and caution in group differences. *Journal of Consulting and Clinical Psychology*, 77(1), 196–201.

Poteat, V. P., Mereish, E. H., DiGiovanni, C. D., and Koenig, B. W. (2011). The effects of general and homophobic victimization on adolescents' psychosocial and educational concerns: The importance of intersecting identities and parent support. *Journal of Counseling Psychology*, 58(4), 597–609.

Poteat, V. P., Sinclair, K. O., DiGiovanni, C. D., Koenig, B. W., and Russell, S. T. (2013). Gay-Straight Alliances are associated with student health: A multi-school comparison of LGBTQ and heterosexual youth. *Journal of Research on Adolescence*, 23(2), 319–330.

Remafedi, G., Farrow, J. A., and Deisher, R. W. (1991). Risk factors for attempted suicide in gay and bisexual youth. *Pediatrics*, 87(6), 869–875.

Rivers, I. (2011). *Homophobic Bullying; Research and Theoretical Perspectives.* New York: Oxford University Press.

Rivers, I., and Noret, N. (2008). Well-being among same-sex and opposite-sex attracted youth at school. *School Psychology Review*, 37(2), 174–187.

Russell, S. T. and Joyner, K. (2001). Adolescent sexual orientation and suicide risk: Evidence from a national study. *American Journal of Public Health*, 91(8), 1276–1281.

Russell, S. T., Sinclair, K. O., Poteat, V. P., and Koenig, B. W. (2012). Adolescent health and harassment based on discriminatory bias. *American Journal of Public Health*, 102(3), 493–495.

Russell, S. T., and Toomey, R. B. (2012). Men's sexual orientation and suicide: Evidence for U. S. adolescent-specific risk. *Social Science and Medicine*, 74(4), 523–529.

Ryan, C., Huebner, D., Diaz, R. M., and Sanchez, J. (2009). Family rejection as a predictor of negative health outcomes in White and Latino lesbian, gay, and bisexual young adults. *Pediatrics*, 123(1), 346–352.

Ryan, C., Russell, S. T., Huebner, D., Diaz, R., and Sanchez, J. (2010). Family acceptance in adolescence and the health of LGBT young adults. *Journal of Child and Adolescent Psychiatric Nursing*, 23(4), 205–213.

Saewyc, E. M. (2011). Research on adolescent sexual orientation: Development, health disparities, stigma, and resilience. *Journal of Research on Adolescence*, 21(1), 256–272.

Savin-Williams, R. C. and Ream, G. L. (2003). Suicide attempts among sexual-minority male youth. *Journal of Clinical Child and Adolescent Psychology*, 32(4), 509–522.

Sue, D. W., Capodilupo, C. M., Torino, G. C., Bucceri, J. M., Holder, A. M., Nadal, K. L., and Esquilin, M. E., (2007). Racial microaggressions in everyday life: Implications for counseling. *The American Psychologist*, 62(4), 271–286.

Suicide Prevention Resource Center [SPRC] (2008). *Suicide Risk and Prevention for Lesbian, Gay, Bisexual, and Transgender Youth*. Newton, MA: Education Development Center, Inc.

Surgeon General (2001). *National Strategy for Suicide Prevention: Goals and Objectives for Action*. Washington, DC: DHHS.

Weiss, J. (1994). The analyst's task. *Contemporary Psychoanalysis*, 30(2), 236–254.

10 Spatial and temporal distribution of suicidal behaviour with a special focus on Hungary

Understanding the variations

Zoltán Rihmer, Xenia Gonda and Peter Dome

Suicidal behaviour (suicidal ideations, attempts and completed suicides) is a major public health problem everywhere in the world, and its prediction and prevention are receiving increasing attention. About 1 million people commit completed suicide in the world every year and the global suicide rate is 14 suicides per 100,000 inhabitants: more specifically 18 suicides per 100,000 males and 11 suicides per 100,000 females (Levi *et al.*, 2003; WHO). Suicide attempts are more prevalent, approximately 3–5 per cent of the adult population have made at least one attempt during his/her lifetime. Attempts are three times more frequent among youths than among people above 30 years of age (Pompili *et al.*, 2008; Goldman-Mellor *et al.*, 2013) In spite of the fact that suicide rates of different countries and continents differ substantially, the rate of completed suicide, in general, is much higher among psychiatric patients, among males, among older people and among Caucasians and among those who have made at least one suicide attempt.

A history of untreated major psychiatric (particularly depressive and alcohol-related) disorders constitutes the most important risk factors for both completed and attempted suicide. However, several environmental, psycho-social and personality factors (given periods of the calendar year, adverse childhood events, psycho-social stressors, financial problems, unemployment, impulsivity, affective temperaments carrying a depressive component, etc.) and other forms of addictive behaviours than drinking (e.g. cigarette smoking) have been also found to be in a statistically significant positive relationship with suicide mortality (Isacsson, 2000; Rihmer *et al.*, 2002, 2007; Rihmer, 2007; Sher, 2006; Almasi *et al.*, 2009; Dome *et al.*, 2010b, 2011; Vázquez and Gonda, 2013). It follows from the above that suicide events are not expected to be homogeneously distributed either in space and in time or in different demographic, social and health-related subpopulations. This fact can lead to the identification of several clinically explorable suicide risk factors and the ability to plan effective preventive strategies.

Distribution of suicide in space and time – geographic and seasonal variations

In the last decade the highest annual suicide rates were reported from Eastern Europe (13–42 suicides per 100,000 persons), some countries (e.g. Japan and the Republic of Korea) of the Western Pacific Region and also from Sri Lanka (with rates higher than 20 suicides/100,000/year) followed by Western/ Nordic European countries (8–21 suicides per 100,000 persons) and North America and Australia/New Zealand (11–13 suicides per 100,000 persons). Latin America as well as 'Latin Europe' (Greece, Spain, Italy), Israel and Central Asian countries report annual suicide rates less than 10 (Wasserman, 2000; Levi *et al.*, 2003; Rihmer and Akiskal, 2006). Spatial differences in European suicide rates have been more or less stable over the last 200 years (Kandrychyn, 2004). It is worthy to note that – in general – immigrants have higher suicide rates than their hosts and also that the rates among immigrants tend to follow those of the country of origin, showing a significant positive correlation between the two rates (Ratkowska and De Leo, 2013; Bursztein Lipsicas *et al.*, 2012).

Reasons for these great differences between national/regional suicide rates have not been fully explained. Geographic (latitude, longitude, altitude), climatic, dietary, religious, socio-cultural and economic differences can be taken into account, but differences in the psychiatric morbidity, as well as the accuracy of the registration of suicide, the stigma associated with suicide possibly influencing reporting rates, the availability of lethal methods, and the availability of the social/health care systems should also be considered (Rihmer *et al.*, 1993, 2002; Lester, 1995; Preti, 2002; Tondo *et al.*, 2006; Voracek and Tran, 2007; Stuckler *et al.*, 2011). Kapusta *et al.* (2011) recently reported that different rates of autopsy between countries and longitudinal changes in the autopsy rate within the same country may also influence official suicide statistics (Kapusta *et al.*, 2011).

It has been repeatedly shown that suicide rates are higher in higher latitudes (with lower levels of illumination) both in the Northern and the Southern Hemispheres (Lester, 1970; Heerlein *et al.*, 2006). In addition, a significant relationship between suicide mortality and longitude has been also reported; suicide rate is significantly higher in the Western than in the Eastern regions of the United States (Lester, 1986; Haws *et al.*, 2009) and also higher in Eastern Europe compared to Western Europe (Wasserman, 2000; Levi *et al.*, 2003; Rihmer and Akiskal, 2006). However, analysing the data from 2584 US counties, recent studies showed that after controlling for the percentage of old people, the percentage of males, the percentage of white, median household income, and population density of each county, the higher-altitude counties had significantly higher suicide rates than the lower-altitude counties (Haws *et al.*, 2009; Brenner *et al.*, 2011). Similar findings have recently been reported from Austria (Helbich *et al.*, 2013). The positive relationship between altitude and suicide mortality can explain some geographic differences, like the Western-Eastern differences in the United States, as higher mountains are situated primarily in the Western part of that country. One group of authors speculated that decreased oxygen saturation at high altitude may exacerbate the bio-energetic dysfunction associated with affective illness and suicide (Haws *et al.*, 2009). However, the picture is much more complicated, because it has been also found that the lithium level in drinking water – that shows a significant negative correlation with the suicide rate in several countries (Blüml *et al.*, 2013; Sugawara *et al.*, 2013) – is significantly lower at higher altitudes (Helbich *et al.*, 2013). In addition, according to the results of a study of the US residents of higher and lower dwelling places, they differed from each other in several sociodemographic factors, proportion of handgun ownership, access to mental health services, etc., and these differences may be at least partially responsible for the differences in suicide rates of places situated on high vs. low altitudes (Betz *et al.*, 2011).

Moreover, dietary tryptophan intake – a precursor of serotonin – also shows a significant negative correlation with national suicide mortality (Voracek and Tran, 2007), and our most recent preliminary findings suggest a positive correlation between the level of arsenic in drinking water and the suicide rate in Hungary (Rihmer *et al.*, unpublished). Considering all the above it is evident that the suicide mortality of a given region is the result of the very complex interplay of several geographic/climatic/dietary, as well as other (psychiatric, economic and cultural) factors.

Suicide rates are high in large parts of Northern and Eastern Europe and some of the highest figures have been reported in Hungary (Levi *et al.*, 2003; Rihmer and Akiskal, 2006). In addition to psycho-social factors, several lines of evidence indicate genetic and biological contributions to the unexpectedly high Hungarian suicide rate (Voracek *et al.*, 2007a; Voracek and Tran, 2007). Within Europe the countries with the highest suicide rates constitute a contiguous J-shaped belt from Finland through the Baltic countries, Russia, Belarus and Ukraine to central Europe (Hungary, Slovenia, Austria) (Voracek *et al.*, 2007a). Genetic similarities observed between populations of these countries led to the Finno-Ugrian Suicide Hypothesis which states that high suicide rates of these countries are the consequence of a shared genetic susceptibility (Voracek *et al.*, 2007a). The genetic background of this phenomenon is very probable because other (e.g. cultural/ socio-political/economic) features of these countries are quite different. Consonant with the theory about the genetic background of the high suicide rate of Hungary, Hungarian immigrants in the United States of America have the highest suicide rates of all immigrant groups (Lester, 1995). In addition, the existence of an unfortunate genetic/cultural susceptibility of Hungarians to sui-cidal behaviour is further bolstered by the fact that suicide rates of those Romanian counties where the proportion of Hungarian people is high (e.g. Harghita, Covasna, Mures) were much higher than of those counties where the population percentages of Hungarians are low (Voracek *et al.*, 2007b). The possible causes of different national/regional suicide rates are listed in Table 10.1.

Between 1960 and 2000 in the vast majority of years the suicide rate of Hungary was the highest in the world. The reason for this very high suicide mor-tality of Hungary is not fully understood. One possibility is that the medical examiners in Hungary certify those deaths as suicide which would otherwise be

Table 10.1 Possible causes of different national/regional suicide rates (after Rihmer *et al.*, 2002)

- Geographic/climatic differences (sunlight, temperature, latitude, longitude, elevation, lithium in the drinking water)
- Socio-cultural differences (alcohol/drugs, religion, alimentation, living place, family structure, media)
- Economic differences (unemployment, availability/quality of social and healthcare, living standard)
- Differences in availability of lethal methods (domestic/car exhaust gas, guns, toxicity of medicines)
- Differences in psychiatric morbidity (depression, substance use disorders)
- Differences in the accuracy of the registration of suicide
- Political situation (war/civil war)

---

labelled as undetermined death or as death related to other causes. However, the highest suicide rate of Hungarian immigrants in the United States (Lester, 1995) and the similarly high suicide rate of ethnic Hungarians living in Romania (Voracek *et al.*, 2007b) contradict this possibility. Political or economic causes are also very unlikely, as between 1960 and 1990 the suicide rates of Poland, Bulgaria, Romania, and former Yugoslavia (countries with similar political and economic systems) were around one-third of the Hungarian figure and during the mentioned period, in the majority of the years, the suicide mortality of Denmark, Finland, Austria, Switzerland and Sweden (with much more advantageous political and economic situations) have been among the top ten in the world. As mentioned above, the most established risk factor(s) of suicide are different forms of (untreated) major affective disorders. Although direct comparison of national epidemiological data on the prevalence of affective disorders is not possible due to some methodological issues (e.g. different studies have frequently used different diagnostic instruments), it can be said that the lifetime prevalence of 'any' bipolar disorder, which carries the highest risk of suicide (Rihmer *et al.*, 1990b; Szadoczky *et al.*, 2000; Rihmer, 2005), is unusually high in Hungary (5.1 per cent) (Pini *et al.*, 2005; Szadoczky *et al.*, 1998). Albeit the lifetime prevalence of major depressive disorder according to DSM-IV criteria in the Hungarian population (15.1 per cent) is similar to corresponding data from other European countries and the USA, a recent study – assessing depressive symptoms using CES-D in the general population of 23 European countries – reported the highest mean scores in Hungary among all the investigated countries (Hasin *et al.*, 2005; Van Velde *et al.*, 2010). In summary, these results raise the possibility that the high prevalence of affective (especially bipolar) disorders (and possibly also the threshold and sub-threshold manifestations of bipolarity and bipolar spectrum disorders) in the Hungarian population may be one of the most important contributors to the markedly high suicide rate of Hungary.

Several epidemiological studies have suggested that the numerical distribution of suicide cases is uneven during the calendar year (Christodoulou *et al.*, 2012). According to the highly replicated results there is a peak in the number of suicide cases in the spring and early summer (and – in some studies – a smaller peak in autumn for females), and a trough in the winter. In general, violent suicide cases (typical for males) are mainly responsible for the seasonal inequality of suicide rates and the seasonality of suicides is more pronounced at higher latitudes and in rural areas (Heerlein *et al.*, 2006; Christodoulou *et al.*, 2012). Studies show that this is the typical seasonal incidence of suicide mortality and is mainly the consequence of the seasonal incidence of depression-related suicides (Reutfors *et al.*, 2009; Postolache *et al.*, 2010). The peak of suicide mortality relates to the rapid increase of environmental light in spring and the number of suicides, particularly violent suicides increase parallel to the duration of daily sunshine (Rocchi *et al.*, 2007). The seasonal variation of suicide also corresponds well to the annual fluctuation of some indices of the central serotonergic metabolism, including brain serotonin transporter binding capacity, indicating significantly lower brain serotonergic activity in spring and summer (Praschak-Rieder *et al.*, 2008). Other links between light exposure and elements of the serotonergic system (e.g. 5-HT$_{1A}$ receptor) were revealed recently (Spindelegger *et al.*, 2012).

The majority of longitudinal investigations have provided some evidence that seasonality in suicidal behaviour has decreased in several countries in the recent decades (Voracek *et al.*, 2004; Mergl *et al.*, 2010; Sebestyen *et al.*, 2010), but some studies from other countries have found either increasing or unchanging trends in suicide seasonality (Christodoulou *et al.*, 2012). As the seasonality of suicide is mostly the reflection of the seasonality of depression-related suicides, some studies suggest that the decreasing seasonality of suicide mortality could be a good marker of the lowering rate of depression-related suicide cases in the population, particularly among males (Rihmer *et al.*, 1998; Mergl *et al.*, 2010; Sebestyen *et al.*, 2010).

Although several investigations aimed to disclose the diurnal pattern of suicidal behaviour, they have been unable to demonstrate a clear and universal pattern as yet (Zakharov *et al.*, 2013; Erazo *et al.*, 2004; Preti and Miotto, 2001; Doganay *et al.*, 2003).

The relatively few studies that have investigated the association between 'season of birth' and the risks of suicidal and other violent behaviours provided somewhat inconclusive results (Dome *et al.*, 2010a).

Geographic and temporal variation of suicide in Hungary

Regional variation and urban–rural differences

Similarly to some other countries, marked regional differences in suicide rates are present in Hungary: the suicide rates are higher in the south-eastern than in the north-western parts of the country (Neeleman *et al.*, 1998; Rihmer *et al.*, 1990a; Zonda *et al.*, 2010; Rihmer *et al.*, 2013a). This pattern is quite stable in time (the first mention of this phenomenon was in the year 1864) (Rihmer *et al.*, 1990a; Zonda *et al.*, 2010; Buda, 2001). Intriguingly, some results suggest that those subjects who were born in Hungarian areas with high-suicide rates have a higher chance of committing suicide after relocating to other regions from their place of birth (Moksony, 2003; Zonda *et al.*, 2010). Although some possible explanations of the spatial inequality of suicide rates have been proposed (e.g. the proportion of Protestants is higher in the south-eastern region; there are regional differences in the reported rates of depression; there are also differences in attitudes towards suicide and levels of social integration in the Durkheimian sense between populations with high vs. low suicide rates), but the exact explanations are still missing (Bálint, 2008; Rihmer *et al.*, 1990a; Zonda *et al.*, 2010). The only study that tried to explore the cause(s) of the marked regional differences in suicide mortality in Hungary based on exact data found a significant negative correlation between the suicide rates and the rates of treated depressions in 19 counties of Hungary; the higher the rate of recognized (treated) depression, the lower the suicide rate in the given county (Rihmer *et al.*, 1990a). However, this cannot be a full explanation, because the mentioned regional difference in suicide mortality of Hungary has been present from the beginning of the twentieth century, several decades before the introduction of antidepressants. However, looking at the severity of depressive symptoms, as measured by the Beck Depression Inventory, in the representative sample of Hungary, it was found that the highest mean total Beck scores were found in North-East Hungary, where the suicide rate was also among the highest (Kopp *et al.*, 1995; Székely and Purebl, 2007).

Although 'urban–rural' differences in suicide rates were negligible in the 1970s, a growing gap between urban and rural suicide rates is observable on the long run in Hungary. Accordingly, a clear trend evolved up to 2010: the greater the level of urbanicity, the lower the level of suicide rate (Rihmer *et al.*, 2013a). This phenomenon is in accordance with observations from several other countries (Kapusta *et al.*, 2008). In females there was an obvious association between domicile and suicide rate in all years examined (1970, 1980, 2010): suicide rates were higher for those females who lived in urban than for those who lived in rural regions (but to the end of the observation period the difference had almost entirely dissipated). A diametrically opposite trend may be observed among males. Very similar results were reported from nearby Austria regarding the same period (Kapusta *et al.*, 2008). Investigating the distribution of suicide mortality across the 175 micro-regions of Hungary between 2005 and 2011, age- and gender-standardized mortality ratios for suicide were significantly associated with the 'political integration' variable (measured by election participation rates) in a negative and with 'lack of religious integration' and 'disability pensionery' variables in a positive manner. These results may draw attention to the relevance and abiding validity of the classic Durkheimian suicide risk factors – such as lack of social integration, a correlate of some mental disorders – with regard to the spatial pattern of Hungarian suicides (Bálint *et al.*, 2013).

Seasonal/circaseptan fluctuation and 'season of birth' effects

Regarding the seasonality of suicide mortality, the Hungarian data are in line with the above-mentioned results from other countries (Rihmer *et al.*, 2013a).

The first Hungarian data set in which the spring peak for suicide was demonstrated derived from the 1930s (a seasonal pattern was similar for both sexes) (Lester and Moksony, 2007). Analyses using data from later years (1980–1999 in one study, 1970–2000 in another study and 1998–2006 in a third study) have also confirmed a peak in the number of suicides in spring–summer and a trough in autumn–winter (Lester and Moksony, 2003; Zonda *et al.*, 2005; Sebestyén *et al.*, 2010). Only one of these studies investigated genders separately, and this one did not find – the above-mentioned – autumn peak for females (Zonda *et al.*, 2005). All three studies reported that seasonal fluctuation of suicide was decreasing during the periods examined (Zonda *et al.*, 2005; Lester and Moksony, 2003; Sebestyén *et al.*, 2010). The one study which investigated seasonal fluctuation of suicide by age (Zonda *et al.*, 2005) found that the decrease pertains only to the young cohorts, while Sebestyén *et al.*, (2010) – investigating a different time period – described how the decrease in suicide seasonality is mainly the consequence of the significant decrease among males. Analysing the relationship between increasing antidepressant utilization and the national suicide rate of Hungary between 1998 and 2006, there was a significant correlation between the steadily increasing antidepressant prescription (113 per cent) and the continuous decline in total national suicide rate (23 per cent) as well as both in females and males (21 per cent and 23 per cent, respectively). Increasing antidepressant utilization was associated with significantly decreased seasonality of suicides only among males. The results suggest that decreasing seasonality of suicides could be a good marker of lowering rate of depression-related suicides in the population particularly among males (Sebestyén *et al.*, 2010).

Another highly confirmed and noteworthy result regarding temporal variations of suicide is that more individuals commit or attempt suicide in the first days of the week than at the weekend ('Blue Monday phenomenon') (Ohtsu *et al.*, 2009; Erazo *et al.*, 2004; Zonda *et al.*, 2008; Zakharov *et al.*, 2013). In contrast to seasonal variation that has strong biological correlates (Rocchi *et al.*, 2007; Praschak-Rieder *et al.*, 2008), this circaseptan fluctuation in completed suicides should have mainly psycho-social determinants. Similarly to results from other countries, the average number of suicides peaked on Monday for both sexes and was lowest on weekend days (for both sexes) in Hungary between 1970 and 2002 (Zonda *et al.*, 2008).

We investigated the effect of 'season of birth' on the risk of completed suicide in a comfortably large sample (78,779 suicide completers and 6,697,361 control individuals) in Hungary. We found that in the whole population investigated, those who were born in the highest risk period (July) have an approximately 13.8 per cent (95 per cent CI: 9.1 per cent–18.6 per cent) higher risk of dying by suicide than those who were born in the lowest risk period (December). Hungarian results on the elevated risk of completed suicide among those who were born in the spring-summer period of the year (compared with those who were born in the autumn-winter period of the year) agree with the majority of relevant previous data (Dome *et al.*, 2010a).

The role of psychiatric disorders in suicidal behaviour in Hungary

Although the traditionally high suicide rate of Hungary is the second highest in the European Community and fifth–sixth highest in Europe, the characteristics of suicidal behaviour (gender, age, and urban-rural distribution, method of suicide, marital status, seasonality, rate of psychiatric morbidity) are very similar to those reported from other countries (Rihmer *et al.*, 2013a). In Hungary – similar to the great majority of developed countries – males consistently show much higher suicide rates than females (Hawton and van Heeringen, 2009; WHO). However, the female suicide rate decreased more markedly between 1983 and 2010 (females: 61 per cent decline, males: 39 per cent decline) and while the male to female suicide ratio was 2.53 in 1983, the same figure was 3.93 in 2010 (Rihmer *et al.*, 2013a).

In a psychological autopsy study conducted more than 25 years ago in Budapest we found that 63 per cent of 200 consecutive suicide victims had current depressive disorders (almost half of them had bipolar depression), 9 per cent schizophrenia and 8 per cent alcoholism (Arato *et al.*, 1988; Rihmer *et al.*, 1990b). More than half of the depressed suicide victims had medical contact during their last depressive episode, but less than 20 per cent of them had received antidepressants and/or mood stabilizers (Rihmer *et al.*, 1990b). In a most recent case-control psychological autopsy study of 194 suicide victims and 194 controls in Budapest (Almasi *et al.*, 2009), we also found that 60 per cent of victims (and 11 per cent of controls) had current affective disorder, 26 per cent of victims (and 38 per cent of controls) had medical contact and 18 per cent of suicides (and 8 per cent of controls) had taken antidepressants in the last four weeks before the suicide or before the interview. This study also identified a number of societal factors that may be important determinants of the suicide risk in individuals. It has been found that a lifetime history of psychiatric illness, separated/divorced/widowed marital status, lower educational level, unemployment or long-term sick/disabled status, adverse life events within the previous three months, alcoholism, and current cigarette smoking was significantly more common among suicide victims, while being responsible for a child less than 18 years of age and practising a religion were significantly less frequent among the victims than among the controls (Almasi *et al.*, 2009).

Two independent studies on nonviolent suicide attempters (drug overdose or poisoning) in Budapest showed that 69–87 per cent of the attempters had a current major depressive episode (in many cases with comorbid anxiety and/or substance-use disorders), and the factors of unemployment, living alone and economically inactive status were overrepresented among them (Balázs *et al.*, 2003; Rihmer *et al.*, 2009). The strong relationship between suicide attempts and agitated/mixed depression has been also found both in population-based epidemiological (Szádóczky *et al.*, 2000) and clinical samples (Balázs *et al.*, 2006).

In spite of the fact that unemployment and alcohol consumption are well-accepted suicide risk factors (Stuckler *et al.*, 2011; Sher, 2006; Almasi *et al.*, 2009;

Razvodovsky, 2011) this two indices do not show a statistical correlation with suicide rate in Hungary between 1992 and 2010. However, a significant positive correlation has been found between tobacco consumption and national suicide rate between 1985 and 2008 (Dome *et al.*, 2011), which may reflect that – as demonstrated also by our studies in Hungary – patients with mood disorders smoke much more frequently than nonpsychiatric persons (Dome *et al.*, 2005) and smoking is a suicide risk factor (Rihmer *et al.*, 2007; Almasi *et al.*, 2009). Moreover, smokers are significantly more impulsive and drink more alcohol than nonsmokers (Mitchell, 2004; Ustacher *et al.*, 2009), and it is well demonstrated that impulsive-aggressive personality features and alcohol-related problems are powerful predictors of suicidal behaviour (Mann *et al.*, 1999; Swann *et al.*, 2005; Razvodovsky, 2011).

Looking at the problem of suicide from the side of a given individual, there is no doubt that suicidal behaviour is the result of the complex interplay between macro-social and personal suicide risk factors, the most powerful of them is the current episode of major depression (Isacsson, 2000; Rihmer *et al.*, 2002; Rihmer, 2007; Hawton and van Heeringen, 2009). In agreement with international findings, several studies demonstrated the important role of depression in suicidal behaviour in Hungary, as we will discuss below. This is particularly important from a practical point of view, as depression is one of most easily amendable suicide risk factor. Accordingly, investigating the regional distribution of recognized and treated depressions and suicide rates in 20 regions of Hungary in 1985, 1986 and 1987, the suicide rate showed a significant negative correlation with the rate of treated depressions in each of the three years: the higher the rate of treated depressions, the lower the suicide rate in the given region. It is also important to note that no such relationship was found regarding treated schizophrenic cases (Rihmer *et al.*, 1990a).

While the suicide rate of Hungary showed a steady (46 per cent) decline between 1983 and 2006, most of the post-communist countries exhibited decrease in their suicide mortality only from the mid-1990s, several years after the big political/economic changes started around 1990. On the other hand, however, the greatest decline in national suicide rate in the world (more than 65 per cent) between the mid-1980s and 2010 was detected in Denmark, that is not a typical post-communist country. This shows that political/economic change was not the main contributor to this favourable trend. However, between 1983 and 2006 the prescription of antidepressants increased by ten-fold. The negative correlation between antidepressant prescription and national suicide rate in Hungary between 1985 and 2011 is well demonstrated in several previously published papers showing that better recognition and more widespread treatment of depressive disorders, as reflected in the increasing antidepressant utilization, seem to be one of the main contributing factors in the markedly declined suicide rate of Hungary in the last three decades (Rihmer *et al.*, 2001; Rihmer, 2004; Berecz *et al.*, 2005; Kalmar *et al.*, 2008; Sebestyén *et al.*, 2010; Dome *et al.*, 2011). Similarly, a statistically significant correlation between increasing antidepressant utilization and decreasing national suicide rates have been reported recently from several countries (Ludwig and Marcotte, 2005; Ludwig *et al.*, 2009), including Sweden, Denmark, Finland, Norway (Bramness *et al.*, 2007; Isacsson, 2000; Søndergård *et al.*, 2006), the United States (Grunebaum *et al.*, 2004), Japan (Nakagawa *et al.*, 2007) and, as mentioned above, from Hungary (Rihmer *et al.*, 2001; Rihmer, 2004; Berecz *et al.*, 2005; Kalmar *et al.*, 2008; Sebestyén *et al.*, 2010, Dome *et al.*, 2011). Although ecological association does not mean causality, consider that:

1. There is a strong relationship between untreated major depression and suicide (Baldessarini *et al.*, 2006; Moller, 2006; Rihmer, 2007).
2. The appropriate acute and long-term treatment of patients with major depressive and bipolar disorders markedly reduces the suicide mortality even in this high-risk patient-population (Baldessarini *et al.*, 2006; Moller, 2006; Rihmer, 2007) and initially suicidal depressives become nonsuicidal with antidepressant treatment (Rihmer, 2007; Tondo *et al.*, 2008).
3. The annual prevalence of major depressive episode in the population is around 6–8 per cent (Rihmer and Angst, 2005; Szadoczky *et al.*, 1998).
4. Studies with more sophisticated methods than the simplest ecological one also supported the theory that antidepressant treatment is protective against suicide on the population level (Isacsson and Ahlner, 2013; Isacsson *et al.*, 2009).

It is logical to assume that more widespread treatment of depression is one of the main causes of declining suicide rates in countries where antidepressant utilization recently increased markedly. On the other hand, however, as national suicide rates are affected by many known (see above) and unknown factors (Gunnell *et al.*, 2003; Preti, 2002), estimating the exact impact of better treatment of depression on declining suicide rates is not easy.

The increase in antidepressant utilization, as reflected in antidepressant prescriptions, is only a proxy marker of greater access of patients to appropriate care, and the higher population density of doctors in general (Rihmer *et al.*, 1993; Tondo *et al.*, 2006) and psychiatrists and psychotherapists in particular (Rihmer, 2004; Tondo *et al.*, 2006; Kapusta *et al.*, 2009) is negatively associated with national and regional suicide rates. It is likely that many patients receiving antidepressants also receive lithium and other mood stabilizers as well as receiving more frequently supportive or specific psychotherapy for depression. Between 1982 and 2000 the number of psychiatrists in Hungary increased from 550 to 850, as well as the number of outpatient psychiatric departments (from 95 to 139), and the number of SOS telephone services (from 5 to 28) (Rihmer *et al.*, 2001). It should be also noted that between 1990 and 2010 the number of telephones (the best mean for rapid communication even in the case of suicidal crisis) increased by five-fold in Hungary and recently the number of ordinary and mobile phones has surpassed the number of individuals in the whole population. Although it is impossible to measure, it seems likely that the new democratic political system since 1990 (including freedom of religion and several newly founded civil organizations) also plays an important role in this favourable process. Therefore, the decrease of suicide rates could reflect a general improvement in mental health care rather than being caused by increasing antidepressant sales alone. The robust increase of antidepressant prescription in Hungary remains the only consistent correlate of a declining suicide rate in Hungary in the last 25–30 years (Rihmer *et al.*, 2001; Rihmer, 2004; Kalmár *et al.*, 2008; Sebestyen *et al.*, 2010; Dome *et al.*, 2011), indicating that better recognition and treatment of depression are one – but not the only – important contributor to this favourable change. On the other hand, however, recently we have suggested that the increasing unemployment rate after 2005 might be one of the contributing factors that accounted for the disappearance of a strong decreasing trend from the suicide rate in 2006 that stabilized around 24/100,000/year between 2006 and 2011 (Rihmer *et al.*, 2013b). The exact causes, the role of possible contributory factors as well as the relationship between them remain to be elucidated. Yet it seems increasingly obvious that patterns and trends in suicide rates in Hungary are determined by a delicate interplay between various genetic, psychiatric, cultural, economic, political, social and treatment-related factors specific to Hungary, determining not only baseline suicide rates but also the rises and falls.

References

Almasi, K., Belso, N., Kapur, N., Webb, R., Cooper, J., Hadley, S., *et al.* (2009). Risk factors for suicide in Hungary: A case-control study. *Bio Med Central Psychiatry*, 9(45), 1–9.

Arato, M., Demeter, E., Rihmer, Z., and Somogyi, E. (1988). Retrospective psychiatric assessment of 200 suicides in Budapest. *Acta Psychiatrica Scandinavica*, 77(4), 454–456.

Balázs, J., Benazzi, F., Rihmer, Z., Rihmer, A., Akiskal, K. K., and Akiskal, H. S. (2006). The close link between suicide attempts and mixed (bipolar) depression: implications for suicide prevention. *Journal of Affective Disorders*, 91(2–3), 133–138.

Balázs, J., Lecrubier, Y., Csiszer, N., Kosztak, J., and Bitter, I. (2003). Prevalence and comorbidity of affective disorders in persons making suicide attempts in Hungary: Importance of the first depressive episodes and of bipolar II diagnoses. *Journal of Affective Disorders*, 76(1–3), 113–119.

Baldessarini, R. J., Tondo, L., Davis, P., Pompili, M., Goodwin, F. K., and Hennen, J. (2006). Decreased risk of suicides and attempts during long-term lithium treatment: A meta-analytic review. *Bipolar Disorders*, 8(5Pt 2), 625–639.

Bálint, L. (2008). Suicides in Hungary: some regional characteristics. [Öngyilkosságok Magyarországon – néhány területi jellegzetesség]. *Spatial Statistics (Területi Statisztika)*, 11(5), 573–591.

Bálint, L., Dome, P., Daroczi, G., Gonda, X., and Rihmer, Z. (2014). Investigation of the marked and long-standing spatial inhomogeneity of the Hungarian suicide rate: A spatial regression approach. *Journal of Affective Disorders*, 155, 180–185.

Berecz, R., Cáceres, M., Szlivka, A., Dorado, P., Bartók, E., Peñas-Lledó, E., *et al.* (2005). Reduced completed suicide rate in Hungary from 1990 to 2001: Relation to suicide methods. *Journal of Affective Disorders*, 88(2), 235–238.

Betz, M. E., Valley, M. A., Lowenstein, S. R., Hedegaard, H., Thomas, D., Stallones, L., and Honigman, B. (2011). Elevated suicide rates at high altitude: Sociodemographic and health issues may be to blame. *Suicide and Life-Threatening Behavior*, 41(5), 562–573.

Blüml, V., Regier, M. D., Hlavin, G., Rockett, I. R. H., König, F., Vyssoki, B., *et al.* (2013). Lithium in the public water supply and suicide mortality in Texas. *Journal of Psychiatric Research*, 47(3), 407–411.

Bramness, J. G., Walby, F. A., and Tverdal, A. (2007). The sales of antidepressants and suicide rates in Norway and its counties 1980–2004. *Journal of Affective Disorders*, 102(1–3), 1–9.

Brenner, B., Cheng, D., Clark, D., and Camargo, C. A. (2011). Positive association between altitude and suicide in 2584 US counties. *High Altitude Medicine and Biology*, 12(1), 31–35.

Buda, B. (2001). Suicide: Medical and sociological studies. [*Az öngyilkosság. Orvosi és társadalomtudományi tanulmányok*]. 2nd Edn; Budapest, Animula Kiadó.

Bursztein, Lipsicas, C., Mäkinen, I. H., Apter, A., De-Leo, D., Kerkhof, A., Lönnqvist, J., *et al.* (2012). Attempted suicide among immigrants in European countries: An international perspective. *Social Psychiatry and Psychiatric Epidemiology*, 47(2), 241–251.

Christodoulou, C., Douzenis, A., Papadopoulos, F. C., Papadopoulou, A., Bouras, G., Gournellis, R., and Lykouras, L. (2012). Suicide and seasonality. *Acta Psychiatrica Scandinavica*, 125(2), 127–146.

Doganay, Z., Sunter, A. T., Guz, H., Ozkan, A., Altintop, L., Kati, C., *et al.* (2003). Climatic and diurnal variation in suicide attempts in the ED. *The American Journal of Emergency Medicine*, 21(4), 271–275.

Dome, P., Kapitány, B., Ignits, G., Porkoláb, L., and Rihmer, Z. (2011). Tobacco consumption and antidepressant use are associated with the rate of completed suicide in Hungary: An ecological study. *Journal of Psychiatric Research*, 45(4), 488–494.

Dome, P., Kapitány, B., Ignits, G., and Rihmer, Z. (2010a). Season of birth is significantly associated with the risk of completed suicide. *Biological Psychiatry*, 68(2), 148–155.

Dome, P., Lazary, J., Kalapos, M. P., and Rihmer, Z. (2010b). Smoking, nicotine and neuropsychiatric disorders. *Neuroscience and Biobehavioral Reviews*, 34(3), 295–342.

Dome, P., Rihmer, Z., Gonda, X., Pestality, P., Kovacs, G., Teleki, Z., and Mandl, P. (2005). Cigarette smoking and psychiatric disorders in Hungary. *International Journal of Psychiatry in Clinical Practice*, 9(2), 145–148.

Erazo, N., Baumert, J., and Ladwig, K. H. (2004). Sex-specific time patterns of suicidal acts on the German railway system. An analysis of 4003 cases. *Journal of Affective Disorders*, 83(1), 1–9.

Goldman-Mellor, S. J., Caspi, A., Harrington, H., Hogan, S., Nada-Raja, S., Poulton, R., and Moffitt, T. E. (2013). Suicide attempt in young people: A signal for long-term health care and social needs. *JAMA Psychiatry*, 71(2), 119–127. doi: 10.1001/jamapsychiatry.2013.2803.

Grunebaum, M. F., Ellis, S. P., Li, S., Oquendo, M. A., and Mann, J. J. (2004). Antidepressants and suicide risk in the United States, 1985–1999. *The Journal of Clinical Psychiatry*, 65(11), 1456–1462.

Gunnell, D., Middleton, N., Whitley, E., Dorling, D., and Frankel, S. (2003). Why are suicide rates rising in young men but falling in the elderly? A time-series analysis of trends in England and Wales, 1950–1998. *Social Science and Medicine*, 57(4), 595–611.

Hasin, D. S., Goodwin, R. D., Stinson, F. S., and Grant, B. F. (2005). Epidemiology of major depressive disorder: Results from the National Epidemiologic Survey on Alcoholism and Related Conditions. *Archives of General Psychiatry*, 62(10), 1097–1106.

Haws, C. A., Gray, D. D., Yurgelun-Todd, D., Moskos, M., Meyer, L. J., and Renshaw, P. F. (2009). The possible effect of altitude on regional variation in suicide rates. *Medical Hypotheses*, 73(4), 587–590.

Hawton, K., and van Heeringen, K. (2009). Suicide. *The Lancet*, 373(9672), 1372–1381.

Heerlein, A., Valeria, C., and Medina, B. (2006). Seasonal variation in suicidal deaths in Chile: Its relationship to latitude. *Psychopathology*, 39(2), 75–79.

Helbich, M., Blüml, V., Leitner, M., and Kapista, N. D. (2013). Does altitude moderate the impact of lithium on suicide? A spatial analysis of Austria. *Geospatial Health*, 7(2), 209–218.

Isacsson, G. (2000). Suicide prevention – a medical breakthrough? *Acta Psychiatrica Scandinavica*, 102(2), 113–117.

Isacsson, G. and Ahlner, J. (2013). Antidepressants and the risk of suicide in young persons – prescription trends and toxicological analyses. *Acta Psychiatrica Scandinavica*. doi: 10.1111/acps.12160.

Isacsson, G., Holmgren, A., Osby, U., and Ahlner, J. (2009). Decrease in suicide among the individuals treated with antidepressants: A controlled study of antidepressants in suicide, Sweden 1995–2005. *Acta Psychiatrica Scandinavica*, 120(1), 37–44.

Kalmar, S., Szanto, K., Rihmer, Z., Mazumdar, S., Harrison, K., and Mann, J. J. (2008). Antidepressant prescription and suicide rates: Effect of age and gender. *Suicide and Life-Threatening Behavior*, 38(4), 363–374.

Kandrychyn, S. (2004). Geographic variation in suicide rates: Relationships to social factors, migration, and ethnic history. *Archives of Suicide Research*, 8(4), 303–314.

Kapusta, N. D., Niederkrotenthaler, T., Etzersdorfer, E., Voracek, M., Dervic, K., Jandl-Jager, E., and Sonneck, G. (2009). Influence of psychotherapist density and antidepressant sales on suicide rates. *Acta Psychiatrica Scandinavica*, 119(3), 236–242.

Kapusta, N. D., Tran, U. S., Rockett, I. R., De Leo, D., Naylor, C. P., Niederkrotenthaler, T., *et al.* (2011). Declining autopsy rates and suicide misclassification: A cross-national analysis of 35 countries. *Archives of General Psychiatry*, 68(10), 1050–1057.

Kapusta, N. D., Zorman, A., Etzersdorfer, E., Ponocny-Seliger, E., Jandl-Jager, E., and Sonneck, G. (2008). Rural-urban differences in Austrian suicides. *Social Psychiatry and Psychiatric Epidemiology*, 43(4), 311–318.

Kopp, M., Skrabski, Á., and Szedmák, S. (1995). Socio-economic factors, severity of depressive symptomatology and sickness absence rate in the Hungarian population. *Journal of Psychosomatic Research*, 39(8), 1019–1029.

Lester, D. (1970). Completed suicide and latitude. *Psychological Reports*, 27(3), 818.

Lester, D. (1986). Faliure to find a U-shaped distribution of suicide rates of USA cities as a function of their longitude. *Psychological Reports*, 59(1), 310.

Lester, D. (1995). Explaining regional differences in suicide rates. *Social Science and Medicine*, 40(5), 719–721.

Lester, D., and Moksony, F. (2003). Seasonality of suicide in eastern Europe: A comment on 'Evidence for lack of change in seasonality of and suicide from Timis County, Romania'. *Perceptual and Motor Skills*, 96(2), 421–422.

Lester, D. and Moksony, F. (2007). The seasonality of suicide in Hungary in the 1930s. *Perceptual and Motor Skills*, 105(3 Pt 1), 714.

Levi, F., La Vecchia, C., Lucchini, F., Negri, E., Saxena, S., Maulik, P. K., and Saraceno, B. (2003). Trends in mortality from suicide, 1965–99. *Acta Psychiatrica Scandinavica*, 108(5), 341–349.

Ludwig, J. and Marcotte, D. E. (2005). Anti-depressants, suicide, and drug regulation. *Journal of Policy Analysis and Management*, 24(2), 249–272.

Ludwig, J., Marcotte, D. E., and Norberg, K. (2009). Anti-depressants and suicide. *Journal of Health Economics*, 28(3), 659–676.

Mann, J. J., Waternaux, C., Haas, G. L., and Malone, K. M. (1999). Toward a clinical model of suicidal behavior in psychiatric patients. *The American Journal of Psychiatry*, 156(2), 181–189.

Mergl, R., Havers, I., Althaus, D., Rihmer, Z., Schmidtke, A., Lehfeld, H., et al. (2010). Seasonality of suicide attempts: association with gender. *European Archives of Psychiatry and Clinical Neuroscience*, 260(5), 393–400.

Mitchell, S. H. (2004). Measuring impulsivity and modeling its association with cigarette smoking. *Behavioral and Cognitive Neuroscience Reviews*, 3(4), 261–275.

Moksony, F. (2003). Region of birth and suicide: does the regional subculture of self-destruction exist?. [Születési régió és öngyilkosság: Létezik-e az önpusztítás területi szubkultúrája.]. *Demográfia*, 46, 203–225.

Möller, H. J. (2006). Evidence for beneficial effects of antidepressants on suicidality in depressive patients: A systematic review. *European Archives of Psychiatry and Clinical Neuroscience*, 256(6), 329–343.

Nakagawa, A., Grunebaum, M. F., Ellis, S. P., Oquendo, M. A., Kashima, H., Gibbons, R. D., and Mann, J. J. (2007). Association of suicide and anti-depressant prescription rates in Japan, 1999–2003. *The Journal of Clinical Psychiatry*, 68(6), 908–916.

Neeleman, J. (1998). Regional suicide rates in the Netherlands: Does religion still play a role? *International Journal of Epidemiology*, 27(3), 466–472.

Ohtsu, T., Kokaze, A., Osaki, Y., Kaneita, Y., Shirasawa, T., Ito, T., et al. (2009). Blue Monday phenomenon among men: Suicide deaths in Japan. *Acta Medica Okayama*, 63(3), 231–236.

Ostacher, M. J., Lebeau, R. T., Perlis, R. H., Nierenberg, A. A., Lund, H. G., Moshier, S. J., et al. (2009). Cigarette smoking is associated with suicidality in bipolar disorder. *Bipolar Disorders*, 11(7), 766–771.

Pini, S., de Queiroz, V., Pagnin, D., Pezawas, L., Angst, J., Cassano, G. B., and Wittchen, H. U. (2005). Prevalence and burden of bipolar disorders in European countries. *European Neuropsychopharmacology*, 15(4), 425–434.

Pompili, M., Innamorati, M., Raja, M., Falcone, I., Ducci, G., Angeletti, G., et al. (2008). Suicide risk in depression and bipolar disorder: Do impulsiveness-aggressiveness and pharmacotherapy predict suicidal intent? *Neuropsychiatric Disease and Treatment*, 4(1), 247–255.

Postolache, T. T., Mortensen, P. B., Tonelli, L. H., Jiao, X., Frangakis, C., Soriano, J. J., and Qin, P. (2010). Seasonal spring peaks of suicide in victims with and without prior history of hospitalization for mood disorders. *Journal of Affective Disorders*, 121(1–2), 88–93.

Praschak-Rieder, N., Willeit, M., Wilson, A. A., Houle, S., and Meyer, J. H. (2008). Seasonal variation in human brain serotonin transporter binding. *Archives of General Psychiatry*, 65(9), 1072–1078.

Preti, A. (2002). Seasonal variation and meteotropism in suicide: Clinical relevance of findings and implications for research. *Acta Neuropsychiatrica*, 14(1), 17–28.

Preti, A. and Miotto, P. (2001). Diurnal variations in suicide by age and gender in Italy. *Journal of Affective Disorders*, 65(3), 253–261.

Ratkowska, K. A., and De Leo, D. (2013). Suicide in immigrants: An overview. *Open Journal of Medical Psychology*, 2, 124–133.

Razvodovsky, Y. E. (2011). Alcohol consumption and suicide in Belarus, 1980–2005. *Suicidology Online*, 2, 1–7.

Reutfors, J., Osby, U., Ekbom, A., Nordström, P., Jokinen, J., and Papadopoulos, F. C. (2009). Seasonality of suicide in Sweden: Relationship with psychiatric disorder. *Journal of Affective Disorders*, 119(1–3), 59–65.

Rihmer, Z. (2004). Decreasing national suicide rates – fact or fiction? *The World Journal of Biological Psychiatry*, 5(1), 55–56.

Rihmer, Z. (2005). Prediction and prevention of suicide in bipolar disorders. *Clinical Neuropsychiatry*, 2(1), 48–54.

Rihmer, Z. (2007). Suicide risk in mood disorders. *Current Opinion in Psychiatry*, 20(1), 17–22.

Rihmer, Z., and Akiskal, H. (2006). Do antidepressants t(h)reat(en) depressives? Toward a clinically judicious formulation of the antidepressant-suicidality FDA advisory in light of declining national suicide statistics from many countries. *Journal of Affective Disorders*, 94(1–3), 3–13.

Rihmer, Z., and Angst, J. (2005). Mood disorders: Epidemiology. In B. J. Sadock and V. A. Sadock (Eds), *Kaplan and Sadock's Comprehensive Textbook of Psychiatry*, 8th Edn (pp. 1575–1581). Philadelphia, PA: Lippincott Williams and Wilkins.

Rihmer, Z., Barsi, J., Arató, M., and Demeter, E. (1990b). Suicide in subtypes of primary major depression. *Journal of Affective Disorders*, 18(3), 221–225.

Rihmer, Z., Barsi, J., Veg, K., and Katona, C. L. (1990a). Suicide rates in Hungary correlate negatively with reported rates of depression. *Journal of Affective Disorders*, 20(2), 87–91.

Rihmer, Z., Belso, N., and Kalmár, S. (2001). Antidepressants and suicide prevention in Hungary. *Acta Psychiatrica Scandinavica*, 103(3), 238–239.

Rihmer, Z., Belso, N., and Kiss, K. (2002). Strategies for suicide prevention. *Current Opinion in Psychiatry*, 15, 83–87.

Rihmer, Z., Dome, P., Gonda, X., Kiss, H. G., Kovács, D., Seregi, K., and Teleki, Zs. (2007). Cigarette smoking and suicide attempts in psychiatric outpatients in Hungary. *Neuropsychopharmacologia Hungarica*, 9(2), 63–67.

Rihmer, Z., Gonda, X., Kapitany, B., and Dome, P. (2013a). Suicide in Hungary-epidemiological and clinical perspectives. *Annals of General Psychiatry*, 12(1), 1–13.

Rihmer, Z., Kapitany, B., Gonda, X., and Dome, P. (2013b). Suicide, recession, and unemployment. *The Lancet*, 381(9868), 722–723.

Rihmer, A., Rozsa, S., Rihmer, Z., Gonda, X., Akiskal, K. K., and Akiskal, H. S. (2009). Affective temperaments, as measured by TEMPS-A, among non-violent suicide attempters. *Journal of Affective Disorders*, 116(1–2), 18–22.

Rihmer, Z., Rutz, W., and Barsi, J. (1993). Suicide rate, prevalence of diagnosed depression and prevalence of working physicians in Hungary. *Acta Psychiatrica Scandinavica*, 88(6), 391–394.

Rihmer, Z., Rutz, W., Pihlgren, H., and Pestality, P. (1998). Decreasing tendency of seasonality in suicide may indicate lowering rate of depressive suicides in the population. *Psychiatry Research*, 81(2), 233–240.

Rocchi, M. B., Sisti, D., Cascio, M. T., and Preti, A. (2007). Seasonality and suicide in Italy: Amplitude is positively related to suicide rates. *Journal of Affective Disorders*, 100(1–3), 129–136.

Sebestyén, B., Rihmer, Z., Balint, L., Szokontor, N., Gonda, X., Gyarmati, B., et al. (2010). Gender differences in antidepressant use-related seasonality change in suicide mortality in Hungary, 1998–2006. *The World Journal of Biological Psychiatry*, 11(3), 579–585.

Sher, L. (2006). Alcoholism and suicidal behavior: A clinical overview. *Acta Psychiatrica Scandinavica*, 113(1), 13–22.

Søndergård, L., Kvist, K., Lopez, A. G., Andersen, P. K., and Kessing, L. V. (2006). Temporal changes in suicide rates for persons treated and not treated with antidepressants in Denmark during 1995–1999. *Acta Psychiatrica Scandinavica*, 114(3), 168–176.

Spindelegger, C., Stein, P., Wadsak, W., Fink, M., Mitterhauser, M., Moser, U., et al. (2012). Light-dependent alteration of serotonin-1A receptor binding in cortical and subcortical limbic regions in the human brain. *The World Journal of Biological Psychiatry*, 13(6), 413–422.

Stuckler, D., Basu, S., Suhracke, M., Coutts, A., and McKee, M. (2011). Effects of the 2008 recession on health: A first look at European data. *The Lancet*, 378(9786), 124–125.

Sugawara, N., Yasui-Furukori, N., Ishii, N., Iwata, N., and Terao, T. (2013). Lithium in tap water and suicide mortality in Japan. *International Journal of Environmental Research and Public Health*, 10(11), 6044–6048.

Swann, A. C., Dougherty, D. M., Pazzaglia, P. J., Pham, M., Steinberg, J. L., and Moeller, F. G. (2005). Increased impulsivity associated with severity of suicide attempt history in patients with bipolar disorder. *The American Journal of Psychiatry*, 162(9), 1680–1687.

Szadoczky, E., Papp, Z., Vitrai, J., Rihmer, Z., and Furedi, J. (1998). The prevalence of major depressive and bipolar disorders in Hungary. Results from a national epidemiologic survey. *Journal of Affective Disorders*, 50(2–3), 153–162.

Szadoczky, E., Vitrai, J., Rihmer, Z., and Furedi, J. (2000). Suicide attempts in the Hungarian adult population: Their relation with DIS/DSM-III-R affective and anxiety disorders. *European Psychiatry*, 15(6), 343–347.

Szekely, A., and Purebl, Gy. (2007). A depresszió területi megoszlása Magyarországon 1995-ben és 2002-ben. In A. Csepe (Ed.), *Összefogás a depresszió ellen. Kézikönyv a segítő foglalkozásúak számára* (pp. 28–46). Budapest: Semmelweis Kiadó.

Tondo, L., Albert, M. J., and Baldessarini, R. J. (2006). Suicide rates in relation to health care access in the United States: An ecological study. *The Journal of Clinical Psychiatry*, 67(4), 517–523.

Tondo, L., Lepri, B., and Baldessarini, R. J. (2008). Suicidal status during antidepressant treatment in 789 Sardinian patients with major affective disorder. *Acta Psychiatrica Scandinavica*, 118(2), 106–115.

Van Velde, S., Bracke, P., and Levecque, K. (2010). Gender differences in depression in 23 European countries. Cross-national variation in the gender gap in depression. *Social Science and Medicine*, 71(2), 305–313.

Vázquez, G. H., and Gonda, X. (2013). Affective temperaments and mood disorders: A review of current knowledge. *Current Psychiatry Reviews*, 9(1), 21–32.

Voracek, M., Loibl, L. M., and Kandrychyn, S. (2007a). Testing the Finno-Ugrian suicide hypothesis: Replication and refinement with regional suicide data from Eastern Europe. *Perceptual and Motor Skills*, 104(3 Pt 1), 985–994.

Voracek, M., and Tran, U. S. (2007). Dietary tryptophan intake and suicide rate in industrialized nations. *Journal of Affective Disorders*, 98(3), 259–262.

Voracek, M., Vintilă, M., and Muranyi, D. (2007b). A further test of the Finno-Ugrian Suicide Hypothesis: Correspondence of county suicide rates in Romania and population proportion of ethnic Hungarians. *Perceptual and Motor Skills*, 105(3 Pt 2), 1209–1222.

Voracek, M., Yip, P. S., Fisher, M. L., and Zonda, T. (2004). Seasonality of suicide in Eastern Europe: A rejoinder to Lester and Moksony. *Perceptual and Motor Skills*, 99(1), 17–18.

Wasserman, D. (Ed.) (2000). *Suicide: An Unnecessary Death*. London: Martin Dunitz.

Zakharov, S., Navratil, T., and Pelclova, D. (2013). Suicide attempts by deliberate self-poisoning in children and adolescents. *Psychiatry Research*, 210(1), 302–307.

Zonda, T., Bozsonyi, K., and Veres, E. (2005). Seasonal fluctuation of suicide in Hungary between 1970–2000. *Archives of Suicide Research*, 9(1), 77–85.

Zonda, T., Bozsonyi, K., Veres, E., Lester, D., and Frank, M. (2008). The impact of holidays on suicide in Hungary. *Omega (Westport)*, 58(2), 153–162.

Zonda, T., Veres, E., and Juhasz, J. (2010). Suicide as the consequences of the regional social anomie. (Az öngyilkosság, mint a társadalmi anomia területi konzekvenciái). *A Falu*, 25, 57–69.

11 Suicide in the United States military

Tracy A. Clemans and Craig J. Bryan

Overview of suicide in United States military

Beginning in 2004, the suicide rate among active duty military personnel in the United States (US) Armed Forces doubled and became the second leading cause of death in the US military (Ramchand *et al.*, 2011). Prior to this time frame, the suicide rate of active duty military personnel was lower than the rates within the US general population, however, it is noteworthy that comparing these two populations can be challenging for a number of reasons. First, the demographic make-up of the military and general population varies considerably, with military personnel generally being younger, male, and Caucasian as compared to the general population (DOD, 2011). This difference in demographics introduces important risk factors such as gender, age, and race, which must be considered and adjusted for when making comparisons between these two populations. Additionally, the procedures utilized regarding how suicide-related data is reported between states within the US and the Department of Defense (DOD), and between states in the US and other geographic regions differ, resulting in statistics on suicidal behaviors that are not derived from standardized surveillance database or methods. For example, the differences in reporting methods is evident as military suicide statistics are generally reported monthly, whereas general population suicide statistics are often reported several years following the actual year being reflected (i.e., 2013 rates reported in 2015). All of these factors make contextualizing trends in US military suicide compared to the US general population a challenge with direct comparisons between US military and US civilian suicide rates generally not feasible.

Regardless of these limitations, it is well documented that the suicide rates between the US military and US general population have closed during the past decade. The suicide rate for the US general population typically is around 19 per 100,000 individuals; whereas the US military suicide rates is traditionally 10 per 100,000 individuals (Ramchand *et al.*, 2011) after adjusting for differences in demographics such as age, gender, and race. However, beginning in 2004 the US military suicide rate began to steadily rise and surpassed the adjusted general population rate by 2008. The increase in this suicide rate occurred within all branches of the US military, however, the Army and Marines experienced the most significant upsurge with the rate being 20 per 100,000 within the Army in 2011 (Department of Army, 2011). As the military suicide rate increased, the US general population suicide rate increased as well (Centers for Disease Control, 2013), although this growth was much smaller in magnitude.

Risk factors for suicide with United States military personnel

There are multiple risk factors and variables that have contributed to the rise in the US military suicide rate. Death by suicide is most likely to occur among Caucasian men using a firearm (DOD, 2011) with the largest proportion of active duty personnel dying by a self-inflicted gunshot wound (Anestis and Bryan, 2013). Other risk factors for suicidal thoughts and attempts among service members include a history of trauma, or being the victim of interpersonal violence (e.g., sexual assault or domestic battery) with multiple victimizations increasing this risk (Bryan McNaughton-Cassill, Osman, and Hernandez, 2013). Likewise, active duty personnel who have a history of childhood physical and sexual abuse and household dysfunction are an increased risk for later suicidal behavior (Brodsky and Stanley, 2008; Bruffaerts *et al.*, 2010; Dube *et al.*, 2001; Joiner *et al.*, 2007; Nock and Kessler, 2006) with this association being partially mediated by the occurrence of mental disorders among survivors of trauma (Dube *et al.*, 2001). A recent systematic review examining military sexual trauma (MST) and suicide (Monteith *et al.*, 2013) found two studies in which MST was significantly associated with an increased risk for suicidal behaviors (Kimerling *et al.*, 2007) and suicide attempts (Gradus *et al.*, 2013). As a result of exposure to trauma, service members can develop post-traumatic stress disorder (PTSD), severe depression, and guilt which are all associated with an increased risk for suicidal thoughts and behaviors (Bossarte *et al.*, 2012; Bryan, Clemans, Hernandez, and Rudd, 2013; Bryan, Morrow, Etienne, and Ray-Sannerud, 2013; Rudd *et al.*, 2011).

Risk factors for suicide attempts and death by suicide among military personnel also include relationship conflicts and interpersonal problems, legal or disciplinary issues, financial problems, and physical injury (DOD, 2011; Bryan and Rudd, 2012), along with non-suicidal self-injury being overrepresented among military personnel with suicidal ideation and suicide attempts (NSSI; Bryan, under review). It is not uncommon for active duty personnel to experience an increased number of stressors upon their return from deployment and when family problems or family conflict result from these reintegration issues, there is an increased risk for suicidal ideation within service members (Kline *et al.*, 2011). Approximately 25 percent of personnel who served in Operation Enduring Freedom (OEF) and Operation Iraqi Freedom (OIF) report psychological problems post-deployment which also increases the risk for suicide (Hoge *et al.*, 2004; Hoge *et al.*, 2006).

Similar to risk factors established within the civilian literature, nearly 25 percent of military personnel who died by suicide were intoxicated or had abused substances at the time of their death (Logan *et al.*, 2012). Sleep disturbances such as very short sleep duration and insomnia are associated with suicidal ideation and future suicide attempts (Luxton *et al.*, 2011; Ribeiro *et al.*, 2012) in military personnel. Cognitive risk factors for military personnel include a perception of being a burden on others (i.e., perceived burdensomeness) (Bryan, 2011; Bryan Clemans, and Hernandez, 2012; Bryan, Morrow, Anestis, and Joiner, 2010) or that no one cares about them (Bryan, 2011; Bryan, McNaughton-Cassill, and Osman, 2013) and hopelessness (Bryan, Ray-Sannerud, Morrow, and Etienne, 2013a).

In recent years, there has been increased attention on the occurrence of active duty personnel with traumatic brain injury (TBI) secondary to combat activities as a significant number of Army personnel who were deployed to Iraq and Afghanistan have experienced a TBI (Hoge *et al.*, 2008; Schneiderman *et al.*, 2008). Within the civilian literature, several studies established an increased risk of suicidal behavior among individuals with TBI (Simpson and Tate, 2002; Teasdale and Engberg, 2001), therefore TBI is thought to be an additional factor contributing to the rise in the suicide rate among active duty military personnel. A recent study by Bryan and Clemans (2013) found that an increased incidence of lifetime and recent suicidal thoughts or behaviors was associated with the number of TBIs, especially among service members with two or more lifetime TBIs. The association between number of TBIs and suicidality existed after controlling for other clinical symptoms (Bryan and Clemans, 2013). Additionally, TBI is associated with an increased risk for PTSD and depression (Hoge *et al.*, 2008; Kreutzer *et al.*, 2001; Schneiderman *et al.*, 2008) and consequently the neuropsychological sequel of TBI may serve as a factor increasing the risk for suicide among military personnel. These findings suggest that service members who have sustained a TBI are an important population to target with appropriate interventions that can reduce their suicide risk.

Combat exposure and United States military suicide

Studies examining the relationship between deployments, in particular, combat exposure, and suicide risk within military personnel have had inconsistent findings. Some studies have established that combat exposure is directly associated with an increased risk for suicidal thoughts and behaviors among military veterans (Fontana, Rosenheck, and Brett, 1992; Rudd, in press; Maguen *et al.*, 2012; Sareen *et al.*, 2007; Thoresen and Mehlum, 2008), despite this relationship being very small in magnitude. Other studies with active duty personnel suggest combat exposure/deployment is not predictive of suicide attempts or death by suicide (DOD, 2011). These studies have been unable to establish a direct relationship between combat exposure with suicidal thoughts and behaviors among active military personnel (Bryan *et al.*, 2013; Griffith and Vaitkus, 2013; Leardmann *et al.*, 2013). Of note, the strongest predictor of suicidal ideation and suicide attempt in the year post-deployment among US personnel is suicidal ideation and suicidal behaviors that occurred prior to the service member's deployment (Griffith and Vaitkus, 2013).

The majority of military personnel, specifically less than one in six individuals, reported thinking about combat on the same day in which they attempted suicide (Bryan and Rudd, 2012). Recent findings have also suggested that an association between suicidal thoughts and behaviors and combat exposure were moderated by the age of individual, with this relationship only occurring among older military veterans and personnel (Bryan Hernandez, Allison, and Clemans, 2013). These studies reflect the complexity of the relationship between combat exposure and suicide, therefore conceptualizing combat exposure as being a chronic predisposition for suicide risk, similar to other types of trauma, may be helpful. As such, combat exposure which can increase an individual's vulnerability to other risk factors like guilt (Bryan, Morrow, Etienne, and Ray-Sannerud, 2013) may serve as a distal or long-term risk factor for suicide instead of a proximal or short-term risk factor for suicide.

United States military culture and suicide

The distinct culture within the US military is one of the most important considerations when looking at how suicide among military personnel differs from the general population. As providers treat suicidal military personnel and veterans, culturally relevant issues to consider during the treatment process include mental toughness, collectivist orientation, self-reliance, self-sacrifice, and fearlessness of death (Bryan, Jennings, Jobes, and Bradley, 2012). In terms of mental toughness, the military culture values courage, strength, and resilience and perceived weakness is often avoided by military personnel even when they experience discomfort, distress, pain, or adversity. The military cultural norm is experiential avoidance and emotional suppression which are two coping strategies that, in actuality, are extremely adaptive for personnel who are in situations that are high-risk or extremely dangerous, like the combat zone (Bonanno, 2004). In the short term, emotional suppression and avoidance are effective; however long-term suppression can lead service members to experience emotional distress (Beck *et al.*, 2006; Shipherd and Beck, 1999) and suicidal thoughts and behaviors (Najmi *et al.*, 2007).

The military culture highly values group membership therefore placing the goals and needs of the group over the individual's needs and goals is reinforced and a normal part of the culture (McGurk *et al.*, 2006). Fortunately, high levels of group cohesion can be a buffer against emotional distress and can reduce the suicide risk of military personnel. This collectivist orientation within the military emphasizes the protection of the group's identity, reputation, and security which can, unfortunately, negatively impact service members who may be seeking help (e.g., mental health treatment) from individuals who are considered to be 'outside' of the group (Chang and Subramaniam, 2008). Providers and clinicians should be mindful of the value placed on military group cohesion and incorporate a system-based perspective as they conceptualize and formulate treatment for suicidal personnel.

The US military culture expects its personnel to competently perform duties and to navigate any obstacles or problems in order to successfully complete the mission at hand. This value of self-reliance within the military views service members who may be experiencing deficiencies in problem solving due to emotional distress to be 'substandard' and, unfortunately, asking for help from others further violates this expectation of self-reliance. If military personnel continue to experience difficulties with self-management secondary to emotional problems (e.g., suicidal service members), then the value of self-reliance can actually undermine the individual's sense of strength and elitism. Providers, therefore, will find it helpful to recognize that suicidal personnel can feel trapped between the desire to improve and the desire to 'fix things' independently. Thus, it may be beneficial for clinicians to frame the treatment process as a means for service members to achieve or recapture their self-reliance and autonomy.

Self-sacrifice and selflessness are two highly respected values within the military culture and are defined when service members sacrifice themselves for the greater good of others. This value means that military personnel will suffer injuries or even death in order to protect others. Therefore, providers can assist suicidal personnel by helping them to understand the distinction between the military value of 'giving' their life for the protection of others (i.e., self-sacrifice) versus 'taking' their own life (i.e., suicide).

The military culture also reinforces fearlessness about death, as service members are explicitly trained to overcome the fear of death. This process occurs via extensive conditioning (Charney, 2004) throughout the course of military training and leads to habituation to the fear of death, which becomes further solidified during combat. The fear of death is considered a protective factor against suicide (Linehan *et al.*, 1983; Osman *et al.*, 1996), thus when this fear is extinguished among military personnel, the risk for suicide of these service members increases. Clinicians would benefit from integrating this notion of fearlessness of death when conceptualizing the cases of military personnel with whom they are working. Of note, military personnel also have the increased ability to make a suicide attempt. in part, due to access to highly lethal weapons (e.g., guns). Therefore, providers can reduce suicide risk of personnel by routinely providing means restriction counseling, especially with service members who have access to or own firearms.

The culture of mental health within the US is very different from that of the US military culture. The US mental health culture is clinically oriented and psychological problems are typically conceptualized as deficiencies or from the perspective of being part of an individual's 'illness'. In contrast, the military culture emphasizes a strength-based perspective (Bryan and Morrow, 2011) and reinforces the values that were described earlier in the chapter (i.e., self-reliance, self-service). The differences in these cultures clash as the typical mental health care approach reinforces individuals being emotionally vulnerable (e.g., 'It's okay to let your guard down and talk about it') versus the military approach which emphasizes service members being strong and mentally tough. One of the contributors to the mental health stigma among military personnel is the disparity of the two cultures (Bryan and Morrow, 2011), as most anti-stigma efforts utilize an approach in which personnel are encouraged to adopt the cultural norms within the traditional mental health care system (e.g., 'It's okay to get help') and abandon the values inherent within the military culture. One way in which anti-stigma efforts can modify this traditional approach is to adopt a multicultural perspective in which mental health services conform to the cultural norms of the military instead of service members being asked to adapt to traditional mental health care norms.

Fluid Vulnerability Theory (FVT) of suicide and the suicidal mode

In addition to providers having a global, multicultural perspective on how mental health stigma and military culture can impact suicidal personnel, it is imperative providers have a theoretical foundation to assist in conceptualizing the suicide risk of service members. Fluid Vulnerability Theory (FVT; Rudd, 2006) is a cognitive theory that can aid in understanding the process of suicide risk over the short (acute) and long (chronic) term with military personnel. Within FVT is the concept of the *suicidal mode* which has four domains: (1) cognitive system or the suicidal belief system; (2) feelings or the affective system; (3) physiological system; and (4) the behavioral-motivational system. These four systems work together when a service member experiences an internal (e.g., thought) or external (e.g., loss of a relationship) precipitant or stressor. The outcome of the activation of these systems is the suicidal state or suicidal episode, in which military personnel can experience cognitions such as 'I am unlovable' or 'I am a burden to others', emotions like shame or guilt, physiological arousal (e.g., agitation, sleep disturbance), and/or associated death-related behaviors (non-suicidal self-injury, rehearsal behaviors) (Rudd, 2006).

FVT conceptualizes that a service member's vulnerability to suicide is variable, although it is still identifiable and can be quantified (Rudd, 2006). FVT has a fundamental assumption that suicidal episodes are time-limited (Litman, 1991; Rudd, 2006). Additionally, FVT hypothesizes that the baseline risk for suicide, or the threshold at which the suicidal mode is activated, varies among individuals. For example, some military personnel may have a threshold that is high in that their suicidal mode is never activated, whereas other service members may have a lower threshold in which an external stressor (e.g., loss of a relationship) can easily trigger the suicidal mode.

The baseline suicide risk level of military personnel is determined by static factors, including developmental and historical factors such as genetic vulnerabilities, previous suicide attempts, history of abuse, and impulsivity (Rudd, 2006). According to FVT, the baseline risk for service members with a history of multiple suicide attempts (e.g., two or more attempts) is higher and endures for a longer period of time (e.g., greater chronic risk) as compared to personnel who have had one or zero suicide attempts (Rudd, 2006; Rudd *et al.*, 1996; Clark and

Fawcett, 1992). Clinically, this increased risk for personnel with multiple suicide attempts is important for providers as they conceptualize the baseline risk level of personnel with whom they are providing care. Likewise, service members with a history of multiple suicide attempts have fewer available protective factors, which ultimately are those variables that reduce the likelihood of suicidal behaviors and death by suicide, such as family support, positive coping skills, problem solving skills, and other interpersonal resources (Rudd, 2006). Therefore, a focus within treatment on increasing a service member's protective factors (e.g., improving problem solving) is imperative in reducing their suicide risk.

Another assumption inherent in FVT is that once military personnel experience the resolution of an acute suicidal episode, they will always return to their baseline risk level (Rudd, 2006). FVT postulates that a service member's suicide risk is elevated by aggravating factors which are internal and/or external precipitant stressors. For example, aggravating factors may include impaired problem solving, cognitive rigidity, or poor emotion regulation with all aggravating factors falling into one of the four suicidal mode domains discussed earlier. When the suicidal mode is activated by one of these aggravating factors, all four of the domains (i.e., cognitive, affective, physiological, and behavioral) are involved via synchrony of action. Despite an increased risk for suicide during this time frame, this risk only occurs for limited periods of time (e.g., hours, days, weeks) as the human body is unable to maintain this type of arousal for indefinite periods of time. When a service member's physiological arousal level eventually decreases, even if only slightly, the service member will no longer be an imminent risk of suicide. This decrease in arousal level typically leads to more balanced thoughts (e.g., 'Maybe I can cope with this and do not need to kill myself') which, fortunately, reduces the service member's risk level.

Another assumption within FVT is the severity of the suicidal episode is dependent on the interaction between baseline suicide risk and the severity of aggravating factors (Rudd, 2006). For example, if a service member experiences a reemergence of anxiety symptoms (affective domain), it is the interpretation or meaning they make of the change in symptoms that is noteworthy (e.g., 'I have no future because I will never get better'). These maladaptive beliefs can activate the suicidal mode thus increasing the service member's suicide risk level. The final assumption within FVT is the acute risk of military personnel will begin to resolve when aggravating factors/stressors are effectively targeted during the crisis period. Therefore, the primary target within treatment should be focused on current symptoms (cognitive, physiological, and affective) and behaviors. In the following section, we will discuss how providers targeting a service member's aggravating factors within treatment can initiate this process.

Interventions to reduce suicide risk with United States military personnel

Despite the significant problem of suicide among US active duty military personnel and veterans, there is a dearth of studies that have evaluated specific interventions for treating suicidality within this population. Recently, brief-cognitive

behavioral therapy for suicidality (BCBT-S) was implemented as part of a randomized control trial with suicidal active duty Army personnel in Fort Carson,
Colorado. As a part of this trial, 152 personnel were randomized to either BCBT-S
or treatment as usual (TAU) and were followed up to 24 months. Preliminary
findings indicate the suicide attempt rate with personnel who received BCBT-S
versus TAU reduced by 50 percent at both 6 and 12 months (Rudd *et al.*, 2013).
Additionally, preliminary results indicate a significant reduction in self-reported
PTSD symptoms with personnel who received BCBT-S versus TAU, at both
6 months and 12 months (Rudd, 2013). Due to the success of BCBT-S, we want
to conclude this chapter by discussing the important components of this treatment which aided in a significant reduction in suicidal behavior of US service
members.

BCBT-S is a modification of a previously tested and empirically supported
approach to treating suicidality (Rudd *et al.*, 1996, 2000). The primary focus of
BCBT-S is the service member's suicidality regardless of their Axis I and/or Axis
II diagnoses, along with the treatment being focused on the suicidal mode
(i.e. cognitive, affective, physiological, and behavioral factors), including core
beliefs and automatic thoughts that increase a service member's suicide risk.
BCBT-S consists of 12 one-hour sessions and is organized into three separate and
sequential phases: emotion regulation, cognitive restructuring, and relapse
prevention. As the service member demonstrates a mastery of skills and concepts
from earlier phases, they then progress to each subsequent stage within the
treatment (Bryan *et al.*, 2012). During BCBT-S, selected interventions are
practiced in-session by personnel with instructions from the therapist and are also
assigned for between-session practice.

Phase I: Emotion regulation skills training

The first phase within BCBT-S has a primary goal of stabilizing and reducing the
service member's emotional distress through the teaching of basic emotion regulation skills. This goal is accomplished through several tasks – describing the
treatment, conducting a narrative review of the index suicidal episode, psychoeducation about the suicidal mode, developing a treatment plan and crisis
response plan (CRP), and teaching emotion regulation skills. During the narrative review of the index suicidal episode, the clinician asks the service member to
'tell the story' of their most recent suicidal episode or attempt with the purpose
of obtaining information about the circumstances surrounding the suicidal crisis.
Before the completion of the first session, the service member is asked to develop
a crisis response plan (CRP) which is a written list of steps they can take during
future emotional crises, in order to reduce the likelihood of engaging in suicidal
behaviors. The CRP is a problem-solving tool that outlines crisis management
steps they should take as soon as they are aware of 'warning signs' which indicate
they are in distress or crisis. Clinicians follow up with service members during
each subsequent session to inquire whether they utilized their CRP, how it was
used, any barriers to using the plan, and any needed modifications to increase the

likelihood they will continue using their plan. Additionally, providers can obtain permission to integrate family members into the service member's crisis management strategies and in limiting or removing their access to lethal methods (e.g., firearms) as a part of the CRP intervention.

During the remainder of the sessions in phase I, clinicians teach the service member emotion regulation skills (e.g., controlled breathing, mindfulness), provide psychoeducation (e.g., sleep optimization), and complete in-session exercises such as the reasons for living list and survival kit. As the service member gains mastery of emotion regulation skills in this first phase, typically emotional distress and suicidal ideation will begin to decrease in severity and subsequently treatment transitions into the second phase, which is focused on cognitively restructuring the suicidal belief system.

Phase II: Cognitive restructuring of the suicidal belief system

The primary goal of the second phase of BCBT-S is to undermine the components of the service member's suicidal belief system that are contributing to and sustaining long-term vulnerabilities for suicidal behavior. This is accomplished through written exercises and worksheets designed to teach service members the essential elements of critically evaluating and reappraising their automatic thoughts, assumptions, and core beliefs about themselves, others, and the world. The worksheets utilized during this phase include: (1) A-B-C worksheets that help service members understand the connection between their thoughts and feelings; (2) challenging questions worksheets which are used to assist in challenging automatic thoughts and core beliefs; and (3) patterns of problematic thinking worksheets that aid the service member in identifying problematic thinking or cognitive distortions. During this stage, service members are also asked to schedule events and activities designed to increase their sense of self-worth, meaning in life, and social connectedness (i.e., activity scheduling or behavioral activation). Likewise, providers work with personnel to create 'coping cards' which are 3×5 index cards that have a suicidal or maladaptive belief on one side of the card and a balanced, positive response to the maladaptive belief on the other side of the card.

In the second phase of treatment, it is common for service members to experience a change in their sense of identity (e.g., 'Maybe I'm not such a bad person after all, and I'm being too hard on myself'). These changes in self-perception indicate their skill mastery and often correspond with improvements in the service member's day-to-day functioning, which signals a readiness to transition to the third and final phase of treatment: relapse prevention.

Phase III: Relapse prevention

The primary goal of the third phase of BCBT-S is to ensure competence and skill mastery of the emotion regulation and cognitive restructuring skills taught during the first two stages of treatment. During this stage, the clinician 'tests' the service member's capacity to flexibly solve problems and effectively implement coping strategies while emotionally aroused. A relapse prevention task is completed with the service member during a purposely emotionally aroused state because, it is in such a state, that a service member's problem solving capacity declines and when they are most vulnerable to suicidal behavior. During the relapse prevention task, the provider asks the service member to recount the sequence of events that occurred during the index suicidal episode from session one. The service member is asked to rehearse the suicidal episode and to change the outcome of the index episode by imagining him or herself using a coping strategy or skill to resolve the crisis instead of engaging in suicidal behavior. This imaginal rehearsal of the index suicidal episode is repeated several times, with the requirement that the service member generate a different solution with every repetition of the task. To further enhance cognitive flexibility, the clinician increases the difficulty of the task with each rehearsal by introducing potential barriers as the service member imagines using self-management or problem-solving skills they identified earlier during treatment. Intentionally escalating the task's difficulty is an important way to teach personnel how to 'think on their feet' when confronted with unexpected challenges or barriers in real life.

After the service member has successfully completed the rehearsal task, the clinician and service member collaboratively generate hypothetical future scenarios that are most relevant to the service member's suicidal mode to further problem solve. The relapse prevention task is then repeated with personnel imagining themselves effectively resolving future crises. Once the service member successfully completes this additional relapse prevention exercise, BCBT-S can be discontinued with the clinician assessing whether additional treatment is necessary (e.g., trauma-focused treatment, marital therapy). Regardless of the ultimate disposition, personnel are informed about the procedures for re-initiating care in the future and how they can receive 'booster sessions' as needed.

Future directions for research in United States military suicide

Despite many challenges described in this chapter regarding the current state of suicide within the US military, civilian and military researchers have focused significant efforts in recent years on evaluating and improving the mental health care of US service members. Many of these research efforts have led to improved suicide prevention programs, increased behavioral health training of providers, and the implementation of a crisis hotline specific for military personnel and veterans. Work continues across several domains within the military including the evaluation of current suicide risk assessment measures, further exploration of suicide-specific psychological interventions, implementation of suicide-specific interventions, utilization of social media to identify at-risk personnel, and the adaptation of interventions across clinical settings (e.g., primary care versus mental health clinics). Although suicide prevention efforts within the US military are still ongoing, results to date have yielded promising findings that will further guide and refine future research.

References

Anestis, M. D. and Bryan, C. J. (2013). Means and capacity for suicidal behavior: A comparison of the ratio of suicide attempts and deaths by suicide in the US military and general population. *Journal of Affective Disorders*, 148(1), 42–47.

Beck, J. G., Gudmundsdottir, B., Palyo, S. A., Miller, L. M., and Grant, D. M. (2006). Rebound effects following deliberate thought suppression: Does PTSD make a difference? *Behavior Therapy*, 37(2), 170–180.

Bonanno, G. (2004). Loss, trauma, and human resilience: Have we underestimated the human capacity to thrive after extremely aversive events? *American Psychologist*, 59(1), 20–28.

Bossarte, R. M., Knox, K. L., Piegari, R., Altieri, J., Kemp, J., and Katz, I. R. (2012). Prevalence and characteristics of suicide ideation and attempts among active military and veteran participants in a national health survey. *American Journal of Public Health*, 102(S1), S38–S40.

Brodsky, B. and Stanley, B. (2008). Adverse childhood experiences and suicidal behavior. *Psychiatric Clinics of North America*, 31(2), 223–235.

Bruffaerts, R., Demyttenaer, K., Borges, G., Haro, J. M., Chiu, W. T., Hwang, I., *et al.* (2010). Childhood adversities as risk factors for onset and persistence of suicidal behaviour. *The British Journal of Psychiatry*, 197(1), 20–27.

Bryan, C. J. (2011). The clinical utility of a brief measure of perceived burdensomeness and thwarted belongingness for the detection of suicidal military personnel. *Journal of Clinical Psychology*, 67(10), 981–992.

Bryan, C. J. (2013). Non-suicidal self-injury in United States military personnel and veterans: Prevalence, socio-demographics, topography, and relationship with suicidal thoughts and behaviors. Unpublished manuscript submitted for review.

Bryan, C. J. and Clemans, T. A. (2013). Repetitive traumatic brain injury, psychological symptoms, and suicide risk in a clinical sample of deployed military personnel. *JAMA Psychiatry*, 70(7), 686–691.

Bryan, C. J., Clemans, T. A., and Hernandez, A. M. (2012). Perceived burdensomeness, fearlessness of death, and suicidality among deployed military personnel. *Personality and Individual Differences*, 52(3), 374–379.

Bryan, C. J., Clemans, T. A., Hernandez, A. M., and Rudd, M. D. (2013). Loss of consciousness, depression, posttraumatic stress disorder, and suicide risk among deployed military personnel with mild traumatic brain injury (MTBI). *Journal of Head Trauma Rehabilitation*, 28(1), 13–20.

Bryan, C. J., Gartner, A. M., Wertenberger, E., Delano, K., Wilkinson, E., Breitbach, J., *et al.* (2012). Defining treatment completion according to patient competency: A case example using Brief Cognitive Behavioral Therapy (BCBT) for suicidal patients. *Professional Psychology: Research and Practice*, 43(2), 130–136.

Bryan, C. J., Hernandez, A. M., Allison, S., and Clemans, T. (2013). Combat exposure and suicidality in two samples of military personnel. *Journal of Clinical Psychology*, 69(1), 64–77.

Bryan, C. J., Jennings, K. W., Jobes, D. A., and Bradley, J. C. (2012). Understanding and preventing military suicide. *Archives of Suicide Research*, 16(2), 95–110.

Bryan, C. J., McNaughton-Cassill, M., and Osman, A. (2013). Age and belongingness moderate the effects of combat exposure on suicidal ideation among active duty military personnel. *Journal of Affective Disorders*, 150(3), 1226–1229.

Bryan, C. J., McNaughton-Cassill, M., Osman, A., and Hernandez, A. M. (2013). The association of physical and sexual assault with suicide risk in nonclinical military and undergraduate samples. *Suicide and Life-Threatening Behavior*, 43(2), 223–234.

Bryan, C. J. and Morrow, C. E. (2011). Circumventing mental health stigma by embracing the warrior culture: feasibility and acceptability of the Defender's Edge Program. *Professional Psychology: Research and Practice*, 42(1), 16–23.

Bryan, C. J., Morrow, C. E., Anestis, M. D., and Joiner, T. E. (2010). A preliminary test of the interpersonal-psychological theory of suicidal behavior in a military sample. *Personality and Individual Differences*, 48(3), 347–350.

Bryan, C. J., Morrow, C. E., Etienne, N., and Ray-Sannerud, B. (2013). Guilt, shame, and suicidal ideation in a military outpatient clinical sample. *Depression and Anxiety*, 30(1), 55–60.

Bryan, C. J., Ray-Sannerud, B. N., Morrow, C. E., and Etienne, N. (2013a). Optimism reduces suicidal ideation and weakens the effect of hopelessness among military personnel. *Cognitive Therapy and Research*, 37(5), 996–1003.

Bryan, C. J. and Rudd, M. D. (2012). Life stressors, emotional distress, and trauma-related thoughts occurring within 24 h of suicide attempts among active duty US soldiers. *Journal of Psychiatric Research*, 46(7), 843–848.

Centers for Disease Control (2013). *Fatal Injury Reports, National and Regional, 1999–2010*. Atlanta, GA: Centers for Disease Control. Retrieved from http://webappa.cdc.gov/sasweb/ncipc/mortrate10_us.html

Chang, T., and Subramaniam, P. R. (2008). Asian and Pacific Islander American men's help-seeking: Understanding the role of cultural values and beliefs, gender roles, and racial stereotypes. *International Journal of Men's Health*, 7(2), 121–136.

Charney, D. S. (2004). Psychobiological mechanisms of resilience and vulnerability: Implications for successful adaptation to extreme stress. *Focus*, 2(3), 368–391.

Clark, D. C., and Fawcett, J. (1992). Review of empirical risk factors for evaluation of the suicidal patient. In. B. Bongar (Ed.), *Suicide: Guidelines for Assessment, Management, and Treatment* (pp. 16–48). New York: Oxford University Press.

DOD (Department of Defense) (2011). *DODSER: Department of Defense Suicide Event Report: Calendar Year 2010 Annual Report*. Washington, DC: Department of Defense.

Dube, S. R., Anda, R. F., Felitti, V. J., Chapman, D. P., Williamson D. F., Giles, W. H. (2001). Childhood abuse, household dysfunction, and the risk of attempted suicide throughout the life span. Findings from the adverse childhood experiences study. *Journal of American Medical Association*, 286(24), 3089–3096.

Fontana, A., Rosenheck, R., and Brett, E. (1992). War zone traumas and post-traumatic stress disorder symptomatology. *Journal of Nervous and Mental Disease*, 180(12), 748–755.

Gradus, J. L., Shiperd, J. C., Suvak, M. K., Giasson, H. L., and Miller, M. (2013). Suicide attempts and suicide among Marines: A decade of follow-up. *Suicide and Life-Threatening Behavior*, 43(1), 39–49.

Griffith, J. E. and Vaitkus, M. (2013). Perspectives on suicide in the Army National Guard. *Armed Forces and Society*, 39(4), 628–653.

Hoge, C. W., Auchterlonie, J. L., and Milliken, C. S. (2006). Mental health problems, use of mental health services, and attrition from military service after returning from deployment to Iraq or Afghanistan. *Journal of American Medical Association*, 295(9), 1023–1032.

Hoge, C. W, Castro, C. A., Messer, S. C., McGurk, D., Cotting, D. I., Koffman, R. L. (2004). Combat duty in Iraq and Afghanistan, mental health problems, and barriers to care. *New England Journal of Medicine*, 351(1), 13–22.

Hoge, C. W., McGurk, D., Thomas, J. L., Cox, A. L., Engel, C. C., and Castro, C. A. (2008). Mild traumatic brain injury in US soldiers returning from Iraq. *New England Journal of Medicine*, 358(5), 453–463.

Joiner, T. E., Sachs-Ericsson, N. J., Wingate, L. R., Brown, J. S., Anestis, M. D, and Selby, E. A. (2007). Childhood physical and sexual abuse and lifetime number of suicide attempts: A persistent and theoretically important relationship. *Behaviour Research and Therapy*, 45(3), 539–547.

Kimerling, R., Gima, K., Smith, M.W., Street, A., and Frayne, S. (2007). The Veterans Health Administration and military sexual trauma. *American Journal of Public Health*, 97(12), 2160–2166.

Kline, A., Ciccone, D.S., Falca-Dodson, M., Black, C.M., and Losonczy, M. (2011). Suicidal ideation among National Guard troops deployed to Iraq: The association with postdeployment readjustment problems. *Journal of Nervous and Mental Disease*, 199(12), 914–920.

Kreutzer, J. S., Seel, R. T., and Gourley, E. L. (2001). The prevalence and symptom rates of depression after traumatic brain injury: A comprehensive examination. *Brain Injury*, 15(7), 563–576.

LeardMann, C.A., Powell, T. M., Smith, T. C., Bell, M. R., Smith, B., Boyko, E. J., Hooper, T. I., *et al.* (2013). Risk factors associated with suicide in current and former US military personnel. *Journal of American Medical Association*, 310(5), 496–506.

Linehan, M. M., Goodstein, J. L., Nielsen, S. L., and Chiles, J. A. (1983). Reasons for staying alive when you are thinking of killing yourself: The Reasons for Living Inventory. *Journal of Consulting and Clinical Psychology*, 51(2), 276–286.

Litman, R. E. (1991). Predicting and preventing hospital and clinic studies. *Suicide and Life-Threatening Behavior*, 21(1), 56–73.

Logan, J., Skopp, N.A., Karch, D., Reger, M.A., and Gahm, G.A. (2012). Characteristics of suicides among US Army active duty personnel in 17 US states from 2005 to 2007. *American Journal of Public Health*, 102(S1), S40–S44.

Luxton, D. D., Greenburg, D., Ryan, J., Niven, A., Wheeler, G., and Mysliwiec, V. (2011). Prevalence and impact of short sleep duration in redeployed OIF Soldiers. *SLEEP*, 34(9), 1189–1195.

Maguen, S., Metzler, T. J., Bosch, J., Marmar, C. R., Knight, S. J., and Neylan, T. C. (2012). Killing in combat may be independently associated with suicidal ideation. *Depression and Anxiety*, 29(11), 918–923.

McGurk, D., Cotting, D., Britt, T., and Adler, A. (2006). Joining the ranks: The role of indoctrination in transforming civilians to service members. In T. W. Britt, A. B. Adler and C. A. Castro (Eds), *Military Life: The Psychology of Service in Peace and Combat Vol. 2, Operational Stress* (pp. 13–32). Westport, CT: Praeger Publishers.

Monteith, L., Matarazzo, B. B, Clemans, T. A., Kimerling, R., and Bahraini, N. H. (2013). Military sexual trauma and suicide: A systematic review. Manuscript submitted for publication.

Najmi, Wegner, D. M., and Nock, M. K. (2007). Thought suppression and self-injurious thoughts and behaviors. *Behaviour Research and Therapy*, 45(8), 1957–1965.

Nock, M. K. and Kessler, R. C. (2006). Prevalence of and risk factors for suicide attempts versus suicide gesture: Analysis of the National Comorbidity Survey. *Journal of Abnormal Psychology*, 115(3), 616–623.

Osman, A., Kopper, B. A., Barrios, F. X., Osman, J. R., Besett, T., and Linehan, M. M. (1996). The Brief Reasons for Living Inventory for Adolescents (BRFL-A). *Journal of Abnormal Child Psychology*, 24(4), 433–443.

Ramchand, R., Acosta, J., Burns, R.M., Jaycox, L.H., and Pernin, C. G. (2011). *The War Within: Preventing Suicide in the US Military*. Santa Monica, CA: The RAND Corporation.

Ribiero, J. D., Pease, J. L., Gutierrez, P. M., Silva, C., Bernert, R. A., Rudd, M. D., and Joiner, T. E. (2012). Sleep problems outperform depression and hopelessness as cross-sectional longitudinal predictors of suicidal ideation and behavior in young adults in the military. *Journal of Affective Disorders*, 136(3), 743–750.

Rudd, M. D. (2006). Fluid vulnerability theory: A cognitive approach to understanding the process of acute and chronic suicide risk. In T E. Ellis (Ed.), *Cognition and Suicide: Theory, Research, and Therapy* (Vol. 17). Washington, DC: American Psychological Association.

Rudd, M.D. (in press). Severity of combat exposure, psychological symptoms, social support, and suicide risk in OEF/OIF veterans. *Journal of Consulting and Clinical Psychology*.

Rudd, M. D., Bryan, C. J., Stone, S., Arne, K., and Williams, S. (2013). Brief cognitive behavioral therapy and treatment of suicide attempters in a military environment. In M. D. Rudd (Chair), *Suicide Prevention, Risk-Management, and Post-intervention Practices in the US Military and the VA*. Symposium conducted at the annual meeting of the American Psychological Association, Honolulu, HI.

Rudd, M. D., Goulding, J., and Bryan, C. J. (2011). Student veterans: A national survey exploring psychological symptoms and suicide risk. *Professional Psychology: Research and Practice*, 42(5), 354–360.

Rudd, M. D., Joiner, T. E., and Rajab, M. H. (1996). Relationships among suicide ideators, attempters, and multiple attempters in a young-adult sample. *Journal of Abnormal Psychology*, 105(4), 541–550.

Rudd, M. D., Joiner, T. E., and Rajab, M. H. (2000). *Treating Suicidal Behavior*. New York: Guilford Press.

Sareen, J., Cox, B. J., Afifi, T. O., Stein, M. B., Belik, S., Meadows, G., and Asmundson, G. J. G. (2007). Combat and peacekeeping operations in relation to prevalence of mental disorders and perceived need for mental health care. *Archives of General Psychiatry*, 64(7), 843–852.

Schneiderman, A. I., Braver, E. R., and Kang, H. K. (2008). Understanding sequalae of injury mechanisms and mild traumatic brain injury incurred during the conflicts in Iraq and Afghanistan: Persistent postconcussive symptoms and posttraumatic stress disorder. *American Journal of Epidemiology*, 167(12), 1446–1452.

Shipherd, J. C. and Beck, J. G. (1999). The effects of suppressing trauma-related thoughts on women with rape-related posttraumatic stress disorder. *Behaviour Research and Therapy*, 37(2), 99–112.

Simpson, G. and Tate, R. (2002). Suicidality after traumatic brain injury: Demographics, injury and clinical correlates. *Psychological Medicine*, 32(4), 687–697.

Teasdale, T. W. and Engberg, A. W. (2001). Suicide after traumatic brain injury: A population study. *Journal of Neurology, Neurosurgery, and Psychiatry*, 71(4), 436–440.

Thoresen, S., and Mehlum, L. (2008). Traumatic stress and suicidal ideation in Norwegian male peacekeepers. *Journal of Nervous and Mental Disease*, 196(11), 814–821.

12 Contribution of alcohol to suicide mortality in Eastern Europe

Yury E. Razvodovsky

Suicide is one of the leading external causes of death in many countries and its burden is expected to rise over the next several decades (Bertolote and Fleishman, 2002; Jagodic *et al.*, 2012). There are a number of possible reasons for this including lessened social integration, increase in psychiatric disorders, alcohol and drug abuse (Lester, 1997; Mäkinen, 2006). There is marked geographic variability in suicide rates globally, with highest rates being found in Eastern Europe (EE) (Jagodic *et al.*, 2012). The reason for high suicide mortality in EE is not fully understood. A number of variables, including socioeconomic factors, religious and biological background, as well as availability of the health care system should be considered (Bertolote and Fleishman, 2002; Lester, 1997; Pray *et al.*, 2013). Although a suicidal act is a multi-causal behavior as a result of an interaction of biological, psychological and socioeconomic factors, alcohol abuse constitutes one of the most important risk factors (Hufford, 2001). Alcohol consumption and suicide rates are considerably higher in the EE countries than in the countries of Western Europe (WE) (Anderson and Baunberg, 2006; Pray *et al.*, 2013). Accumulated evidence suggests that the mixture of cultural acceptance of heavy drinking, the high rate of distilled spirits consumption, and binge drinking pattern is a major contributor to the suicide mortality burden in EE (Anderson and Baunberg, 2006). Both aggregate- and individual level studies reported a positive association between alcohol and suicide in different parts of the region (Wasserman *et al.*, 1994; Landberg, 2008). This chapter summarizes the evidence of the relationship between alcohol and suicide in the Eastern European countries.

Alcohol and suicide

Alcohol abuse has long been considered an important and probably causal factor of suicidal behavior (Pompilli *et al.*, 2010). It is generally accepted now that both acute and chronic alcohol use are among the major behaviorally modifiable factors that are associated with suicidal behavior (Cherpitel *et al.*, 2004). The exact mechanism for the association, however, is unclear. Hufford (2001) presents a conceptual framework of distal and proximal risk factors relating alcohol to suicidal behavior. According to this concept distal risk factors create a statistical potential for suicide. Alcohol dependence, as well as associated comorbid psychopathology and negative life events, act as distal risk factors for suicidal behavior. Proximal risk factors determine the timing of suicidal behavior by translating the statistical potential of distal risk factors into action. The acute effects of alcohol intoxication act as important proximal risk factors for suicidal behavior among alcoholics and nonalcoholics alike. Acute alcohol intoxication may trigger self-destructive behavior by provoking depressive thoughts, decreasing self-control and constricting cognition that impairs the generation of an effective coping strategy to avoid psychosocial distress (Hufford, 2001; Pompilli *et al.*, 2010). In their rigorous review of studies of acute alcohol use and suicidal behavior published over a 10-year period (1991–2001), Cherpitel *et al.* (2004) found a wide range of alcohol-positive cases for both completed suicide (10–69 percent) and suicide attempts (10–73 percent). Several case-control studies at the individual level have shown a high prevalence of alcohol abuse and dependence among suicide victims (Kõlves *et al.*, 2006).

The international literature provides increasing evidence of an association between alcohol consumption and suicide rates at the aggregate level (Pompilli *et al.*, 2010). In his classic work, Norström (1995) argues that the effect of alcohol consumption on suicide rate is stronger in a 'dry' drinking culture, characterized by a low per capita consumption with the bulk of consumption concentrated on a few occasions, than in a 'wet' drinking culture with a high average consumption which is more evenly distributed throughout the week. The reason for this is that heavy drinkers in the 'dry' culture are more likely to experience weakened family and community bonds because their behavior is viewed as marginal. In his comparative time-series analysis based on the data for the period from 1950–1995 covering 14 European Union countries, Ramstedt (2001) has shown that an increase in population drinking had a greater impact on suicide in northern Europe (8.6 percent per liter for men and 11.4 percent for women) than in mid-Europe and southern Europe (0.6 percent per liter for men and 0.5 percent for women).

Suicide in Eastern Europe

Suicides rates in the EE countries are among the highest in the world (Jagodic *et al.*, 2012; Razvodovsky and Stickley, 2009). Suicide mortality rates in the region are highly variable (Pray *et al.*, 2013). The reasons for these differences have not been fully explained. The variability of socioeconomic, cultural and biological factors might contribute to the regional differences in suicide rates (Pray *et al.*, 2013). High suicide rates across EE have been associated with the dramatic societal changes during the post-Soviet transitional period (Lester, 1998; Mäkinen, 2006). Most of the post-communist countries exhibited a decrease in their suicide mortality rates from the mid-1990s (Landberg, 2008). Despite a gradual decline in suicide mortality over the past decade, the former Soviet republics still have the highest suicide rates in the world (Pray *et al.*, 2013). In his well-designed study Mäkinen (2000) has presented the following clusters of EE countries according to the values of the main suicide mortality variables:

1. The 'high suicide, unequal sex distribution' group consisted of Belarus, Estonia, Kazakhstan, Latvia, Lithuania, Russia, Slovenia, and Ukraine. Characteristic of this group of countries was a higher-than-average suicide rate, high sex quota, and a low age quota.
2. The 'high suicide, unequal age distribution' group consisted of Croatia, East Germany, and Hungary. This group was distinguished from the first one by its relatively low sex quota and a high age quota.
3. The 'low-suicide, unequal sex distribution' group was made up of Poland, Romania, and Slovakia. These countries showed a lower-than-average suicide rate together with a high sex quota and a low age quota.
4. The 'low suicide, unequal age distribution' group included Bulgaria, the Czech Republic, Macedonia, Serbia, and Montenegro. In these countries, a lower than average suicide rate was accompanied by a low sex quota but also by a higher than average age quota.
5. The 'low suicide, equal distribution' group demonstrated lower than average values of the suicide rate, its sex quota, and the age quota. It consisted of Albania, Armenia, Azerbaijan, Georgia, Tajikistan, Turkmenistan, and Uzbekistan.

Alcohol in Eastern Europe

Although alcohol is a major risk factor in many parts of the world, EE has the highest alcohol-attributable burden of disease and mortality (Rehm *et al.*, 2006). Alcohol makes a large contribution to the difference in mortality observed between the East and West parts of Europe (Anderson and Baunberg, 2006). In particular, its effects on health seem to have been especially acute in the countries of the former Soviet Union where it has recently been identified as one of the most important factors underpinning the alarming rise in mortality that has occurred in the post-communist period (Stickley *et al.*, 2007). According to the estimates alcohol consumption is responsible for 13.6 percent of premature mortality cases among men aged 20 to 64 years in Poland; this figure is 16.3 percent in the Czech Republic, 22.8 percent in Lithuania, and 25.2 percent in Hungary (Rehm *et al.*, 2006). Its contribution is especially striking in Russia, where alcohol may be responsible for more than 30 percent of all deaths (Nemtsov and Razvodovsky, 2008). The overall volume of alcohol consumption in EE region is the highest in the world. As reported by the WHO (2003), in 2003 the average total level of recorded consumption in the region was 14.2 liters, which is 2.3 times higher than global estimates (6.2 liters). There were also considerable variations in the levels of total per capita alcohol consumption among the EE countries. The highest average level of total alcohol was reported in Moldova (25.2 liters), and the lowest was in Bulgaria (15.0 liters). Countries with relatively high levels of total alcohol consumption included Hungary (17.6 liters), Croatia

(16.8 liters), Ukraine (16.6 liters), Russia (15.2 liters), Belarus 15.0 liters), and Lithuania (14.8 liters).

Despite ongoing homogenization of alcohol consumption within Europe in recent decades, EE represents three historically distinct alcohol cultures: spirits-drinking countries with a detrimental drinking pattern (Russia, Belarus, Poland, Lithuania, Latvia and Estonia); wine-drinking countries, characterized by regular consumption of wine with food and the general acceptance of alcohol as part of the diet (Hungary, Bulgaria, Romania, Slovenia); beer-drinking countries (the Czech Republic, Slovakia), although recent trends there betray a notable rise in the consumption of distilled spirits (Anderson and Baunberg, 2006). Due to differences in consumption level and drinking cultures, EE countries cannot be regarded as a homogeneous region with regard to how alcohol affects suicide rates.

Alcohol and suicide in Eastern Europe: individual level studies

The empirical literature provides evidence of an association between alcohol and suicide at the individual level in many EE nations. The official autopsy reports of the Estonian Bureau of Forensic Medicine for the period from 1981 to 1992 show that 48.7 percent of males and 22.0 percent of females were BAC-positive (blood alcohol concentration) at the time of suicide (Värnik *et al.*, 2006). Research shows that 74.6 percent of suicide victims in Slovenia were under the influence of alcohol (Bilban and Skibin, 2005). In this study, men were drunk in 87.1 percent of cases, women only in 12.9 percent and the given alcohol levels were substantially higher for men (0.65:0.26 g/kg). The shares of BAC-positive suicides reach its peak in the 35–54 age group (Bilban and Skibin, 2005). In Croatia, the average blood alcohol concentration at the moment of suicide was 0.68 g/kg in male, and 0.29 g/kg in female victims (Coklo *et al.*, 2008). According to the results of the autopsy, 60 percent of men and 27 percent of women in Romania were BAC-positive at the time of death (Jung *et al.*, 2009).

In a Polish sample Binczycka-Anholcer (2006) found that 47.5 percent of men and 36.0 percent of women who committed suicide had a positive BAC at the time of death. In a similar study alcohol was found in 39.5 percent of individuals autopsied in the Department of Forensic Medicine at the Medical University of Warsaw (Fudalej *et al.*, 2009). In this study, the rates of alcohol-positive suicides were 43 percent in men and 31.3 percent in women, while the average BAC was 0.17 g/dL and did not differ between genders. Additionally, the researchers found an association between the selected polymorphism of TPH2 and alcohol-related suicide phenotype under the recessive model of inheritance. It was also reported, that alcohol dependence was the stronger predictor of suicide under the influence of alcohol (Fudalej *et al.*, 2009). Similarly, in a psychological autopsy study in Budapest, alcoholism was identified as an important determinant of suicide risk (Coklo *et al.*, 2008). A more recent retrospective psychological autopsy study has reported that 68 percent of males and 29 percent of females who committed suicide met criteria for alcohol abuse or dependence (Kölves *et al.*, 2006).

The findings suggest that alcohol is an important determinant of suicide rates at the individual level in Belarus (Razvodovsky, 2006a, 2006b, 2010, 2012, 2013). A psychological autopsy study revealed that alcohol abuse and alcohol dependence were diagnosed in 70 percent of male and 71.4 percent of female suicide victims (Razvodovsky, 2013). A recent study based on the autopsy reports of the Bureau of Forensic Medicine of Belarus revealed that 61 percent of males and 30.6 percent of females were BAC-positive at the time of death (Razvodovsky, 2010). Positive blood alcohol cases were found more frequently in men aged 30–59 (66 percent) and women aged 19–39 (48 percent). The average BAC was 2.2 g/L for males and 2.1 g/L for females (Razvodovsky, 2010). So, there is growing evidence that a substantial number of suicides in EE are related to alcohol.

Alcohol and suicide in Eastern Europe: population level studies

Most of the evidence linking excessive drinking and suicide in EE is based on population data. Both longitudinal and cross-sectional aggregate-level studies usually report a significant and positive association between alcohol consumption and suicide (Landberg, 2008; Mäkinen, 2000; Razvodovsky, 2007). On the basis of the multivariate analysis, Marusic (1999) concluded that the prevalence of alcohol psychoses appears to be among the most important predictors of regional suicide rates in Slovenia. Further, Pridemore (2006) has highlighted a close cross-sectional link between alcohol and suicide in Russian regions during the mid-1990s.

Recent studies addressing the alcohol-suicide relationship at the aggregate level applied the sophisticated statistical modeling technique developed by Box and Jenkins (1976) often referred to as ARIMA (autoregressive integrated moving average) time-series analysis. This technique minimizes the risk of spurious correlation. An additional advantage of this approach is that ARIMA time-series analysis provides a base for comparing the relationship between alcohol and suicide across countries. In their time-series analysis Bielinska-Kwapisz and Mielecka-Kubien (2011) reported that alcohol consumption is strongly and significantly positively related to the suicide rate in Poland: an increase in consumption by 1 liter of pure alcohol per capita would increase the suicide rate by 0.83.

Several studies highlighted a significant aggregate level association between alcohol and suicide in the former republics of Soviet Union. In their pioneering work Värnik and Wasserman (1992) revealed a positive and statistically significant association between alcohol consumption per capita and suicide rates in the former Soviet Slavic and Baltic republics between 1984 and 1992. Alcohol appeared to have a lower explanatory value for female suicides compared with male suicides (Värnik *et al.*, 1998a, 1998b). It was reported that in all the republics, alcohol can explain a large proportion of suicides: 85 percent in Belarus, 77 percent in Ukraine, 75 percent in the Russian Federation, 65 percent in Estonia, 63 percent in Latvia, 60 percent in Lithuania (Wasserman *et al.*, 1994).

In his time series analysis data for the period 1965–1999 Nemtsov (2003) has reported that a 1-liter increase in alcohol consumption is expected to increase suicide rates by 11.4 percent for the total population (13.1 percent for men and 6.6 percent for women). A more recent update suggests that 1-liter increase in per capita consumption is associated with an increase in overall suicide rates of 7.2 percent (8 percent for males and 4.3 percent for females) (Landberg, 2008). In another study based on the Russian time series data between 1980 and 2005, Razvodovsky (2011b) found that overall alcohol consumption is significantly associated with both male and female suicides: a 1-liter increase in alcohol consumption would result in an increase in the suicide rate of 7.0 percent for males and 3.2 percent for females. The estimated effects of alcohol consumption on the age-specific suicide rate for men range from 0.029 (75+ age group) to 0.084 (30–44 age group) and for women range from 0.008 (60–74 age group) to 0.036 (15–29 age group). The estimates of AAF (alcohol-attributable fraction) for females (35 percent) were lower than the estimates for males (61 percent). The estimated AAF for men range from 33 percent (75+ age group) to 68 percent (30–44 age group) and for women range from 10 percent (60–74 age group) to 39 percent (15–29 age group) (Razvodovsky, 2011b). These findings indicate that the relationship between overall alcohol consumption and suicide rates was stronger for working-age males. The author argues that it is not surprising, given that the previous studies identified an unhealthy lifestyle among middle-aged working-class Russian males with the high level of alcohol consumption (Cockerham, 2000). Moreover, this shows a harmful pattern of drinking featuring big doses of vodka in a short period of time with a small snack. An analysis of frequency of drinking by male age groups indicates that the frequency climbs steadily to a peak between ages 30 and 39, before decreasing slightly in the ages 40–44 and 45–49 years and from age 50 declines significantly (Cockerham, 2000).

Several researchers have focused on the role of drinking culture as a possible explanation of the extremely high suicide rates in Russia (Pridemore and Chamlin, 2006; Razvodovsky, 2009a). The distinctive traits of Russian drinking culture are the heavy episodic (binge) drinking pattern, the preference for distilled spirits, and sociocultural tolerance for heavy drinking (Nemtsov and Razvodovsky, 2008). A worldwide assessment of drinking patterns showed that Russia and the former Soviet republics had the most hazardous pattern of drinking (Rehm *et al.*, 2006). The findings suggest that binge drinking and suicide mortality are positively related phenomena in Russia. In their time series analysis employing ARIMA technique Pridemore and Chamlin (2006) found a positive association between suicide and proxy for heavy drinking in Russia from 1956 to 2002. The results from another study based on Russian data from 1956 to 2005 showed a positive association between fatal alcohol poisoning (as a proxy for binge drinking) and suicide rate (Razvodovsky, 2009b). In their recent time series analysis Stickley *et al.* (2011) concluded that binge drinking had a significant association with the occurrence of suicide in Russia and the magnitude of the relation is the same across the course of the later-Tsarist, Soviet, and post-Soviet periods.

Additional support for the hypothesis that an unfavorable mixture of higher overall level of alcohol consumption and binge drinking of spirits is a major risk factor for suicide mortality in Russia provides the results of time-series analysis focused on the relation between the sale of different alcoholic beverages and suicide rates. It was reported that vodka consumption as measured by sale was significantly associated with both male and female suicide rate: 1 liter change in per capita vodka sale was associated with an increase in suicide rates by 9.3 percent for men and by 6 percent for women (Razvodovsky, 2009a). Instead, the consumption of beer and wine were not associated with suicide rate. The estimates of the age-specific models for men were positive (except for the 75+ age group) and range from 0.069 (60–74 age group) to 0.123 (30–44 age group). The estimates for women were positive for the 15–29 age group (0.08), the 30–44 age group (0.096) and the 45–59 age group (0.057) (Razvodovsky, 2009a).

This research evidence replicates previous findings from other settings, which highlighted that the relationship between alcohol and suicide is stronger for distilled spirits relative to total alcohol and wine/beer consumption. On the basis of pooled cross-sectional time series analysis of US data, Gruenewald *et al.* (1995) found that only spirits' sales displayed a significant relationship with suicide rate whereas wine and beer sales were not associated with suicide. Similarly, in their time series analysis Norström and Rossov (1999), based on data from Norwegian and Sweden, reported that in both countries the suicide rate was related to spirits sales but not to wine sales: a 1-liter increase in spirits sales in Norway was associated with a 11 percent increase in the male suicide rate; the corresponding figure for Sweden, was 14 percent. The strong aggregate level association between vodka sales, and suicide rate in Russia might be an outcome of a preference for spirits among heavy drinkers (Nemtsov and Razvodovsky, 2008). The effects of drinking spirits may also be exacerbated by the way they are drunk as a heavy episodic drinking pattern is widespread. The heavy drinking of spirits in Russia may result in high suicide rates due to so-called 'Mellanby effect' i.e. the more rapid rise of blood alcohol concentration and thus intake of spirits implies a large extent of immediate impairment (Stickley *et al.*, 2011). In addition, the expectations of aggressive behavior associated with spirits intake might trigger auto-aggressive behavior (Gruenewald *et al.*, 1995). It appears that acute alcohol intoxication may act as a disinhibitor in people predisposed to suicide for social and economic reasons.

The results of aggregate-level studies highlighted that alcohol is among the most consistent predictors of the suicide rates in Belarus. For example, results from a time-series analysis based on the data from 1970–2005 suggest a positive correlation between fatal alcohol poisoning/alcohol-related psychosis morbidity (as a proxy for alcohol consumption) and suicide rates (Razvodovsky, 2007). The results of another study covering the period 1980–2005 show that population-level alcohol consumption has a positive and statistically significant association with the suicide rate, with a 1-liter change in per capita consumption being associated with a 7.4 percent increase in the suicide rate among males and a 3.1 percent increase among females (Razvodovsky, 2009c); the estimated effects of alcohol consumption on the age-specific suicide rates for men range from 0.024 (15–29 age group) to 0.082 (30–44 and 45–59 age groups). The estimated effects of alcohol consumption on age-specific rates for women were positive for age groups 15–29 (0.017), 30–44 (0.047), 45–59 (0.039) and 60–74 (0.017) (Razvodovsky, 2009c). In yet another study, Razvodovsky (2001) demonstrated a stronger association between alcohol and suicide with the consumption of distilled spirits (vodka) relative to the total level of alcohol consumption. Finally, the results of time-series analysis indicated a statistically significant relationship between fatal alcohol poisoning rates and number of BAC-positive suicides (Razvodovsky, 2011a).

The role of alcohol as major contributor to a high rural/urban gradient in suicide rate was highlighted in a recent study indicating the presence of a close association between suicide and fatal alcohol poisoning rates for rural men and women in Belarus (Razvodovsky, 2012). Furthermore, the findings on the spatial relationship between suicides and alcohol psychoses incidence rates suggest that a regional pattern of alcohol-related problems is a major factor responsible for suicides rate regional variations in Belarus (Razvodovsky, 2013).

In his time-series analysis Landberg (2008) showed a significant association between alcohol and suicide in seven eastern European countries. Most importantly, he revealed that the sizes of the effects were stronger in spirits drinking countries with a detrimental drinking pattern. The estimates for females were markedly smaller than those for men in most countries and did not differ between the two country groups. The pooled alcohol effect for men in the spirits countries was similar to that found for northern Europe, while the pooled effect for the non-spirits countries was larger than those for southern and mid-Europe. The female pooled effects for both countries' groups were similar to the pooled effect for mid-Europe. The spirits-drinking countries obtained higher overall and male AAF estimates than did the non-spirits countries. For example, Russian and Polish males stand out with an AAF of 70 percent and 45 percent respectively, whereas the non-spirits countries range between 31 percent and 37 percent. The female estimates were lower than the estimates for males in all countries except Bulgaria (Landberg, 2008).

Collectively, these findings provided support for Norstrom's hypothesis suggesting that the suicide rate was strongly influenced by alcohol consumption in the countries where the drinking culture was characterized by heavy drinking episodes. Furthermore, these findings add to the growing evidence that the binge drinking pattern (i.e. excessive consumption of alcohol in the form of spirits) results in a quicker and deeper level of intoxication, increasing the propensity for autodestructive behavior. This may be especially true, as the level of per capita vodka sales in Russia and Belarus seems to be a better predictor of suicide rate than the overall level of alcohol sales (Razvodovsky, 2001, 2009).

It is important to point out that the size of the bivariate association between alcohol and suicide for men in EE is substantially greater than for women. This means that alcohol-related suicide is mainly a male phenomenon. For example, Wasserman *et al.* (1994) estimated for the former USSR that the attributable fraction of alcohol for male suicides (more than 70 percent) exceeded considerably that for females (24 percent). A more recent estimate suggests that alcohol may be responsible for 61 percent of male suicides and 35 percent of female suicides in Russia (Razvodovsky, 2011h). Beverage preference and harmful drinking patterns might be responsible for the gender difference in the suicide rate as vodka continues to be the drink of choice for the majority of men in Russia, while women not only drink less often than men, but those who do drink, consume vodka less frequently than men. Indeed, according to a population survey, 44 percent of men and only 6 percent women reported that they drink an equivalent of 25 cl of vodka or more at one occasion (Bobak *et al.*, 1999). According to a more recent study 28 percent of men and 4 percent of women consume at least 200g (86+ g of pure alcohol) on one occasion at least once every 2–3 weeks (Pomerleau *et al.*, 2008).

In contrast to the studies, presented above, it was shown that the suicide rate in Hungary declined from 46 per 100,000 in 1984 to 32 per 100,000 in 1998 (–32 percent), in spite of the fact that between 1989 and 1996 there was a 25 percent rise in the alcohol-dependence prevalence rates and a six-fold increase in unemployment (Kovács, 2008). Similarly, Rancaris *et al.* (2001) concluded that the alcohol psychoses incidence rate (as a proxy for alcohol consumption) could not sufficiently explain the rapid increase in suicide rate in Latvia during the years 1980–1998. The inconsistent results of epidemiological studies of the relation between alcohol and suicide suggest that multiple sociocultural factors influence suicide rates.

Thus, most of the research evidence presented here suggests that alcohol consumption is a significant determinant of suicide mortality at the population level in EE.

Natural experiments

Natural experiments, such as sudden and large changes in alcohol consumption level, provide an opportunity to test the efficacy of policy attempts to reduce the rate of alcohol-related problems in the population. These types of experiments are being used in social epidemiology and allow a rigorous evaluation of the efficacy of public health interventions. Russia, due to its high overall level of consumption, hazardous drinking patterns and its high suicide rate, provides an important contextual setting for this type of analysis. In recent decades, Soviet and later Russian governments have adopted a series of restrictive measures in an attempt to curb the alcohol-related burden. Gorbachev's anti-alcohol campaign in 1985–1988 is the most well-known natural experiment in the field of alcohol policy.

A few studies have examined the effect of the Soviet anti-alcohol campaign on the suicide rate. For example, Värnik *et al.* (2006) found that the restrictive alcohol policy in Estonia led to a 39.4 percent reduction in suicides in which alcohol was presented in the blood of the victims, BAC-negative suicides showed a 3 percent increase. Mean BAC-positive suicides decreased by 39.2 percent for males and 41.4 percent for females from the baseline period to the intervention.

In his study Nemtsov (2003) examined trends in per capita alcohol consumption and suicide rate in Russia from 1965 to 1999 and found that the anti-alcohol campaign was accompanied by a substantial decline in suicide mortality: in 1984–1986 there was a drop of 39.1 percent (from 37.9 to 23.1 per 100,000 of the population), while alcohol consumption decreased by 26.8 percent (from 14.2 to 10.5 liters). Most importantly, it was shown that the number of BAC-positive suicides sank by 55 percent (from 22.0 per 100,000 in 1984 to 9.9 per 100,000) between 1984 and 1986 (Nemtsov, 2003). The potential benefits of the restrictive policy were clearly demonstrated during Gorbachev's anti-alcohol campaign in Belarus when a reduction in the per capita consumption of alcohol from 13.3 to 6.7 liters between 1984 and 1986 was accompanied by a fall in the suicide rates from 15.4 to 7.0 per 100,000 of residents (Razvodovsky, 2001). In another study Razvodovsky (2011a) highlighted that alcohol-related suicides were more affected by the restriction of alcohol availability during the anti-alcohol campaign: between 1984 and 1996 the number of BAC-positive suicide cases dropped by 54.2 percent, while the number of BAC-negative suicides decreased by 7.1 percent.

It seems obvious that the sudden decline in suicide rate appears to be entirely due to the anti-alcohol campaign of 1985–1988 that significantly reduced alcohol consumption by limiting its manufacture and availability. However, despite such circumstances in which all the newly independent states of the former Soviet Union have been going through similar transformations, any general trend of suicide mortality cannot be identified in this country. Such Eastern European republics as Belarus, Estonia, Latvia, Lithuania, Russia, or Ukraine belong to the 'high-suicide, unequal sex distribution' group (Mäkinen, 2000). This group experienced a substantial drop in suicide rates in 1985–1989, especially for middle-aged males, followed by a large increase in 1989–1993. It should be noted, that this country has highest level of alcohol consumption compared to any other country of the former USSR. Azerbaijan, Georgia, Tajikistan, Turkmenistan, and Uzbekistan, that belong to the 'low suicide, equal sex distribution' group, demonstrate another pattern of suicide. These republics demonstrated falling rates of suicide rate for the entire period 1985–1993. It was shown that changes in the level of alcohol consumption were significantly correlated with those in suicide in the first group of countries only (Mäkinen, 2000). This evidence conflicts with the theory of 'social correlates of suicide', and confirms the intermediating role of culture in relation to suicides.

Some researchers argue that alcohol is unlikely to provide the universal explanation for the mortality fluctuations during the 1980s in Russia (Wasserman *et al.*, 1994). They believe that the decrease in suicide mortality rate in Russia in the mid-1980s could have been related to the political and social liberalization during the period known as 'perestroika', which gave rise to social optimism and new hope. One can argue, however, that social changes should also have resulted in increased anomie, which according to Durkheim, is associated with a high suicide rate (Durkheim, 1966). In addition, Nemtsov has highlighted that in Russia the number of BAC-positive suicides shrank by 55 percent, while the number of BAC-negative suicides did not change substantially during Gorbachev's perestroika (Nemtsov, 2003). He argues that 'so-called national optimism was more likely a projection of the emotions of the more intelligent sections of the population (including scientists) than of the Russian population as a whole'. Moreover, it has been shown that the oldest age groups of both men and women did not experience a reduction in their suicide rates during the anti-alcohol campaign, while working-age males faced the greater decreases in suicide mortality in the mid-1980s and the subsequent increases in the late 1980s and early 1990s (Pridemore and Spivak, 2003). Decrease in suicide rates in the Slavic and Baltic republics during the anti-alcohol campaign occurred to a greater degree for ages 25–54, averaging a drop of 45 percent for men and 33 percent for women between 1984 and 1986–1988 (Värnik *et al.*, 1998b). In contrast to a pattern of age-specific suicide rates for women, a distinctive pattern of male suicide rates in the Slavic and Baltic republics converged with those found in other parts of Europe during 1986–1988 (Värnik *et al.*, 1998b). It appeared that the anti-alcohol campaign contributed to a unique pattern of male suicide mortality in this region, especially in the 25–54 age group. Similarly, it was shown that the pattern of the age-specific distribution of suicides and fatal alcohol poisonings coincided during the anti-alcohol campaign (Nemtsov, 2003).

There is strong evidence for the key role of alcohol in explaining the Russian suicide mortality crisis in the early-1990s. In his well-designed study Mäkinen (2000) has reported that alcohol consumption was a powerful predictor of suicide rates in 'high-suicide, unequal sex distribution' group of Eastern Bloc countries (including Russia) which experienced a large drop in suicide rates in 1985–1989, especially for middle-age males, followed by a large general increase in 1989–1993. This evidence supports the hypothesis that the increase in alcohol consumption was the main determinant of suicide mortality crisis in Russia in the early-1990s.

Several scholars have argued that psychosocial distress resulting from the 'shock therapy' economic reform and sudden collapse of the Soviet paternalist system was the main determinant of the suicide mortality crisis in the former Soviet republics in the 1990s (Andreeva *et al.*, 2008). A recent cross-sectional time-series analysis focused on suicide rates and socioeconomic factors in Eastern European countries after the collapse of the Soviet Union suggests that changes in suicide rates were related to socioeconomic disruptions experienced during the transition period (Kõlves *et al.*, 2013). Instead, suicide rates in EE were not associated with alcohol consumption during the transitional period. Similarly, Lester (1998) suggested that the increase in suicide rates in this period may be a result of the disappointment over the changes in the standard of living after the initial hope that social conditions would improve rapidly. So, psychosocial distress may have been an important underlying factor of the suicide mortality crisis in the former Soviet republics in the 1990s. However, close aggregate level association between alcohol consumption and suicide rates, as well as the recent findings from Belarus highlighting the fact that the number of BAC-suicides dramatically jumped in the 1990s (Razvodovsky, 2011a), strongly supports an alcohol-related hypothesis and suggests that rather than playing a major causal role, psychosocial distress may represent a confounding factor.

The key point in debates on alcohol and suicide in Russia relates to the causes of increase of alcohol consumption in the early 1990s. There is evidence that alcohol is often used as medication for stress-related discomfort (Koposov *et al.*, 2002). A prior study revealed that heavy drinking was most common among men who experienced loss in social standing during the transition (Yukkala *et al.*, 2008). This suggests that heavy drinking and psychosocial distress are closely linked since distress increases involvement in binge drinking that heightens the risk of suicide.

It seems plausible that the psychosocial distress resulting from the reforms were the main causes of increased demand for alcohol at this time. This demand was met by factors that increased supply. Following the repeal of the state alcohol monopoly in January 1992, the alcohol market fragmented, including many private producers and importers operating without a license or registration (Nemtsov and Razvodovsky, 2008). The country was practically flooded by a wave of home-made, counterfeit, and imported alcohol, mainly spirits (Stickley *et al.*, 2007). The negative outcomes of an increase of alcohol consumption during this period included a sharp rise in suicide mortality.

One of the most interesting features of suicide mortality crisis in Russia in the early-1990s is the gender difference in spite of the fact that men and women share the same socioeconomic circumstances (Andreeva *et al.*, 2008). It seems that males were most vulnerable to the stressful experience resulting from abrupt socioeconomic changes, political instability, unemployment and impoverishment. This disproportionately affects the working-age male population because their work and family roles rendered them more vulnerable to socioeconomic disruption (Cornia and Poniccia, 2000). Several studies have suggested that men in Russia, as a result of traditional masculine norms, are more prone to respond to stressful situations with maladaptive behavior such as increased alcohol consumption, while women have a more adaptive stress response. Based on interviews conducted with a stratified random sample of 1190 Muscovites Yukkala *et al.* (2008) concluded that experiencing several kinds of economic problems is positively related to the risk of binge drinking among men. In contrast, women seemed less likely to binge drink when experiencing manifold economic problems. Cockerham *et al.* (2006) found that in Russia psychological distress promotes frequent drinking among men, but not among women, even though women reported significantly more distress.

In contemporary Russia, recognizing the central role of alcohol in the mortality crisis, President Putin signed a law regulating production and sale of alcohol production in 2005 (Nemtsov and Razvodovsky, 2008). The law contained regulations aimed at controlling the volume and quality of alcohol products and requiring the registration of alcohol production and distribution facilities. In a recent study Predimore *et al.* (2013) took advantage of this natural experiment to assess the impact on suicide mortality of a suite of Russian alcohol policies. They used autoregressive integrated moving average (ARIMA) interrupted time series techniques to model the effect of the alcohol policy on monthly male and female suicide counts between January 2000 and December 2010. They revealed that the alcohol policy in Russia led to a 9 percent reduction in male suicide mortality, meaning the policy was responsible for saving 4000 male lives annually that would otherwise have been lost to suicide.

Another piece of evidence suggesting the close link between alcohol and suicide at the population level comes from Slovenia. Recognizing the high level of alcohol-related problems, the Slovenian National Assembly passed new legislation in January 2003 that aimed to reduce alcohol-related harm by restricting alcohol's availability. The law established a minimum age of 18 years for drinking and purchasing alcoholic beverages and limited where and when alcohol can be purchased. There is evidence that this new alcohol policy has had an impact on suicide mortality. In particular, Pridemore and Snowden (2009) assessed the effect of a national alcohol policy on suicide mortality using interrupted time-series techniques, and found that the implementation of alcohol policy was followed by an immediate and permanent reduction in male suicide mortality. More specifically, there was an immediate and permanent reduction of 3.6 male suicides per month, or approximately 10 percent of the pre-intervention average. In contrast, the new policy had no statistically significant effect on female suicides.

In a more recent study Zupanc *et al.* (2013) reported that during the period before the implementation of the measures which limited the availability of alcohol in Slovenia, the BACs of BAC-positive suicide victims were higher than those tested in the period after the implementation of the act. This evidence suggests that legislation measures restricting alcohol availability may be an effective means of BAC reduction in BAC-positive suicide victims. Together with similar findings elsewhere, these results suggest an important role for public health interventions, including restrictive alcohol policy, in reducing alcohol-related suicide deaths.

Nevertheless, the impact of natural experiments on suicide mortality is not always unequivocal. In particular, increasing awareness concerning the rising level of alcohol-related problems was the main reason behind the implementation of a new alcohol policy in Lithuania during 2007–2009 (Sauliune *et al.*, 2012). The major policy innovations included strict regulation of advertising, raising the excise tax on alcohol, controlling drunk driving, and curtailing illegal alcohol imports and sales. Implementation of these alcohol control measures resulted in a significant reduction in the alcohol-attributable burden of violent mortality. However, despite the successful implementation of the anti-alcohol policy, suicide rates and YPLL (years of potential life lost) due to alcohol-related suicides had a tendency to increase among males, while among women it remained rather stable throughout 2006–2009 (Sauliune *et al.*, 2012). The authors hypothesized that the increase in suicide rates in this period might be affected by the economic recession and large rises in unemployment followed by increased psychological distress.

Collectively, most of the empirical evidence indicates that a restrictive alcohol policy appears to be one of the most effective suicide prevention policies in EE. Together with similar findings elsewhere, this evidence suggests an important role for public health interventions in reducing alcohol-related suicide deaths.

Policy implications

In a number of studies using various designs, alcohol consumption has been found to be important risk factor for suicide in EE. The high level of alcohol consumption in combination with detrimental drinking patterns in the EE countries results in a high level of alcohol-related suicides and a strong association between alcohol consumption and suicide rates in EE. The proportion of suicide victims who were under the influence of alcohol at the time of death in EE is higher than in WE. This evidence is in accordance with aggregate-level studies that show that the association between alcohol consumption and suicide rates is stronger in EE countries compared to WE countries. Studies of natural experiments have also demonstrated a significant impact of alcohol consumption on suicide rate in EE. In particular, a fairly close aggregate-level match between alcohol consumption and suicide mortality during Gorbachev's anti-alcohol campaigns may be used as evidence suggesting that alcohol is responsible for a substantial number of suicide deaths. This empirical evidence indicates that a restrictive alcohol policy can be considered an effective measure of suicide prevention in countries where rates of both alcohol consumption and suicide are high. The studies presented here suggest that the suicide rate in several EE nations in addition to overall level of consumption is related to the beverage preference and drinking pattern. Assuming that drinking spirits is usually associated with intoxication episodes, these findings provide additional evidence that the drinking pattern is an important determinant in the alcohol-suicide relationship in EE countries. These findings support the hypothesis that the association between alcohol consumption and suicide rates in EE countries is stronger than in WE countries due to a more detrimental drinking pattern and preference of strong spirits. This compelling evidence has important policy implications suggesting that any attempts to reduce overall consumption should also be linked efforts through differential taxation to shift beverage preference away from spirits.

References

Anderson, P. and Baunberg, B. (2006). *Alcohol in Europe*. London: Institute of Alcohol Studies.

Andreeva, E., Ermakov, S., and Brenner, H. (2008). The socioeconomic etiology of suicide mortality in Russia. *International Journal of Environment and Sustainable Development*, 7(1), 21–48.

Bertolote, J. M. and Fleishman, A. (2002). A global perspective in the epidemiology of suicide. *Suicidology*, 7(2), 6–8.

Bielinska-Kwapisz, A. and Mielecka-Kubien, Z. (2011). Alcohol consumption and its adverse effects in Poland in years 1950–2005. *Economic Research International*, Article ID 870714.

Bilban, M. and Skibin, L. (2005). Presence of alcohol in suicide victims. *Forensic Science International*, 147(Suppl.), S9–S12.

Binczycka-Anholcer, M. (2006). Alcohol as a significant factor in women's suicidal behavior, *Suicidologia*, 2, 57–63.

Bobak, M., McKee, M., Rose, R., and Marmot, M. (1999). Alcohol consumption in a sample of the Russian population. *Addiction*, 94(6), 857–866.

Box, G. E. P. and Jenkins, G. M. (1976). *Time Series Analysis: Forecasting and Control*. London: Holden-Day Inc.

Cherpitel, C. J., Borges, L. G. and Wilcox, H. C. (2004). Acute alcohol use and suicidal behavior: A review of the literature. *Alcoholism: Clinical and Experimental Research*, 28(5), 18–28.

Cockerham, C. W. (2000). Health lifestyle in Russia. *Social Science and Medicine*, 51(9), 1313–1324.

Cockerham, C. W., Hinote, B. P., and Abbot, P. (2006). Psychological distress, gender, and health lifestyles in Belarus, Kazakhstan, Russia, and Ukraine. *Social Science and Medicine*, 63(9), 2381–2394.

Coklo, M., Stemberga, V., Cuculić, D., Sosa, I., Jerković, R., and Bosnar, A. (2008). The methods of committing and alcohol intoxication of suicides in Southwestern Croatia from 1996 to 2005. *Collegium Antropologicum*, 32(Suppl. 2). 123–125.

Cornia, G. A. and Poniccia, P. (2000). The transition mortality crisis: Evidence, interpretation and policy response. In G. A. Cornia and P. Poniccia (Eds), *The Mortality Crisis in Transitional Economies* (pp. 4–37). Oxford: Oxford University Press.

Durkheim, E. (1966). *Suicide*. New York: The Free Press.

Fudalej, S., Ilgen, M., Fudalej, M., Wojnar, M., Matsumoto, H., Barry K. L., *et al.* (2009). Clinical and genetic risk factors for suicide under the influence of alcohol in a Polish sample. *Alcohol and Alcoholism*, 44(5), 437–442.

Gruenewald, P., Ponicki, W. R. and Mitchell, P. R. (1995). Suicide rates and alcohol consumption in the United States, 1970–89. *Addiction*, 90(8), 1063–75.

Hufford, M. R. (2001). Alcohol and suicidal behavior. *Clinical Psychology Review*, 21(5), 797–811.

Jagodic, H. K., Agius, M. and Pregeli, P. (2012). Inter-regional variations in suicide rates. *Psychiatria Danubina*, 34(2), 1–20.

Jung, H., Matei, D. B., and Hecser, L. (2009). Biostatistical study of suicide features in Mures Country (Romania). *Legal Medicine*, Suppl.1, 95–97.

Kõlves, K., Milner, A. and Värnik, P. (2013). Suicide rates and socioeconomic factors in Eastern European countries after the collapse of the Soviet Union: Trends between 1990 and 2008. *Sociological Health Illness*, 35(6), 956–970.

Kõlves, K., Värnik, A., Tooding, L. M., and Wasserman, D. (2006). The role of alcohol in suicide: A case-control psychological autopsy study. *Psychological Medicine*, 36(7), 923–930.

Koposov, R. A., Ruchkin, V. V., Eeisemann, M., and Sidorov, P. I. (2002). Alcohol use in adolescents from northern Russia: The role of social context. *Alcohol and Alcoholism*, 37(3), 297–303.

Kovács, K. (2008). Suicide and alcohol-related mortality in Hungary in the last two decades. *International Journal of Public Health*, 53(5), 252–259.

Landberg, J. (2008). Alcohol and suicide in Eastern Europe. *Drug and Alcohol Review*, 27(4), 361–373.

Lester, D. (1997). Suicide in an international perspective. *Suicide and Life-Threatening Behavior*, 27(1), 105–111.

Lester, D. (1998). Suicide and homicide after the fall of communist regimes. *European Psychiatry*, 13(2), 98–100.

Mäkinen, I. H. (2000). Eastern European transition and suicide mortality. *Social Science and Medicine*, 51(9), 1405–1420.

Mäkinen, I. H. (2006). Suicide mortality of Eastern European regions before and after the communist period. *Social Science and Medicine*, 63(2), 307–319.

Marusic, A. (1999). Suicide in Slovenia: Lessons from cross-cultural psychiatry. *International Review of Psychiatry*, 11(2–3), 212–218.

Nemtsov, A.V. (2003). Suicide and alcohol consumption in Russia, 1965–1999. *Drug and Alcohol Dependence*, 71(2), 161–168.

Nemtsov, A. V. and Razvodovsky, Y. E. (2008). Alcohol situation in Russia, 1980–2005. *Social and Clinical Psychiatry*, 2, 52–60.

Norström, T. (1995). Alcohol and suicide: A comparative analysis of France and Sweden. *Addiction*, 90(11), 1465–1469.

Norström, T. and Rossov, I. (1999). Beverage specific effects on suicide. *Nordic Studies Alcohol Drugs*, 16, 109–118.

Pomerleau, J., McKee, M., Rose, R., Haerpfer, C. W., Rotman, D., and Tumanov, S. (2008). Hazardous alcohol drinking in the former Soviet Union: A cross-sectional study of eight countries. *Alcohol and Alcoholism*, 43(3), 351–359.

Pompilli, M., Serafini, G., Innamorati, M., Dominici, G., Ferracuti, S., Kotzalidis G. D., *et al.* (2010). Suicide behavior and alcohol abuse. *International Journal Environment Research, Public Health*, 7(4), 1392–1431.

Pray, L., Cohen, C., Makinen, I. H., Varnik, A., and MacKellar, F. L. (Eds). (2013). *Suicide in Eastern Europe, the Commonwealth of Independent States, and the Baltic Countries: Social and Public Health Determinants*. Vienna: Remaprint.

Pridemore, W. A. (2006). Heavy drinking and suicide in Russia. *Social Forces*, 85(1), 413–430.

Pridemore, W. A. and Chamlin, M. B. (2006). A time-series analysis of the impact of heavy drinking on homicide and suicide mortality in Russia, 1956–2002. *Addiction*, 101(12), 1719–1729.

Pridemore, W. A., Chamlin, M. B. and Andreev, E. (2013). Reduction in male suicide mortality following the 2006 Russian alcohol policy: An interrupted time series analysis. *American Journal Public Health*, 103(11), 2021–2026.

Pridemore, W. A. and Snowden, A. J. (2009). Reduction in suicide mortality following a new national alcohol policy in Slovenia: An interrupted time-series analysis. *American Journal of Public Health*, 99(5), 915–920.

Pridemore, W. A. and Spivak, A. L. (2003). Pattern of suicide mortality in Russia. *Suicide and Life-Threatening Behavior*, 33(2), 132–150.

Ramstedt, M. (2001). Alcohol and suicide in 14 European countries. *Addiction*, 96(Suppl 1), 59–75.

Rancans, E., Salander-Renberg, E., Jacobsson, L. (2001). Major demographic, social and economic factors associated to suicide rates in Latvia 1980–98. *Acta Psychiatrica Scandinavica*, 103(4), 275–281.

Razvodovsky, Y. E. (2001). The association between the level of alcohol consumption per capita and suicide rate: Results of time-series analysis. *Alcoholism*, 2, 35–43.

Razvodovsky, Y. E. (2006a). Some socioepidemiological correlates of suicides in Belarus. *Psychiatria Danubina*, 18(Suppl.1), 145.

Razvodovsky, Y. E. (2006b). Alcohol consumption and suicide rate in Belarus. *Psychiatria Danubina*, 18(Suppl.1), 64.

Razvodovsky, Y. E. (2007). Suicide and alcohol psychoses in Belarus 1970–2005. *Crisis*, 28(2), 61–66.

Razvodovsky, Y. E. (2008). A comparative analysis of dynamic of suicides in Belarus and Russia. *Journal of Belarusian Psychiatric Association*, 14, 15–19.

Razvodovsky, Y. E. (2009a). Beverage-specific alcohol sale and suicide in Russia. *Crisis*, 30(4), 186–191.

Razvodovsky, Y. E. (2009b). Suicide and fatal alcohol poisoning in Russia, 1956–2005. *Drugs: Education, Prevention and Policy*, 16(2), 127–139.

Razvodovsky, Y. E. (2009c). Alcohol and suicide in Belarus. *Psychiatria Danubina*, 21(3), 290–296.

Razvodovsky, Y. E. (2010). Blood alcohol concentration in suicide victims. *European Psychiatry*, 25(Supplement 1), 1374.

Razvodovsky, Y. E. (2011a). Alcohol consumption and suicide in Belarus. *Suicidology Online*, 2, 1–7.

Razvodovsky, Y. E. (2011b). Alcohol consumption and suicide rates in Russia. *Suicidology Online*, 2, 67–74.

Razvodovsky, Y. E. (2012). *Alcohol and Suicide in Belarus.* Saarbrucken: LAP, LAMBERT Academic Publishing.

Razvodovsky, Y. E. (2013). Suicide trends in Belarus, 1980–2008. In L. Pray, C. Cohen, I. H. Makinen, A. Varnik and F. L. MacKellar (Eds), *Suicide in Eastern Europe, the CIS, and the Baltic Countries: Social and Public Health Determinants* (pp. 21–28). Vienna: Remaprint.

Razvodovsky, Y. E. and Stickley, A. (2009). Suicide in urban and rural regions of Belarus, 1990–2005. *Public Health*, 123(1), 120–126.

Rehm, J., Taylor, B. and Patra, J. (2006). Volume of alcohol consumption, pattern of drinking and burden of disease in the European region. *Addiction*, 101(8), 1086–1095.

Sauliune, S., Petrauskiene, J. and Kalediene, R. (2012). Alcohol-related injuries and alcohol control policy in Lithuania: Effects of the year of sobriety. *Alcohol and Alcoholism*, 47(4), 458–463.

Stickley, A., Jukkala, T. and Norström, T. (2011). Alcohol and suicide in Russia, 1870–1894 and 1956–2005: Evidence for the continuation of a harmful drinking culture across time? *Journal of Studies on Alcohol and Drugs*, 72(2), 341–347.

Stickley, A., Leinsalu, M., Andreew, E., Razvodovsky, Y. E., Vagero, D., and McKee, M. (2007). Alcohol poisoning in Russia and the countries in the European part of the former Soviet Union, 1970–2002. *European Journal of Public Health*, 17(5), 444–449.

Värnik, A., Kõlves., K., Vali, M., Tooding, L., and Wasserman, D. (2006). Do alcohol restrictions reduce suicide mortality? *Addiction*, 102(2), 251–256.

Värnik, A. and Wasserman, D. (1992). Suicides in the former Soviet republics. *Acta Psychiatrica Scandinavica*, 86(1), 76–78.

Värnik, A., Wasserman, D., Dankowicz M., and Eklund G. (1998a). Marked decrease in suicide among men and women in the former USSR during perestroika. *Acta Psychiatrica Scandinavica*, 98(Suppl. 394), 13–19.

Värnik, A., Wasserman, D., Dankowicz, M., and Eklund, G. (1998b). Age-specific suicide rates in the Slavic and Baltic regions of the former USSR during perestroika in comparison with 22 European countries. *Acta Psychiatrica Scandinavica*, 98(Suppl.394), 20–25.

Wasserman, D., Värnik, A., and Eklund, G. (1994). Male suicides and alcohol consumption in the former USSR. *Acta Psychiatrica Scandinavica*, 89(5), 306–313.

Yukkala, T., Mäkinen, I. H., Kislitsyna, O., and Ferlander, S. (2008). Economic strain, social relations, gender, and binge drinking in Moscow. *Social Science and Medicine*, 66(3), 663–674.

Zupanc, T., Agius, M., Videtič Paska, A., and Pregelj, P. (2013). Reduced blood alcohol concentration in suicide victims in response to a new national alcohol policy in Slovenia. *European Addiction Research*, 19(1), 7–12.j184

13 Media content representation of suicide in various societies

A critical review

Qijin Cheng and Paul S. F. Yip

Suicide is a serious problem worldwide but shows significant differences between national/regional suicide rates. Reasons for these great differences between national/regional suicide rates have been investigated from various aspects. Socio-cultural contexts, economic conditions, climate, religions, psychiatric morbidity, accuracy of the registration of suicide, availability of lethal methods, and the availability of the social/health care system have been taken into account (O'Connor *et al.*, 2011; Wasserman and Wasserman, 2009).

Media are a crucial part of the socio-cultural context regarding the suicide problem in society. Ecological studies have provided evidence to demonstrate that mass media, especially prominent news reports of suicide, can facilitate the increase in suicide rates at the population level (Fu and Yip, 2007; Gould *et al.*, 2003; Niederkrotenthaler *et al.*, 2012; Stack, 2003). Also mass media's prominent reporting of a new suicide method can facilitate a rapid increase of the prevalence of the method (Chen *et al.*, 2013; Lee *et al.*, 2005; Yip *et al.*, 2013). In addition, in survey studies and qualitative interviews, some suicidal individuals reported that they were influenced by media content, including non-fictional and fictional media, in terms of suicidal ideation or choice of a suicide method (Biddle *et al.*, 2012; A. T. A. Cheng *et al.*, 2007; Tsai, 2010), which endorsed the media content's impacts.

The media's effects on suicide are believed to be related with how the media represents suicide. The term 'media representation' is different from 'media report' as the former is rooted in the theory of social construction of reality and the theory of mass-mediated depiction of reality. Modern sociology and cultural studies commonly emphasize that individuals can only process symbolic reality which is a representation of the objective reality embedded in the institutional fabric of society (Adoni and Mane, 1984; Gamson *et al.*, 1992). The process of reality representation is referred to as the *social construction of reality*, where the mass media play an important role. Starting from Walter Lippmann, a famous writer and journalist in the US, an argument has been raised and supported that the mass media were not simply *reporting* the reality but representing the reality based on their own publishing policies, agenda, and interpretations (Schudson, 1997).

As far as we know, no study has been conducted to systematically review how the media represent suicide in different societies and what factors possibly influence the differences. Furthermore, many previous studies only examined frequency or density of suicide news reports as a quantitative representation of suicide issues but fewer studies specifically examined the content of suicide reports. Therefore, the present study aims to fill these gaps through a systematic literature review. Previous studies found non-fictional media reports, rather than fictional content, have stronger and more consistent effects on real suicide, and the effects are often observable in the short term (Gould, 2001; Pirkis and Blood, 2001a, 2001b; Stack, 2005). Hence, the present study limited its review scope to contemporary non-fictional media content.

Methods

The conduct of this systematic literature screening followed the principles of the PRISMA statement (Liberati *et al.*, 2009). A demonstration of the review procedure is shown in Figure 13.1. A literature search was conducted in October 2013 using ISI Web of Knowledge, Academic Search Premier (via EBSCO), Communication and Mass Media Complete (via EBSCO), and Scopus. The search terms combine 'suicide' and a set of keywords relating to the media (media OR newspaper OR press OR print OR television OR radio OR film OR movie OR music OR book OR fiction OR internet OR web OR online), which were searched in article titles. In total, 1028 records were identified through database searching (ISI = 322, EBSCO = 384, Scopus = 322). After removing duplicates, 786 records remained for first stage screening.

Records that did not meet the following criteria were excluded from the review: (1) it must be published in English or Chinese so that they are readable by the authors; (2) it must use 'suicide' to refer to human suicidal thoughts or behaviors; (3) it must be an academic publication but not news articles, book reviews, film reviews, nor ads; (4) it must be an original research paper but not letters, commentaries, or conference abstracts; (5) its study objectives must include analyzing suicide-related media content; (6) it is not about suicide bombing or terrorism; (7) the media content in the study is neither historical nor fictional; and (8) it has full-text available for retrieval. Eventually, 61 papers remained for review.

Although previous review papers about suicide and the media often constructed their review by different media types (Blood and Pirkis, 2001; Gould, 2001), the present review is more concerned with similarities and differences in various societies. Therefore, we primarily grouped these papers by which countries'/regions' media were studied. Furthermore, we critically reviewed these papers to identify what factors possibly influenced media content of suicide in a society, broadly citing from relevant suicide research and media studies.

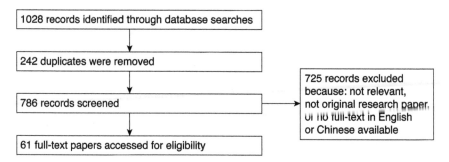

Figure 13.1 Procedure of the systematic literature screening (proposed by authors).

Results

Only 61 papers published from 1988 to 2013 were identified as relevant to the research topic, which suggests that the study of media content representation is still young and developing. These papers were published in journals from various disciplines, including suicide research, mental health research, public health research, journalism and media research, sociology, anthropology, and cultural studies, which demonstrates a broad concern with this research topic.

According to the World Health Organization and other research summaries (Levi *et al.*, 2003; World Health Organization, 2011), the highest annual suicide rates are reported from Eastern Europe (e.g. Lithuania, Hungary, Ukraine, Estonia, etc.) and some Eastern Asian countries (i.e. South Korea, Japan, China), followed by some Nordic/Western European countries (e.g. Finland, Belgium, Austria), Southeastern countries/regions (e.g. Hong Kong, Taiwan, Sri Lanka), and then English-speaking countries (i.e. the United States, the United Kingdom, Canada, Australia, New Zealand). Latin America and Islamic countries report lower annual suicide rates, whereas no official suicide data are available at all in some African countries.

As shown in Table 13.1, there is no clear association between the number of papers and the suicide rates in the country/region. Rather, a country/region's socio-economic development level seems to be more influential on the number of papers. Media content representation in developed countries/regions, such as the United States, Australia, and Hong Kong SAR, has been studied more; whereas there are very few studies conducted in developing countries, such as the Eastern European countries and China, despite high suicide rates there. No study has been conducted in South America and Africa, which might be related to low suicide rates or unavailability of suicide data in these countries.

Based on our review of the literature, we summarized similarities and differences between studies conducted in different countries/regions and discussed what factors possibly lead to these similarities and differences.

Table 13.1 Composition of the reviewed papers by country/region*

Composition of the articles	Number of papers	Suicide rates per 100,000 per year in most recent year available**	
		males	*females*
US	17	17.7	4.5
Australia	8	12.8	3.6
Hong Kong SAR	6	19.0	10/7
Japan	6	36.2	13.2
UK	4	10.9	3.0
Canada	3	17.3	5.4
Switzerland	3	24.8	11.4
Austria	3	23.8	7.1
New Zealand	2	18.1	5.5
Sweden	2	18.7	6.8
Finland	1	29.0	10.0
Belgium	1	28.8	10.3
Germany	1	17.9	6.0
Netherlands	1	13.1	5.5
Italy	1	10.0	2.8
Hungary	1	40.0	10.6
Estonia	1	30.6	7.3
Mexico	1	7.0	1.5
Mainland China	2	13.0	14.8
Taiwan	2	20.8***	11.5***
India	1	13.0	7.8
Israel	1	7.0	1.5

Notes:
*　Comparative study of more than one country's media representation is counted as one study for each of the countries.
**　Data obtained from the World Health Organization (2011). www.who.int/mental_health/prevention/suicide_rates/en/
**　Data obtained from Taiwan Ministry of Health and Welfare (2012), Cause of death statistics. www.mohw.gov.tw/EN/Ministry/Statistic.aspx?f_list_no=474&fod_list_no=4092

Similarities of media representation across countries

Some common features representing suicide in traditional media were noticed, when we compared findings from relevant papers. Most of these papers assessed the quality of traditional media reporting suicide by whether the reports were compliant with guidelines for responsible suicide reporting that were recommended by suicide prevention organizations, or whether suicide stories reported by the media match their counterparts in official records of suicides, such as coroners' reports or psychological autopsy. These studies were conducted in

Switzerland (Frey *et al.*, 1997; Michel *et al.*, 2000), Austria (Niederkrotenthaler and Sonneck, 2007; Niederkrotenthaler *et al.*, 2010), the US (Edwards-Stewart *et al.*, 2011; Jamieson *et al.*, 2003; Tatum *et al.*, 2010), Australia (Pirkis *et al.*, 2002, 2009), New Zealand (Thom *et al.*, 2012), India (Ramadas and Kuttichira, 2011), Israel (Weimann and Fishman, 1995), Hong Kong (Au *et al.*, 2004; Cheng and Yip, 2012; Fu and Yip, 2008), Taiwan (Chen *et al.*, 2012), and Mainland China (Fu *et al.*, 2011).

These papers found that the media in different countries commonly tend to over-report youth suicides and under-report elderly suicide (Au *et al.*, 2004; Chen *et al.*, 2012; Fu *et al.*, 2011; Niederkrotenthaler *et al.*, 2009; Pirkis *et al.*, 2002). In terms of the suicide person's background, celebrities or well-known names, famous or infamous, often attracted prominent reporting (Frost, 2011; Fu and Yip, 2008; Hamilton *et al.*, 2011; Michel *et al.*, 1995; Pirkis *et al.*, 2002; Stack, 1996; Tatum *et al.*, 2010; Van den Bulck and Claessens, 2013). In terms of suicide method, rare or novel methods, such as charcoal burning (Au *et al.*, 2004; Cheng and Yip, 2012), and violent methods, such as shooting and jumping (Frey *et al.*, 1997; Niederkrotenthaler *et al.*, 2009; Niederkrotenthaler *et al.*, 2010; Thom *et al.*, 2012; Weimann and Fishman, 1995), were associated with a higher likelihood of reporting than suicides by a common method – hanging (Chen *et al.*, 2012; Pirkis *et al.*, 2002).

Specifically, four studies, published in forensic journals, examined newspaper reports of homicide-suicide as an approach to monitor this issue in the United States (Malphurs and Cohen, 2002; Warren-Gordon *et al.*, 2010), the Netherlands (Liem and Koenraadt, 2007), and Italy (Roma *et al.*, 2012). These studies assumed that homicide-suicide incidences would highly likely be captured by the mass media. Therefore, when there is no national surveillance system for homicide-suicide, they suggested that media surveillance can be an alternative approach to monitor the incidence. These studies all found that the perpetrators were predominantly males and the victims were most often women and children. Firearms/guns were involved in most of the incidents.

In terms of attributes of what led to the suicides, they commonly found that suicide causes were over-simplified and pre-diagnosed mental disorder or depression was under-reported (Au *et al.*, 2004; Jamieson *et al.*, 2003; Niederkrotenthaler *et al.*, 2009; Pirkis *et al.*, 2002; Ramadas and Kuttichira, 2011; Tatum, *et al.*, 2010; Weimann and Fishman, 1995). There is an interesting case study of the representation of website-related suicides among various media, including traditional news outlets and news websites, in New Zealand (Thom *et al.*, 2011). The study found that these news reports often over-emphasized the role of online technology as 'enablers' or 'preventers' of suicide but largely overlooked the contribution of mental well-being to suicide.

The media's selective reporting patterns are not surprising, given that rare events are more newsworthy. However, when the readers are not aware of the media's selective reporting, the phenomenon may create a myth in their readers that youth suicides are more severe problems or novel suicide methods are more popular.

Certainly, we also noticed different findings between these studies and will report the differences in later sections. Nevertheless, the similarities of media representation cross-nationally suggest that there are common patterns in terms of the media's selective reporting of suicide. These findings supported the statement that the mass media were not simply *reporting* the reality but representing the reality based on their own selection and interpretation.

In addition, common patterns of online representation of suicide were also observed. When comparing first-three-page search results in Mainland China (Cheng *et al.*, 2011) and Hong Kong (Cheng, 2011) with those in the US (Recupero *et al.*, 2008) and the UK (Biddle *et al.*, 2008), the proportion of anti-suicide search results was all around 32.3 percent to 40 percent, higher than pro-suicide content. Chronologically, Westerlund (2012) compared first 100 Google search results when using 'suicide' as a keyword in 2005, 2009, and 2012 in English. It found that the majority of search results in all of the three years were suicide-preventive and provided by institutions such as government departments, NGOs, or associations, whereas there was no pro-suicide result found in 2012. The findings suggest that online representation of suicide is mainly formulated by anti-suicide content, in terms of quantity. However, when assessing the quality of online representation of suicide risk factors or warning signs by whether they are compliant with scientific research findings, two studies of English content (Mandrusiak *et al.*, 2006; Szumilas and Kutcher, 2009) both found that over half of the online content was not evidence-based or too vague to be useful.

The findings of online representation of suicide show that online platforms allow organizations and individuals to publish more anti-suicide information, which break the traditional mass media's monopoly of media representation. However, the quality of online anti-suicide content, as well as the quality of traditional media's suicide reports, still need to be improved.

Cultural tradition and different media representation

Besides similarities, more research findings demonstrate that media represent-ation of suicide varies from country to country, or even within the same country. Cultural tradition is often referred to as the primary reason to explain these differences.

A cross-cultural study compared suicide reports in Hungary, Japan, the United States, Germany, Austria, and Finland in 1981 and 1991 (Fekete *et al.*, 2001) and found significant differences. They observed that the Hungarian media, compared with the other five counterparts, significantly more often represented suicide as an effective 'communicative force' that evoked positive valuations in the mass media. Meanwhile, the Hungarian media did not clearly present positive attitudes toward suicide but ambivalence. In the Japanese media, suicide was more often framed as related to group affiliation, attachment, and traditional methods and less frequently with psychopathol-ogy and abnormality. Meanwhile, the American, Finnish, and German media represented suicide more unambiguously, emphasizing pain and the painful circumstances of suicide, highlighting the consequent sufferings of other people, and the association with mental illness or criminality. The report was rather brief and did not provide detailed data of their findings. Nonetheless, it demonstrated the cross-country differences and warranted more studies on this topic.

We know that Hungary and Japan both suffer from high suicide rates (World Health Organization, 2011). Suicide rates in Hungary are comparable with Japan, and were even the highest in the world in the years between 1960 and 2000 (Rihmer et al., 2013). However, the reason for the high suicide rates in Hungary is not fully understood and the media content of suicide in this country was rarely studied. By contrast, five papers about media content in Japan were identified through our literature screen. Previous studies have noticed that Japanese culture contains norms to tolerate suicide as a way to fulfill one's responsibility or duty as a member of highly formal and tightly-knit human groups and classes (Fusé, 1980), which was consistent with Fekete et al.'s findings of Japanese media content. Furthermore, four studies in our review pool (Ikunaga et al., 2013; Ozawa-De Silva, 2008, 2010; Seko, 2008), through analyzing suicide content in online groups, forums, or bulletin boards, demonstrated that the traditional collective culture in Japan is still represented in suicide-related online content. Ozawa-De Silva (2008, 2010) argued that the emerging phenomenon of forming suicide groups/pacts through the internet are still reflecting Japanese traditional conceptions of self, in which the dominant cultural rhetoric ties selfhood closely to the social self that is the object of perception and experience by others. In other words, individuals in such a society often perceive a need for social connectedness and the fear of social rejection and isolation, which was also represented in their participation in online suicide groups and wish to die together. Seko (2008) argued that online discussion forums about suicide not only facilitated individuals to look for suicide companions but also served as a social outlet to freely disclose their pent-up struggles. However, no matter on which side of the forum, Seko noticed that forum participants' discourses reflect the collective culture, collectively committing suicide or collectively transgressing social taboos of suicide. Ikunaga and colleagues (Ikunaga et al., 2013) found that the posts on the online BBS contained themes related to those identified in western psychological theories of suicide (e.g., psychological pain, mental illness, hopelessness, and escape). However, when analyzing the content more closely, they found that these themes still represented individuals' interpersonal concerns (e.g., seeking connection online, interpersonal conflict, lack of support, and group suicide wish), which are deeply embedded in Japanese culture.

Japanese researchers' findings are interestingly contrasted with another study of online pro-suicide content in Sweden (Westerlund, 2012). Westerlund conducted a qualitative content analysis with a typical Swedish pro-suicide website and found that the pro-suicide content on this website was produced as a critique of the whole of society and its institutions and strongly emphasized individualism and anti-social currents, which have their roots in Western cultural and civilization history.

Cultural tradition is not only influencing the media representation of attitudes towards suicide, but also is influencing media stereotypes of certain suicide phenomena. Both in Hong Kong (Cheng and Yip, 2012) and Taiwan (Chen *et al.*, 2012), male suicides were stereotyped as being associated with work-related issues, unmanageable debt, or legal problems, whereas female suicides were often attributed to mental illness or relationship breakups. These gender-specific stereotypes were considered to be related to traditional Chinese culture that men should be stronger and are the breadwinners in the family while women are weaker and more fragile (Chen *et al.*, 2012). A study from Mexico (Reyes-Foster, 2013) highlighted ethnic stereotypes regarding suicide in the Yucatecan media. It observed that the local media stereotyped suicides as associated with young, poor, alcoholic men with Mayan last names and by hanging. The author argued that the stereotyping is rooted in the local society's discrimination against Mayan natives and reinforced the stigma of suicide.

Media ecology and different media representation

Besides Fekete *et al.*'s cross-national comparison, another paper conducted a comparison of media content in three societies sharing Chinese cultural traditions, namely, Hong Kong, Taiwan, and Guangzhou (Fu *et al.*, 2011). Suicide rates in the three societies are all over 13 per 100,000, which can be considered relatively high. The study screened suicide news articles published in Hong Kong, Taiwan, and Guangzhou, which are all Chinese societies but have different political and legal systems, in 2006. The study adopted WHO media guidelines for suicide reporting to assess suicide news reports in the three societies. It found that Hong Kong newspapers reported suicide news significantly more frequently and sensationally (e.g. more often publicizing photos or graphics but less often including preventive advice) than Guangzhou ones. In addition, the Hong Kong media more often reported attempted suicide than completed suicide, which was the reverse of the Guangzhou and Taiwan media. The study did not discuss much of what led to the differences among the three societies. Nonetheless, its findings demonstrated that media representation of suicide might be influenced by complex factors, besides cultural traditions. The media ecology, as well as the political and legal systems that the media are monitored by, are distinct in Hong Kong, Taiwan, and Mainland China.

Even within the same society, studies have noticed that tabloid-type media often represented suicide stories more frequently and sensationally than others (Cheng and Yip, 2012; Frey, *et al.*, 1997). When the media ecology in a society includes more tabloid-type media and vigorous media competition, the overall media representation of suicide news may tend to be more sensational (Chen *et al.*, 2011; Cheng, *et al.*, in press; Weimann and Fishman, 1995).

The differences between tabloid-type media and the others can be significant when they are faced with a dilemma of taste versus news value. One example was when Pennsylvania State Treasurer R. Budd Dwyer invited the media to a press conference and committed suicide there, the media had to choose whether or not to publish graphic photos of the event (Kochersberger, 1988). While tabloid-type media would maximize news values and represent suicide dramatically, some media chose to put taste over news values and report suicide with respect for the bereaved (Blood *et al.*, 2007; Etzersdorfer *et al.*, 2001; Kochersberger, 1988).

To counterbalance the media's selective and sensational reporting of suicide, as mentioned in the previous section, media guidelines for responsible reporting suicide have been developed and implemented in various countries (Bohanna and Wang, 2012; Pirkis *et al.*, 2006). However, the implementation of these guidelines in different societies has faced different effectiveness (Bohanna and Wang, 2012). In Austria (Niederkrotenthaler and Sonneck, 2007; Niederkrotenthaler *et al.*, 2010), Switzerland (Frey *et al.*, 1997; Michel *et al.*, 2000), and Australia (Pirkis *et al.*, 2009), the media representation of suicide has improved significantly in terms of less sensational and prominent coverage and more often portrayal of suicide as related to mental illness. However, in Hong Kong (Fu and Yip, 2008) and the US (Tatum *et al.*, 2010), the effectiveness of the media guidelines was found to be slight, which was believed to be related to the highly competitive media ecology in these societies.

Several qualitative studies have conducted an in-depth investigation of the process of how a suicide event was represented by the media in a certain media context. These studies demonstrated that journalists and opinion leaders played important roles in framing suicide stories or problems (Chesebro and McMahan, 2006; Cover, 2012; Frost, 2011; Siu, 2008). In addition, the representation can be more preventive if the bereaved ones can honestly tell the public that the deceased suffered from mental illness and suicide prevention professionals can actively provide suicide prevention information to the media (Jobes and Berman, 1996; Tousignant *et al.*, 2005).

Interaction between online and offline representation

As reported previously, a few studies examined what kinds of content are accessible online when a person uses a popular search engine to look for suicide-related information. Besides the similarity that the majority of online content shows anti-suicide tendency, the proportion of pro-suicide search results in Hong Kong (Cheng, 2011) (2.8 percent) and Mainland China (4.2 percent) (Cheng *et al.*, 2011) were much fewer than the figures reported by the US study (Recupero *et al.*, 2008) (11.7 percent) and the UK study (Biddle, *et al.*, 2008) (9 percent). In addition, anti-suicide websites in Chinese provided less information on seeking help and there were fewer government or professional mental health websites in Chinese. Furthermore, the Hong Kong study noticed that when using search terms such as 'suicide method', 'charcoal burning suicide', and 'painless suicide', the first page search results were often pro-suicide information, which suggests that the online representation of suicide might be different when the internet users are looking for the information for different purposes. These findings suggest that the quality of online anti-suicide information is related to offline availability and quality of mental health services in a society (Cheng *et al.*, 2011).

In addition, one paper about online discussion of a murder-suicide case in Estonia (Sisask *et al.*, 2012) showed that online comments on this suicide case were initiated by traditional media's reports of the case and many of them stemmed from dominant topics provided by newspaper articles. On the other hand, the authors also noticed that some online comments were not directly related to newspaper articles' content but individuals' own value judgments.

Discussion

The study of non-fictional media representation of suicide is relatively young but developing rapidly and attracting interest from a broad range of disciplines around the world. However, the development of the field has shown uneven distribution in various aspects. In terms of geographic regions, more studies were conducted in developed regions than developing regions, despite the severe level of suicide rates in the regions. In terms of medium types, textual media content was more studied than video and audio content. More studies are needed to fill these gaps.

Our review shows that non-fictional media representation of suicide case or suicide problems is based on real incidence and can, to a certain extent, reflect the real incidence. This is why some forensic studies proposed using newspaper surveillance as an alternative approach to understand homicide-suicide problem when a national surveillance system is not available. However, when official records are available to compare with media reports, researchers commonly observed that the media representation of suicide is different from official records or professional psychological autopsy findings of suicide, no matter in traditional media or online media. The media's selective representation of suicide is related to some common news values shared by the media across the world. Celebrity suicides, youth suicides, and suicides using rare or violent methods are commonly more appealing to the media. The phenomenon reminds us not to under-estimate how challenging it is if we want to engage the media in suicide prevention efforts. Meanwhile, the process of media representation of suicide is not only manipulated by the media, but also by various stakeholders such as opinion leaders, bereaved ones, suicide prevention professionals, and some readers. The involvement of various stakeholders can shape or change the media representation of suicide. One example is the effectiveness of the implementation of media guidelines in some countries. The other example is the framing of Kurt Cobain's suicide led to more suicide prevention when the bereaved ones shared their experiences with the public and suicide prevention professionals actively engaged with the media. The implication of these findings is that we need to work with diverse stakeholders, not merely media professionals, to change the media representation of suicide toward being more preventive.

In addition, the process of constructing media representation is dynamic and evolving within a certain social context, where cultural traditions are still powerfully influential. Our review shows that the media often interpret or frame suicide stories following traditional attitudes toward suicide and social stereotypes of gender, ethnicity, and so on. The media's representation, furthermore, reinforces these social norms and stereotypes. Some of these social norms and stereotypes are actually myths or stigma about suicide and would hinder suicide prevention. Our review warrants further investigation on the relationships between cultural traditions, the media representation of suicide, and actual suicide incidence.

In addition, our review identifies that interactions between online and offline media lead to more diverse media representation of suicide. For example, in our review, one study showed that individuals' online comments on a suicide story that was reported by traditional media were sometimes not directly influenced by the media framing but more rooted in cultural traditions. In other words, traditional media's function as a gatekeeper of information is weakened by the accessibility of new media. The online diversity allows suicide prevention organizations and professionals to contribute more content to represent a more preventive reality. However, the diversity also allows the traditional stigma regarding suicide, which might have been restrained in traditional media because of journalism ethics or implementation of media guidelines, to be represented through individuals' representation. Therefore, one can predict that we may observe more cross-cultural differences rather than similarities of media representation of suicide on the internet, compared with traditional media. Whether the prediction is true needs to be tested by future studies. If it is true, it means that the new media are not only allowing information to flow around the world but also facilitating local culture or minority culture to regain a voice. Therefore, our future efforts to promote suicide prevention through the media will have to be more localized and pay more attention to local culture.

Our review generates a comprehensive and dynamic process of producing media representation of suicide in various societies. There are still numerous gaps on this research topic. Besides the uneven distribution of studies in different societies and different media types, there is also a lack of comparative studies of media representation, cross-regionally as well as longitudinally.

In summary, our review demonstrates that, for suicide research, examining media representation of suicide can be a useful research approach to decode social contexts and norms of suicide at both population and individual levels. For suicide prevention practices, our review suggests that professionals play a more proactive role in constructing the media representation of suicide and lead the evolution of media representation to a more preventive one.

References

Adoni, H. and Mane, S. (1984). Media and the social construction of reality: Toward an integration of theory and research. *Communication Research*, 11(3), 323–340.
Au, J. S. K., Yip, P. S. F., Chan, C. L. W., and Law, Y. W. (2004). Newspaper reporting of suicide cases in Hong Kong. *Crisis*, 25(4), 161–168.

Biddle, L., Donovan, J., Hawton, K., Kapur, N., and Gunnell, D. (2008). Suicide and the Internet. *British Medical Journal*, 336(7648), 800–802.

Biddle, L., Gunnell, D., Owen-Smith, A., Potokar, J., Longson, D., Hawton, K., *et al.* (2012). Information sources used by the suicidal to inform choice of method. *Journal of Affective Disorders*, 136(3), 702–709.

Blood, R. W., and Pirkis, J. (2001). Suicide and the media. *Crisis: Journal of Crisis Intervention and Suicide*, 22(4), 163–169.

Blood, R. W., Pirkis, J., and Holland, K. (2007). Media reporting of suicide methods: An Australian perspective. *Crisis: Journal of Crisis Intervention and Suicide Prevention*, 28(S1), 64–69.

Bohanna, I., and Wang, X. (2012). Media guidelines for the responsible reporting of suicide: a review of effectiveness. *Crisis*, 33(4), 190–198.

Chen, Y. Y., Chen, F., and Yip, P. S. F. (2011). The impact of media reporting of suicide on actual suicides in Taiwan, 2002–05. *Journal of Epidemiology and Community Health*, 65(10), 934–940.

Chen, Y. Y., Chen, F., Gunnell, D., and Yip, P. S. F. (2013). The impact of media reporting on the emergence of charcoal burning suicide in Taiwan. *PLoS One*, 8(1).

Chen, Y. Y., Yip, P. S. F., Tsai, C. W., and Fan, H. F. (2012). Media representation of gender patterns of suicide in Taiwan. *Crisis*, 33(3), 144–150

Cheng, A. T. A., Hawton, K., Chen, T. H. H., Yen, A. M. F., Chang, J. C., Chong, M. Y., *et al.* (2007). The influence of media reporting of a celebrity suicide on suicidal behavior in patients with a history of depressive disorder. *Journal of Affective Disorders*, 103(1–3), 69–75.

Cheng, Q. (2011). Online suicide-related information in Hong Kong: Perspectives from youth suicide prevention. *Journal of Youth Studies* (in Chinese), 14(1), 74–85.

Cheng, Q., Fu, K. W., Caine, E., and Yip, P. S. (2014). Why do we report suicides and how can we facilitate suicide prevention efforts? Perspectives from Hong Kong media professionals. *Crisis*, 35(2), 74–81.

Cheng, Q., Fu, K. W., and Yip, P. S. (2011). A comparative study of online suicide-related information in Chinese and English. *Journal of Clinical Psychiatry*, 72(3), 313–319.

Cheng, Q. and Yip, P. S. F. (2012). Suicide news reporting accuracy and stereotyping in Hong Kong. *Journal of Affective Disorders*, 141(2), 270–275.

Chesebro, J. W. and McMahan, D. T. (2006). Media constructions of mass murder-suicides as drama: The *New York Times'* symbolic construction of mass murder-suicides. *Communication Quarterly*, 54(4), 407–425.

Cover, R. (2012). Mediating suicide: Print journalism and the categorization of queer youth suicide discourses. *Archives of Sexual Behavior*, 41(5), 1173–1183.

Edwards-Stewart, A., Kinn, J. T., June, J. D., and Fullerton, N. R. (2011). Military and civilian media coverage of suicide. *Archives of Suicide Research*, 15(4), 304–312.

Etzersdorfer, E., Voracek, M., and Sonneck, G. (2001). A dose-response relationship of imitational suicides with newspaper distribution. *Australian and New Zealand Journal of Psychiatry*, 35(2), 251–255.

Fekete, S., Schmidtke, A., Takahashi, Y., Etzersdorfer, E., Upanne, M., and Osvath, P. (2001). Mass media, cultural attitudes, and suicide. Results of an international comparative study. *Crisis*, 22(4), 170–172.

Frey, C., Michel, K., and Valach, L. (1997). Suicide reporting in Swiss print media: Responsible or irresponsible? *European Journal of Public Health*, 7(1), 15–19.

Frost, J. (2011). Movie star suicide, Hollywood gossip, and popular psychology in the 1950s and 1960s. *Journal of American Culture*, 34(2), 113–123.

Fu, K. W., Chan, Y. Y., and Yip, P. S. F. (2011). Newspaper reporting of suicides in Hong Kong, Taiwan and Guangzhou: Compliance with WHO media guidelines and epidemiological comparisons. *Journal of Epidemiology and Community Health*, 65(10), 928–933.

Fu, K. W., and Yip, P. S. F. (2007). Long-term impact of celebrity suicide on suicidal ideation: Results from a population-based study. *Journal of Epidemiology and Community Health*, 61(6), 540–546.

Fu, K. W. and Yip, P. S. F. (2008). Changes in reporting of suicide news after the promotion of the WHO media recommendations. *Suicide and Life-Threatening Behavior*, 38(5), 631–636.

Fusé, T. (1980). Suicide and culture in Japan: A study of seppuku as an institutionalized form of suicide. *Social Psychiatry*, 15(2), 57–63.

Gamson, W. A., Croteau, D., Hoynes, W., and Sasson, T. (1992). Media images and the social construction of reality. *Annual Review of Sociology*, 18, 373–393.

Gould, M., Jamieson, P., and Romer, D. (2003). Media contagion and suicide among the young. *American Behavioral Scientist*, 46(9), 1269–1284.

Gould, M. S. (2001). Suicide and the media. In H. Hendin and J. J. Mann (Eds), *Suicide Prevention: Clinical and Scientific Aspects* (Annals of the New York Academy of Sciences, pp. 200–224). New York: New York Academy of Sciences.

Hamilton, S., Metcalfe, C., and Gunnell, D. (2011). Media reporting and suicide: A time-series study of suicide from Clifton Suspension Bridge, UK, 1974–2007. *Journal of Public Health*, 33(4), 511–517.

Ikunaga, A., Nath, S. R., and Skinner, K. A. (2013). Internet suicide in Japan: A qualitative content analysis of a suicide bulletin board. *Transcultural Psychiatry*, 50(2), 280–302.

Jamieson, P., Jamieson, K. H., and Romer, D. (2003). The responsible reporting of suicide in print journalism. *American Behavioral Scientist*, 46(12), 1643–1660.

Jobes, D. A. and Berman, A. L. (1996). The Kurt Cobain suicide crisis: Perspectives from research, public health, and the news media. *Suicide and Life-Threatening Behavior*, 26(3), 260–269.

Kochersberger, J. R. C. (1988). Survey of suicide photos use by newspapers in three states. *Newspaper Research Journal*, 9(4), 1–12.

Lee, D. T. S., Chan, K. P. M., and Yip, P. S. F. (2005). Charcoal burning is also popular for suicide pacts made on the internet. *British Medical Journal*, 330(7491), 602.

Levi, F., La Vecchia, C., Lucchini, F., Negri, E., Saxena, S., Maulik, P. K., and Saraceno, B. (2003). Trends in mortality from suicide, 1965–99. *Acta Psychiatrica Scandinavica*, 108(5), 341–349.

Liberati, A., Altman, D. G., Tetzlaff, J., Mulrow, C., Gøtzsche, P. C., Ioannidis, J. P. A., *et al.* (2009). The PRISMA statement for reporting systematic reviews and meta-analyses of studies that evaluate health care interventions: Explanation and elaboration. *PLoS Med*, 6(7), e1000100.

Liem, M. C. A. and Koenraadt, F. (2007). Homicide-suicide in the Netherlands: A study of newspaper reports, 1992–2005. *Journal of Forensic Psychiatry and Psychology*, 18(4), 482–493.

Malphurs, J. E. and Cohen, D. (2002). A newspaper surveillance study of homicide-suicide in the United States. *American Journal of Forensic Medicine and Pathology*, 23(2), 142–148.

Mandrusiak, M., Rudd, M. D., Joiner, T. E., Berman, A. L., Van Orden, K. A., and Witte, T. (2006). Warning signs for suicide on the Internet: A descriptive study. *Suicide and Life-Threatening Behavior*, 36(3), 263–271.

Michel, K., Frey, C., Schlaepfer, T. E., and Valach, L. (1995). Suicide reporting in the Swiss print media: Frequency, form and content of articles. *European Journal of Public Health*, 5(3), 199–203.

Michel, K., Frey, C., Wyss, K., and Valach, L. (2000). An exercise in improving suicide reporting in print media. *Crisis*, 21(2), 71–79.

Niederkrotenthaler, T., Fu, K. W., Yip, P. S. F., Fong, D. Y. T., Stack, S., Cheng, Q., and Pirkis, J. (2012). Changes in suicide rates following media reports on celebrity suicide: A meta-analysis. *Journal of Epidemiology and Community Health*, 66(11), 1037–1042.

Niederkrotenthaler, T. and Sonneck, G. (2007). Assessing the impact of media guidelines for reporting on suicides in Austria: Interrupted time series analysis. *Australian and New Zealand Journal of Psychiatry*, 41(5), 419–428.

Niederkrotenthaler, T., Till, B., Herberth, A., Voracek, M., Kapusta, N. D., Etzersdorfer, E., *et al.* (2009). The gap between suicide characteristics in the print media and in the population. *European Journal of Public Health*, 19(4), 361–364.

Niederkrotenthaler, T., Voracek, M., Herberth, A., Till, B., Strauss, M., Etzersdorfer, E., *et al.* (2010). Role of media reports in completed and prevented suicide: Werther v. Papageno effects. *British Journal of Psychiatry*, 197(3), 234–243.

O'Connor, R. C., Platt, S., and Gordon, J. (2011). *International Handbook of Suicide Prevention: Research, Policy, and Practice.* Chichester: Wiley-Blackwell.

Ozawa-De Silva, C. (2008). Too lonely to die alone: Internet suicide pacts and existential suffering in Japan. *Culture, Medicine and Psychiatry*, 32(4), 516–551.

Ozawa-De Silva, C. (2010). Shared death: Self, sociality and internet group suicide in Japan. *Transcultural Psychiatry*, 47(3), 392–418.

Pirkis, J. and Blood, R. W. (2001a). Suicide and the media. Part I: Reportage in nonfictional media. *Crisis*, 22(4), 146–154.

Pirkis, J., and Blood, R. W. (2001b). Suicide and the media. Part II: Portrayal in fictional media. *Crisis*, 22(4), 155–162.

Pirkis, J., Blood, R. W., Beautrais, A., Burgess, P., and Skehan, J. (2006). Media guidelines on the reporting of suicide. *Crisis: Journal of Crisis Intervention and Suicide Prevention*, 27(2), 82–87.

Pirkis, J., Dare, A., Blood, R. W., Rankin, B., Williamson, M., Burgess, P., and Jolley, D. (2009). Changes in media reporting of suicide in Australia between 2000/01 and 2006/07. *Crisis*, 30(1), 25–33.

Pirkis, J., Francis, C., Blood, R. W., Burgess, P., Morley, B., Stewart, A., and Putnis, P. (2002). Reporting of suicide in the Australian media. *Australian and New Zealand Journal of Psychiatry*, 36(2), 190–197.

Ramadas, S. and Kuttichira, P. (2011). The development of a guideline and its impact on the media reporting of suicide. *Indian Journal of Psychiatry*, 53(3), 224–228.

Recupero, P. R., Harms, S. E., and Noble, J. M. (2008). Googling suicide: Surfing for suicide information on the internet. *Journal of Clinical Psychiatry*, 69(6), 878–888.

Reyes-Foster, B. (2013). He followed the funereal steps of ixtab: The pleasurable aesthetics of suicide in newspaper journalism in Yucatán, Mexico. *Journal of Latin American and Caribbean Anthropology*, 18(2), 251–273.

Rihmer, Z., Gonda, X., Kapitany, B., and Dome, P. (2013). Suicide in Hungary-epidemiological and clinical perspectives. *Annals of General Psychiatry*, 12(1), 21

Roma, P., Spacca, A., Pompili, M., Lester, D., Tatarelli, R., Girardi, P., and Ferracuti, S. (2012). The epidemiology of homicide-suicide in Italy: A newspaper study from 1985 to 2008. *Forensic Science International*, 214(1–3), e1–e5.

Schudson, M. (1997). The sociology of news production. In D. A. Berkowitz (Ed.), *Social Meanings of News: A Text-Reader* (pp. 7–22). Thousand Oaks, CA: Sage Publications.

Seko, Y. (2008). 'Suicide machine' seekers: Transgressing suicidal taboos online. *Learning Inquiry*, 2(3), 181–199.

Sisask, M., Mark, L., and Värnik, A. (2012). Internet comments elicited by media portrayal of a familicide-suicide case. *Crisis*, 33(4), 222–229.

Siu, W. L. W. (2008). News discourse of teachers' suicide: Education and journalism: Media coverage of an educational crisis. *Journal of Asian Pacific Communication*, 18(2), 247–267.

Stack, S. (1996). The effect of the media on suicide: Evidence from Japan, 1955–1985. *Suicide and Life-Threatening Behavior*, 26(2), 132–142.

Stack, S. (2003). Media coverage as a risk factor in suicide. *Journal of Epidemiology and Community Health*, 57(4), 238–240.

Stack, S. (2005). Suicide in the media: A quantitative review of studies based on nonfictional stories. *Suicide and Life-Threatening Behavior*, 35(2), 121–133.

Szumilas, M., and Kutcher, S. (2009). Teen suicide information on the internet: A systematic analysis of quality. *Canadian Journal of Psychiatry*, 54(9), 596–604.

Tatum, P. T., Canetto, S. S., and Slater, M. D. (2010). Suicide coverage in US newspapers following the publication of the media guidelines. *Suicide and Life-Threatening Behavior*, 40(5), 524–534.

Thom, K., Edwards, G., Nakarada-Kordic, I., McKenna, B., O'Brien, A., and Nairn, R. (2011). Suicide online: Portrayal of website-related suicide by the New Zealand media. *New Media and Society*, 13(8), 1355–1372.

Thom, K., McKenna, B., Edwards, G., O'Brien, A., and Nakarada-Kordic, I. (2012). Reporting of suicide by the New Zealand media. *Crisis*, 33(4), 199–207.

Tousignant, M., Mishara, B. L., Caillaud, A., Fortin, V., and St-Laurent, D. (2005). The impact of media coverage of the suicide of a well-known Quebec reporter: The case of Gaetan Girouard. *Social Science and Medicine*, 60(9), 1919–1926.

Tsai, J. F. (2010). The media and suicide: Evidence-based on population data over 9 years in Taiwan. *Suicide and Life-Threatening Behavior*, 40(1), 81–86.

Van den Bulck, H., and Claessens, N. (2013). Celebrity suicide and the search for the moral high ground: Comparing frames in media and audience discussions of the death of a Flemish celebrity. *Critical Studies in Media Communication*, 30(1), 69–84.

Warren-Gordon, K., Byers, B. D., Brodt, S. J., Wartak, M., and Biskupski, B. (2010). Murder followed by suicide: A newspaper surveillance study using the New York *Times* index. *Journal of Forensic Sciences*, 55(6), 1592–1597.

Wasserman, D. and Wasserman, C. (2009). *Oxford Textbook of Suicidology and Suicide Prevention*. Oxford and New York: Oxford University Press.

Weimann, G., and Fishman, G. (1995). Reconstructing suicide: Reporting suicide in the Israeli press. *Journalism and Mass Communication Quarterly*, 72(3), 551–558.

Westerlund, M. (2012). The production of pro-suicide content on the internet: A counter-discourse activity. *New Media and Society*, 14(5), 764–780.

World Health Organization. (2011). *Mental Health: Suicide Prevention (SUPRE)*. Retrieved from www.who.int/mental_health/prevention/suicide/suicideprevent/en/

Yip, P. S., Kwok, S. S., Chen, F., Xu, X., and Chen, Y. Y. (2013). A study on the mutual causation of suicide reporting and suicide incidences. *Journal of Affective Disorders*, 148(1), 98–103.

14 The formal assessment of suicide risk

Bruce Bongar, Elvin Sheykhani,
Uri Kugel and David Giannini

This chapter examines data and findings on the formal assessment of suicide risk, and provides recommendations for the consideration of risk factors, protective factors, and symptoms presentation. In addition, common obstacles for mental health providers in approaching clients exhibiting suicide risk are examined and recommendations for a variety of formal and structured approaches in the assessment of suicide are discussed.

What is formal risk and suicide assessment?

The formal assessment of suicide risk is a practice in which medical professionals, mental health practitioners, and at times peace officers assess an individual for the potential to harm the self, others, or for grave disability. If risk is deemed to meet medical necessity, safety procedures such as safety planning and hospitalization may be utilized. This chapter will focus on formal risk assessment as it pertains to suicidal risk. Formal risk assessments include integrating a clinical interview, behavioral observations such as a mental status exam, historical and contextual factors, as well as evidence-based practice (Jacobs, 2007). Formal risk assessment varies depending on the setting (such as a hospital, mental health clinic, or jail), the population at hand, the nature of the disorder, as well as factors such as severity of psychopathology, and history of past suicidal behavior. Accurate risk assessment requires a clinician to skillfully integrate clinical judgment with evidence-based practice to accurately predict behavior. This practice is inherently difficult, and prone to false positives (Bongar, 1991). Suicide risk assessment is necessary to establish the likelihood of lethal behavior within the immediate future. Suicide risk management is an ongoing and collaborative process in the treatment of suicidal clients. It is conducted systematically and on the availability of clinically relevant information (Jacobs, 2007).

Why is formal risk assessment important?

Mental health practitioners and health care professionals who lack competence and training treating individuals with suicidality are shown to hinder recovery, as well as the disclosure of suicidal thoughts and behaviors. Furthermore, clinicians without adequate training often promote stigma, and contribute to poor clinical outcomes (Meerwijk *et al.*, 2010; Pauley, 2008; Registered Nurses' Association of Ontario, 2009). The severity of the suicidal risk informs decisions in terms of the interventions employed to maintain an individual's safety, as well as scope of the treatments going forward. Treatment, including screening and assessment for suicidality, needs to be considered at all points of entry into the mental health care system, in day-to-day clinical practice, or at frequent intervals of care, depending on the treatment setting. The severity of suicide risk assessed should inform the care interventions, levels of observation, ongoing screening and treatment approaches (Registered Nurses' Association of Ontario, 2009). Utilizing formal risk assessment allows clinicians to begin the stepwise process of assessing the severity of risk, and target their interventions directly at stabilization and safety planning for a client.

Suicide rate statistics

Suicide is a major concern for mental health professionals, regardless of the setting in which they are employed. A mere 5 percent of clinical psychologists reported that they had never treated a suicidal client. Suicidality is not only the most common psychological emergency, but also is distinct in its potential for fatality (Packman *et al.*, 2004). Despite the many deaths due to suicide, prediction is still quite difficult (Packman *et al.*, 2004). In the United States, each year there are over 713,000 emergency department visits due to self-inflicted injuries. Since 1950, completed suicides have risen by 60 percent, and within the United States over 38,000 people die from suicide each year. (Centers for Disease Control and Prevention [CDC], 2010a). Research states that one in three practicing clinical psychologists have lost a patient to suicide, and over half of all practicing psychiatrists have experienced a similar loss (Bersoff, 1999; McAdams and Foster, 2000; McIntosh, 1993). According to the CDC, suicide remains the second leading cause of death of individuals 25–34, and is the third leading cause of death overall for people 15–24. In 2009, 8.3 million Americans reported having suicidal ideation, and an estimated 2.2 million Americans reported having made suicidal plans within the last year. An overall estimated 1 million Americans (0.5 percent of the US adult population) reported making a suicide attempt (CDC, 2012).

Critical areas and screening of suicidality

The Risk Management Foundation of the Harvard Medical Institution (RMFHMI) (1996) states that adequate assessment of potentially suicidal clients begins with a comprehensive psychiatric and psychological evaluation, which includes a detailed mental status examination, relevant psychosocial history, and the integration of physical/laboratory examinations. The RMFHMI notes that suicide risk assessment should occur across four domains: (1) identifying risk factors, and distinguishing chronic and acute stressors; (2) identifying protective factors; (3) conducting an open, nonjudgmental, and comprehensive inquiry into the client's suicidal ideation; and (4) the use of information gathering within the clinical interview and assessment to distinguish client's level of risk, treatment and/or safety planning (Jacobs, 2007; RMFHMI, 1996; Shea, 2002).

Clinical diagnosis and relation to risk

Shea (2002) discussed critical areas of exploration within a risk assessment across five domains. A client's current functioning in terms of mental illness is important in terms of co-morbid disorders as well as co-occurring substance use. Severity and onset of a mental disorder such as schizophrenia often impact a client's propensity toward suicidal behavior (Gliatto and Rai, 1999). Understanding a disorder's course and baseline behaviors proves fruitful for clinicians assessing for potential harm to the self. Disorders such as Borderline Personality Disorder and Post Traumatic Stress Disorder have been shown to have high rates of suicidal behavior, and baseline knowledge of tendencies of individuals diagnosed with these disorders proves helpful to clinicians in understanding predilections toward such behaviors (Gliatto and Rai, 1999). Substance use disorders are often comorbid with mental illness; which further impact a client's functioning. Substances such as alcohol have a disinhibiting effect, which often lead to suicidal behavior. In study conducted by the CDC (2010b), 33.3 percent of all individuals who completed suicide tested positive for alcohol.

History of suicidal behaviors

During the clinical interview, it is imperative for a clinician to assess a client's history of suicidal behaviors. Understanding prior attempts, aborted attempts, and family history of suicidal behaviors proves crucial in treatment and safety planning. Being able to view past antecedents to a behavior, and provide possible coping strategies if similar situations arise are the essence of proper safety planning (Jacobs, 2007; RMFHMI, 1996; Shea, 2002). Assessing suicide-related symptomatology provides a basis on which the client and clinician may collaborate and address risk accordingly. Assessing past and present suicidal ideation, hopelessness, and low positive emotions are thought to be crucial during the initial phase of assessment. Degree of hopelessness is one of the best correlates to attempted and complete suicidal behaviors (Centre for Applied Research in Mental Health and Addiction [CARMHA], 2007). This further highlights the need of clinicians at large to understand the contextual and symptomatic factors that lead to suicidal behaviors. Arming a clinician with baseline knowledge of suicidal behaviors and symptoms provides utility in the assessment process. Without this bench-to-bedside approach, a clinician may find themselves overlooking pertinent and clinically relevant data. Being well read on the current scientific literature provides a clinician with the ability to provide competent and comprehensive services.

Client strengths and vulnerabilities

Understanding a client's strengths and vulnerabilities provides a clinician further information within the formal risk assessment process. Suicidal behaviors are often employed due to inadequate coping abilities. If an individual demonstrates inadequate coping abilities, these will often become a target of an intervention. An individual may see their situation as obdurate, or irreconcilable. These negative cognitions are often compounded by hopelessness, and suicide is viewed as the only option to escape intolerable distress. These distorted cognitions are often the root of suicidal behavior, and arming individuals with a means of coping with their negative situation may bolster hope, and alleviate some of the distress (Baumeister, 1990; Gliatto and Rai, 1999; Jacobs, 1997; RMFHMI, 1996). Low distress tolerance has also been identified as vulnerability for suicidal behaviors. An individual with low distress tolerance may be more likely to underestimate their ability to cope, and view their psychological distress as unavoidable by means other than suicidal behaviors (Jacobs, 2007; RHFHMI, 1996; Shea, 2002). Furthermore, understanding a client's ability for reality testing provides clinical utility, which is crucial in risk assessment often suicidal behaviors partly stem from cognitive distortions. Assessing a client's ability to put these cognitive distortions to a test of reality provides some alleviation of distress and may be an individual strength.

Risk factors of self-harm

There is no single predictor that assesses for suicidality with 100 percent certainty. Assessment of acute and chronic suicidality appreciates the complexity of correlation between risk factors and their compounding effect that predispose an individual to suicidal behaviors (Bongar, 1991; Sullivan and Bongar, 2009; Shea, 2002). Individuals afflicted by multiple risk factors are often at the greatest risk for suicidal behaviors. Individuals who express low positive emotions, have had past suicidal behaviors and express a high degree of hopelessness are thought to be at the highest risk of self-injurious behavior. Although individuals who are most likely to complete suicide are the least likely to explicitly endorse suicidal ideation (Baumeister, 1990; Dean and Range; 1999; Jacobs, 2007). It is important to note that often stressful life events act as an antecedent to suicidal ideation and behaviors. Individuals with co-morbid psychological and medical disorders are thought of as vulnerable populations. As individuals who are currently in distress experience further distress, a compounding effect occurs, and often leads to increased hopelessness and may spur ideation and/or action. Synthesis of clinically relevant information is required to accurately predict an individual's potential for self-harm. A multitude of contextual factors such as an individual's current support structure (or lack thereof), socio-economic status, and ability to utilize resources such as impatient or outpatient psychological services further impact completed and attempted suicide rates (Hughs, 1996).

Protective factors

Although suicidal ideation is prevalent, less than 1 percent of those who endorse suicidal ideation go on to complete suicide (CDC, 2010). A multitude of protective factors have been identified that often act as a boon to distressed individuals that prevent them from attempting or completing suicide. Strong religious beliefs and fear of social disapproval act as a strong deterrent toward suicidal behavior (CARHMA, 2007; Jacobs, 2007; Malone *et al.*, 2000). The notion that one will negatively affect those they care about, acts as both a deterrent and a means for individuals to seek treatment. Within the scientific literature, a positive social support group has often been indicted as a protective factor (Bongar, 1991; CARMHA, 2007; Grob, 1992; Jacobs, 2007; RMFHMI, 1996). A study of individuals diagnosed with major depression who attempted suicide found that those with positive 'reasons for living' were more likely to abstain from suicidal behaviors. Those with positive coping abilities, positive family structure, positive peer supports, and lower levels of hopelessness were less likely to attempt suicide. These protective factors are theorized to restrain or guard individuals from attempts. It is important to note that these individuals would endorse recurrent suicidal ideation, but no suicidal behaviors were reported or observed (Malone *et al.*, 2000).

Risk assessment based on setting

Suicide assessment protocols vary depending on the population at hand, as well as the rules, regulations and laws of where an agency or mental health clinic is located. Examining Veterans Administration (VA) hospitals, general hospitals, and community mental health centers helps to illuminate the many different protocols employed when clinical emergencies occur. Emergency rooms in VA hospitals are frequently the primary contact within the health care system for suicidal clients (Knox *et al.*, 2012). General hospitals offer a distinct opportunity in this field of research. Due to the variety of demographics in suicidal clients, health care professionals in hospitals must be attentive to assessing for suicidal risk (Mitchell *et al.*, 2005). A majority of individuals with mental illness in the United States are served in community mental health settings (Chu *et al.*, 2012).

Suicide assessment in VA hospitals

One particular area of concern regarding suicide is that of military veterans. It is estimated that current and former military members account for 20 percent of the known suicides in the United States (Bakst *et al.*, 2010). Recent estimates note that prior and current military service members may account for 22 percent of those who attempt and complete suicide (Haney *et al.*, 2012). In order to obtain detailed information about veteran suicidality, researchers have attempted, via a retrospective study, to determine the content of the health care visits leading up to completed suicides (Denneson *et al.*, 2010). Denneson and his colleagues

(2010) reported that 41 percent of the veterans who completed suicide were assessed for suicidal ideation one year before death. Sixteen percent of these veterans were assessed for suicide in their final medical or mental health visit. This information may suggest that screening for suicidal thoughts is not sufficient. Fear of stigma within the military community may make it difficult for clients to answer such questions honestly (Langford *et al.*, 2013). Traditionally, formal assessment of suicide risk has been limited to individual factors such as age, gender, and ethnicity. These assessments have not included numerous factors which have been shown to be linked with suicidality, such as family structure, religiosity, and level of personal happiness (Bah *et al.*, 2011).

According to the Department of Veterans' Affairs (VA) official report (Haney *et al.*, 2012), a Suicide Risk Assessment Pocket Card has been developed to assist clinicians to make care decisions regarding individuals who present with suicidal ideation. The pocket card begins with major warning signs including threatening suicide, seeking access to pills or weapons, and talking about death and dying. Other warning signs including hopelessness, rage, increasing substance abuse, and dramatic changes in mood are of important note (Haney *et al.*, 2013). Next, there are risk factors and protective factors listed. Risk factors include current ideation, previous suicide attempts, substance abuse, demographics, and sexual orientation. Protective factors include social support, spirituality, children, and a positive therapeutic relationship. This pocket guide recommends asking a set of screening questions regarding suicide, but only when the clinical situation or presentation warrants risk of suicidality (Haney *et al.*, 2012).

Suicide assessment in hospitals

In 1998, the Joint Commission issued an alert regarding preventing suicides in inpatient settings. In 2010, there was an update to this alert which included patients in general hospitals, surgical units, and emergency departments (Bagian and Cohen, 2010). Suicide has been particularly difficult to assess for in these environments. According to a study by Bostwick and Rackley (2007), many patients who complete suicides have no history of either psychiatric conditions or previous suicide attempts. It is important to note that in comparison to inpatient settings, those in general hospital settings have more access to items with which to complete suicides. In addition, these patients are given more privacy and time alone; therefore they have more opportunities to attempt suicide (Bagian and Cohen, 2010). Patients in general hospitals attempt to commit suicide both more quickly and with smaller amounts of warning as compared to psychiatric patients (Tseng *et al.*, 2011). Suicides completed in general hospitals also tend to be of more violent in nature. These include hanging, jumping, and self-inflicted gunshot wounds (Suominen *et al.*, 2002). Many of the risk factors mentioned in the Joint Commission report are similar to those mentioned by the VA. However, there are risk factors which are specific to the health care environment. These environmental risk factors include intentional drug overdose and means provided by the hospital such asphyxiation via plastic bags, elastic tubing, and restraint belts

(Bostwick and Rackley, 2007). Tishler and Reiss (2009) noted that poor staff training, communication issues, low staffing, and a lack of information about suicide prevention have led to an increased number of attempted and completed suicides in hospital settings. Suicide is often difficult to assess due to time constraints. Many hospitals do not have the resources to implement many risk prevention strategies due to many patients being admitted for a short duration. For this reason, there is a lack of consistency across hospital settings. General hospitals must each decide which risk prevention strategies would be the most effective in their particular facility (Bagian and Cohen, 2010).

The Joint Commission report noted all hospitals were required to identify patients who were at risk for suicide (Bagian and Cohen, 2010). The three aspects of this identification were: (1) conducting a risk assessment which includes individual characteristics and environmental features which increase or decrease the chances of a suicide attempt; (2) assessing the individual's immediate safety; and (3) providing suicide prevention information to the individual when they leave the facility (Bagian and Cohen, 2010). The commission suggested two main additions to these assessment measures. First, the hospital must educate the staff about risk factors for suicide. Education includes obtaining help in emergencies, overcoming stigma, and understanding behavioral health. The most important aspects of this education include particular warning signs and changes in behavior. When behavioral changes are noticed or warning signs are noted, staff must be empowered to contact a mental health professional and make appropriate referrals when warranted. The second addition is implementing risk reduction strategies provided in the report and decide which would be the most effective in that particular hospital. These include providing medical professionals with a list of medications known to be associated with suicidal thoughts, utilizing a suicide assessment measure, the Suicide Assessment Five-Step Evaluation and Triage (SAFE-IT); a five-step evaluation which identifies risk factors, and education in the form of Mental Health First Aid USA; which educates health professionals regarding myths about suicide (Bagian and Cohen, 2010).

Despite the detail of the Joint Commission Report, these guidelines are not always followed. Miret *et al.* (2009) examined the documentation of suicide risk assessment in clinical records. The researchers found documentation of 907 patients who were seen in emergency rooms after suicide attempts. Nearly a quarter of these reports have been considered incomplete. Using more stringent methods, only 53 percent of these records are seen as adequate (Miret *et al.*, 2009).

Suicide assessment in community mental health

Generally speaking, within the last ten years there has been a significant increase in patients who receive care via community mental health clinics (Yoon *et al.*, 2013). Community mental health clinics refer to an agency, which provides mental health services to individuals within a community who may not have the means to afford it otherwise. These services are largely outpatient, but can include inpatient wards (Bentley, 1994). A growing proportion of those with severe mental illness are seen within these community-based clinics (Grob, 1992). Nearly 14 million individuals have received care in over 1000 community-based facilities in the United States (Yoon *et al.*, 2013). Professionals working in community mental health encounter many of the same problems as those in larger hospital settings. Specifically, staff in the same location attend differing training programs, use different assessment strategies, and do not have a consistent definition of risk (McAuliffe and Perry, 2007).

There is a paucity of research available on the assessment of suicide in community mental health. In Canada, however, there are particular benchmarks set for health organizations. This research, summarized by McAuliffe and Perry (2007), emphasizes the fact that a suicide assessment tool is not sufficient. They have since instituted training programs for mental health professionals. Another important aspect is that all professionals were given the same training protocol, known as Applied Suicide Intervention Skills Training (ASIST). This program focuses on enhancing clinicians' comfort in therapeutic discussion regarding suicide and self-harm (McAuliffe and Perry, 2007). This study showed that due to these programs, there has been a reduction in hospital admission rates and the length of hospital stays (McAuliffe and Perry, 2007). Farrow (2002) in a study of New Zealand nurses, found the nurses tended to use suicide assessment tools, such as No Suicide Contracts (NSCs), even when they are contraindicated. Many nurses stated that they were never formally taught to assess for suicide and/or risk (Farrow, 2002).

Implications

As evident through this review of the formal assessment of suicide risk in three distinct mental health care settings, more research is needed regarding the methods employed for suicide assessment. All three mental health care settings are at great risk for suicidal clients. The rise in military and veteran suicides has been well documented both in research and in the mass media. Additionally, due to the difficulty in predicting suicidality, detailed research is necessary regarding which assessment measures accurately predict risk in suicidal clients (Packman *et al.*, 2004). One option for further research is studying areas where there is a distinct protocol which is consistently followed, such as the research created by McAuliffe and Perry (2007). In the future it may be possible to determine the success of these programs, as detailed by Miret *et al.* (2009). This will enable researchers to determine which particular methods for suicide assessment are effective in limiting false negatives.

Assessing suicidal risk can be difficult for even the most skillful clinicians. If clinicians are not properly trained or well versed in the subject, they often fail to ask pertinent questions and use client-friendly language. Suicide is often viewed with stigma across cultures, and using blunt or accusatory statements may hinder proper suicide assessment as well as the therapeutic alliance. Pragmatic approaches in which the therapeutic alliance is used to approach the sensitive topic and the use of collaboration and de-escalation lead to clinical outcomes in which the client may understand the nature of their distress. Avoiding an adversarial and suspicious tone and approaching suicidal ideation with curiosity, non-judgment, and a calm-accepting demeanor may aid in developing a clinically accurate perspective on the client's level of functioning. Furthermore assessing a client's functioning using a diathesis-stress model may prove fruitful, as stressful life events often act as an antecedent to suicidal ideation and behaviors. Utilization of formal tests to evaluate a person's likelihood of attempting or completing suicide remains elusive, yet important discoveries continue to be made. The application of proper training, baseline knowledge, adequate clinical interview, and integration of a psychosocial history provides the best prognosis for an individual endorsing suicidality. Although the practice may appear daunting, accurate risk assessment provides a crucial role within mental health treatment as a whole.

References

Bagian, J. P., and Cohen, M. (2010). A follow-up report on preventing suicide: Focus on medical/surgical units and the emergency department. *The Joint Commission Sentinel Event Alert*, 46, 1–5.

Bah, A., Wilson, C., Fatkin, L., Atkisson, C., Brent, E., and Horton, D. (2011). Computing the prevalence rate of at-risk individuals for suicide within the army. *Military Medicine*, 176(7), 731–742.

Bakst, S., Rabinowitz, J., and Bromet, E. J. (2009). Antecedents and patterns of suicide behavior in first-admission psychosis. *Schizophrenia Bulletin*, 36(4), 880–889.

Baumeister, R. F. (1990). Suicide as an escape of the self. *Psychological Review*, 97(1), 90–113.

Bentley, K. J. (1994). Supports for community-based mental health care: An optimistic view of federal legislation. *Health and Social Work*, 19(4), 288–294.

Bersoff, D. N. (1999). *Ethical Conflicts in Psychology* (2nd edn). Washington, DC: American Psychological Association.

Bongar, B. (1991). *The Suicidal Patient: Clinical and Legal Standards of Care.* Washington, DC: American Psychological Association.

Bostwick, J. M., and Rackley, S. (2007). Completed suicide in medical/surgical patients: Who is at risk? *Current Psychiatry Reports*, 9(3), 242–246.

Centers for Disease Control and Prevention. (2010a). *National Hospital Ambulatory: Emergency Department Summary Tables.* Washington: DC.

Centers for Disease Control and Prevention (2010b), *National Center for Injury Prevention and Control. Web-based Injury Statistics Query and Reporting System (WISQARS).* Washington, DC. Retrieved from www.cdc.gov/injury/wisqars/index.html

Centers for Disease Control and Prevention. (2012). Surveillance for violent deaths: National violent death reporting system, 16 States, 2009. *MMWR Surveillance Summary*, 61(ss06), 1–43.

Centre for Applied Research in Mental Health and Addiction. (2007). Working with the client who is suicidal: A tool for adult mental health and addiction services. *British Columbia Ministry of Health.* Retrieved from www.health.gov.bc.ca/library/publications/year/2007/MHA_WorkingWithSuicidalClient.pdf

Chu, J. P., Emmons, L., Wong, J., Goldblum, P., Reiser, R., Barrera, A. Z., and Byrd-Olmstead, J. (2012). Public psychology: A competency model for professional psychologists in community mental health. *Professional Psychology: Research and Practice*, 43(1), 39–49.

Dean, J. R. and Range, L. M. (1999). Testing the escape theory of suicide in an outpatient clinical population. *Cognitive Therapy and Research*, 23(6), 561–572.

Denneson, L. M., Basham, C., Dickinson, K. C., Crutchfield, M. C., Millet, L., Shen, X., and Dobscha S. K. (2010). Suicide risk assessment and content of VA health care contacts before suicide completion in Oregon. *Psychiatric Services*, 61(12), 1192–1197.

Farrow, T. L. (2002). Owning their expertise: Why nurses use 'no suicide contracts' rather than their own assessments. *International Journal of Mental Health Nursing*, 11(4), 214–219.

Gliatto, M. F. and Rai, A. K. (1999). Evaluation and treatment of individuals with suicidal ideation. *American Family Physician*, 59(6), 1500–1506.

Grob, G. N. (1992). Mental health policy in America: Myths and realities. *Health Affairs*, 11(3), 7–22.

Haney, E. M., O'Neil, M. E., Carson, S., Low, A., Peterson, K., Denneson, L. M., *et al.* (2012). Suicide risk factors and risk assessment tools: A systematic review. *Department of Veteran Affairs*, 1, 1–137.

Hughs, D. H. (1996). Suicide and violence assessment in psychiatry. *General Hospital Psychiatry*, 18(6), 416–421.

Jacobs, D. (2007). *Suicide Assessment*. Ann Arbor, MI: University of Michigan Depression Centre Colloquium Series.

Knox, K. L., Stanley, B., Currier, G. W., Brenner, L., Ghahramanlou-Holloway, M., and Brown, G. (2012). An emergency department-based brief intervention for Veterans at Risk for Suicide (SAFE VET). *Field Action Report*, 102(Suppl. 1), 33–37.

Langford, L., Litts, D., and Pearson, J. L. (2013). Using science to improve communications about suicide among military and veteran populations: Looking for a few good messages. *American Journal of Public Health*, 103(1), 31–38.

Malone, K. M., Oquendo, M. A., Haas, G. L., Ellis, S. P., Shuha, L., and Mann, J. J. (2000). Protective factors against suicidal acts in major depression: Reasons for living. *American Journal of Psychiatry*, 157(7), 1084–1088.

McAdams, C. R., III and Foster, V. A. (2000). Client suicide: Its frequency and impact on counselors. *Journal of Mental Health Counseling*, 22(2), 107–121.

McAuliffe, N. and Perry, L. (2007). Making it safer: A health centre's strategy for suicide prevention. *Psychiatry Quarterly*, 78(4), 295–307.

McIntosh, J. L. (1993). Control group of suicide survivors: A review and critique. *Suicide and Life-Threatening Behavior*, 23(2), 141–162.

Meerwijk, E. L., van Meijel, B., van den Bout, J., Kerkhof, A., de Vogel, W. and Grypdonck, M. (2010). Development and evaluation of a guideline for nursing care of suicidal patients with schizophrenia. *Perspectives in Psychiatric Care*, 46(1), 65–73.

Miret, M., Nuevo, R., and Ayuso-Mateos, J. (2009). Documentation of suicide risk assessment in clinical records. *Psychiatric Services*, 60(7), 994.

Mitchell, A. M., Garand, L., Dean, D., Panzak, G., and Taylor, M. (2005). Suicide assessment in hospital emergency departments: Implication for patient satisfaction and compliance. *Topics in Emergency Medicine*, 27(4), 302–312.

National Institutes of Mental Health. (2010). *Suicide in the US: Statistics and Prevention*. Washington, DC: Federal Printing Office.

Packman, W. L., Marlitt, R. E., Bongar, B., and Pennuto, T. O. (2004). A comprehensive and concise assessment of suicide risk. *Behavioral Sciences and the Law*, 22(5), 667–680.

Pauley, B. (2008). Shifting moral values to enhance access to health care. Harm reduction as an ethical context for nursing practice. *International Journal of Drug Policy*, 19(3), 195–204.

Registered Nurses' Association of Ontario (RNAO). (2009). *Assessment and Care of Adults with Suicidal Ideation and Behaviour*. [Online]. Retrieved from www.rnao.org/Storage/58/5263_Sucide_-Final-web.pdf.

Risk Management Foundation, Harvard Medical Institutions (RMFHMI). (1996). *Guidelines for Identification, Assessment, and Treatment Planning for Suicidality*. Retrieved from https://www.rmf.harvard.edu/Guidelines-Algorithms/2011/~/media/Files/_Global/KC/PDFs/suicideAs

Shea, S. C. (2002). *The Practical Art of Suicide Assessment: A Guide for Mental Health Professionals and Substance Abuse Counselors* (2nd edn). Hoboken, NJ: John Wiley and Sons.

Sullivan, G. R., and Bongar, B. (2009). Assessing suicide risk in the adult patient. In P. M. Kleespies (Ed.), *Behavioral Emergencies: An Evidence-based Resource for Evaluating and Managing Risk of Suicide, Violence, and Victimization* (pp. 59–78). Washington, DC: American Psychological Association.

Suominen, K., Isometsa, E., Heila, H., Lonnqvist, J., and Henriksson, M. (2002). General hospital suicides: A psychological autopsy study in Finland. *General Hospital Psychiatry*, 24(6), 412–416.

Tishler, C. L. and Reiss, N. S. (2009). Inpatient suicide: Preventing a common sentinel event. *General Hospital Psychiatry*, 31(2), 103–109.

Tseng, M. M., Cheng, C., and Hu, F. C. (2011). Standardized mortality ratio of inpatient suicide in a general hospital. *Journal of Formosan Medical Association*, 10(4), 267–269.

Yoon, J., Bruckner, T. A., and Brown, T. T. (2013). The association between client characteristics and recovery in California's comprehensive community mental health programs. *American Journal of Public Health*, 103(10), 89–95.

15 Culturally competent suicide assessment

Uri Kugel, Lori Holleran, Kasie Hummel, Joyce Chu, Peter Goldblum and Bruce Bongar

Cultural identity and suicidality

The concept of cultural identity is crucial for the focus of this chapter. Cultural identity is an individual's perception of their position in varying dimensions of life such as race, sexual orientation, ethnicity, gender, religious belief, and age (Tatum, 1997). Additional examples of cultural identity include subgroups such as military veterans, college students, and people with disabilities. Due to the multidimensional nature of one's identity, one's core sense of self and belief system may be influenced by numerous factors at once. With regard to suicidality, aspects of cultural identity could include symptomatic presentation, and risk and protective factors. These various elements can be impacted in different pathways dependent on the interaction between the cultural identity of the individual and unique stressors existing in their life.

It is quite evident that there is great variety in suicide rates and risk factors across cultural groups and individuals with different cultural identities (Chu *et al.*, 2010). In 2010, US completed suicide rates were the highest among American Indians (25.85 per 100,000), followed by 25.65 for White males, 9.32 for Asian/Pacific Islanders, 9.10 for African Americans, and 5.27 for Hispanics (Centers for Disease Control and Prevention [CDC], 2010). When specifically considering individuals who have served in the military, it is estimated that 22 Veterans commit suicide per day, contributing to approximately 21 percent of the total US suicide rate (Kemp and Bossarte, 2012).

While no national data is currently available regarding suicide rates in sexual minorities within the US, a national registry study conducted in Denmark found that among sexual minority males, suicide rates are nearly eight times higher, and 1.5 times higher in sexual minority females, relative to their heterosexual peers (Mathy *et al.*, 2011). Additionally, in a comprehensive literature review, an increase in suicidal behaviors was seen among sexual minorities across the globe (Plöderl *et al.*, 2013). While risk is seen to vary based on group membership related to both ethnic and other cultural factors, common suicide risk assessment practices often lack systematic incorporation of these unique risk factors for suicide (Chu *et al.*, 2010). Some additional examples for such groups in the US include Transgender people, Latina high school students, and African American adolescent males.

Suicidal ideation

Research has demonstrated that symptoms of suicidal ideation vary between ethnicities, gender, and sexual orientation. Suicidal ideation is a critical symptom of depression (American Psychiatric Association, 2000, 2013). However, as data indicates, symptoms of depression can vary based on one's cultural background. For example, in developing Eastern countries, such as Iran, speaking about emotions is forbidden and seen as an indication of weakness (Seifsafari *et al.*, 2013). As a result, somatic symptoms (e.g., headache, irritability, and pain) might be articulated instead (Tryon, 2008). The idea that certain emotional states are substituted by somatic symptoms is based on a psychodynamic view and was originally proposed by Freud (Tryon, 2008). However, more recently, stigmatization and fear of appearing psychologically ill have been postulated as possible reasons for this somatic manifestation (Dere *et al.*, 2013). The expression of emotional complaints through somatic symptoms is not unique to Eastern countries, it is also commonly found among Asian, Hispanic, and Latino patients (Dere *et al.*, 2013; Organista, 2008; Seifsafari *et al.*, 2013; Zhou *et al.*, 2011).

Unlike in western cultures, suicide in Japan does not carry with it any association of shame or guilt (Kawanishi, 2008). On the contrary, it is commonly utilized as a method of problem solving and is viewed as the highest form of apology for an unforgivable mistake. In a sense, taking one's life to demonstrate genuine repentance negates the individual's mistake and restores honor to the family. Even though this tolerant or even encouraging attitude toward suicide within the Japanese culture is an ongoing obstacle for suicide prevention efforts, suicide rates continue to be higher elsewhere in the globe (Kawanishi, 2008). Furthermore, like Iranians, Japanese individuals are more likely to endorse somatic complaints and to seek the advice of general practitioners (Waza *et al.*, 1999).

Suicide method

The choice of method in suicide has also been found to vary across cultural groups. Means for committing suicide often differ across the globe due to social acceptability and availability. In a study conducted by De Leo *et al.* (2013) in which 14 different countries (the Commonwealth of Australia, New Zealand, Philippines, Mongolia, French Polynesia, Hong Kong (two sites), Guam, Tonga, Vanuatu, Fiji, Italy, China, and Brazil) participated, the preferred method of suicide was hanging. Moreover, data indicated that more than 13 percent of suicides in Fiji were attributed to fire and flames. In regards to nonfatal suicidal behavior, overdosing on drugs, cutting, and poisoning were the most common among the entire sample.

Furthermore, in 2004, over half of all suicides in Japan were completed by individuals most likely to be affected by the financial recession, specifically middle-aged men (Beautrais, 2006). In a work-centered society like Japan, *karo-jisatsu* or 'suicide by overwork' has been recognized as a societal issue (Kawanishi, 2008,

p. 65). A distinct characteristic of this method of suicide is the significant self-blame that the individual feels regarding an inability to meet work demands (as evidenced by suicide notes). In line with the Japanese view of suicide as a method of problem resolution, individuals who engage in *karo-jisatsu* are often attempting to save face. Lastly, in traditional China, hanging is the dominant method because of the belief that the soul of the individual who dies by hanging will return to Earth to plague the living, specifically those who caused harm (Braun and Nichols, 1997). As a result, suicide by hanging carries with it the association of wrath and vengeance.

According to De Leo *et al.* (2013), completed suicide across all countries is more common among males; whereas nonfatal suicidal behaviors are more common among females. Seifsafari *et al.* (2013) found related results among an Iranian sample. Suicidal ideation was more common among females and attempts were more common among males. Furthermore, both genders implement harmful behaviors that are consistent with their culture's gender scripts (De Leo *et al.*, 2013). However, two exceptions to the gender pattern of suicide have been demonstrated. The suicide rates in Fiji are equal between genders and men in the Philippines engage in a higher rate of nonfatal suicidal behavior. In regards to rate differences between age groups, past data from the World Health Organization indicated that suicide is generally completed by middle-aged to older individuals. Inconsistent with these findings, De Leo *et al.* (2013) found that younger individuals in the Pacific Island countries were more likely to commit suicide.

Risk and protective factors

Cultural identities such as ethnicity and gender are not necessarily the sole influences on an individual's beliefs about suicide. Risk and protective factors that are unique to each cultural identity affect an individual's belief system. Gibbs (1997) found that religiosity, social support, old age, and residing in the southern region of the United States were protective factors among African Americans that could reduce the risk of suicide. Conversely, Rowell *et al.* (2008) established that exposure to violence, being HIV positive, substance use, and negative interactions with law enforcement were associated with an increased risk of suicide for this same population.

Meyer *et al.* (2008) studied how social stress contributes to the overall stress that an individual might experience. The social stress theory is a 'framework as a sociological paradigm that views social conditions as a cause of stress for members of disadvantaged social groups' (Meyer *et al.*, 2008, p. 368). Their findings demonstrated that consistent with the social stress theory, sexual orientation and race/ethnic minority statuses are associated with an increase in overall stressors and prejudice-related stressors. According to O'Donnell *et al.* (2011), risk factors for suicide among African American and Latino lesbian, gay, and bisexual (LGB) individuals include minority stress (prejudice, stigma, discrimination), family rejection, early age of self-labeling, race/ethnicity, and gender-atypical behavior. In regards to protection against suicide for LGB individuals, a strong social support system and a cohesive family can help decrease an individual's level of vulnerability to engage in suicidal behavior (Wilder and Wilder, 2012).

Suicidality assessment

Currently there are numerous measures utilized to assess for suicide risk including the Scale for Suicide Ideation (SSI; Beck *et al.*, 1979), which was subsequently translated into the Beck Scale for Suicide Ideation (BSI; Beck and Steer, 1991), the Beck Depression Inventory (BDI; Beck and Steer, 1987), the Beck Hopelessness Scale (BHS; Beck and Steer, 1988), and the Suicide Ideation Scale (SIS; Rudd, 1989). The SSI is a 19-item scale, scored from 0–2, assessing suicidal thoughts and attitudes toward suicide, which originally were ascertained by a clinician through a semi-structured interview, but was adapted into a self-report measure during the transition into the BSI. The BDI is a self-report questionnaire consisting of 21 items, scored from 0–3, assessing depression symptoms and severity. The BHS is a self-report measure comprised of 20 true-false items, examining hopelessness through pessimistic beliefs regarding the future. The SIS is a self-report measure consisting of 10 items, scored upon a five-point Likert scale, assessing suicidal ideation along a continuum 'ranging from covert suicidal thoughts to more overt or intense ideation and, ultimately, actual suicide attempts' (Rudd, 1989, p. 175).

While these measures are widely regarded to be reliable and valid in assessing risk within the majority population (Beck *et al.*, 1979; Beck *et al.*, 1990; Beck and Steer, 1987; Beck and Steer, 1988; Luxton *et al.*, 2011; Steer *et al.*, 1993), there is a paucity of information regarding their utility when assessing culturally diverse populations. During the initial development and validation of the SSI, identifying risk level was based mainly on psychological factors 'as opposed to demographic variables' due to the belief that these variables lacked 'practical utility' in assessing an individual's suicide risk (Beck *et al.*, 1979, p. 344). In a study seeking to validate the use of the BHS and BDI within an outpatient population, neither ethnicity nor other cultural factors, beyond age, gender, and diagnosis, were considered (Beck *et al.*, 1990). While these assessment measures were found to be suitable for use in assessing risk in an outpatient population, it is impossible to ascertain how appropriate they are for use with culturally diverse populations.

In a study validating the use of the BDI, BHS, Beck Anxiety Inventory (BAI), and SSI as a battery to assess risk in an outpatient setting, only the roles of gender, age, and diagnosis on risk profiles were examined (Steer *et al.*, 1993). While race was recorded, its implications on risk were not investigated, and with 32 African-American participants (2.7 percent) and 13 Asian participants (1.1 percent), out of 1172 participants, it is notably uncharacteristic of the current broader population (13.6 percent and 5.6 percent, respectively, US Census Bureau, 2010). More recently a study examining risk factors in a non-clinical population, utilizing the SSI, BHS, BAI, and BDI among other measurements, similarly recorded race but failed to consider its influence on results (Brown *et al.*, 2000). In addition to not examining the specific findings related to minority participants, only a small percentage of participants represented minority populations. Out of 6891 participants, 354 identified as African American (5.14 percent), 40 as Hispanic (0.58 percent), and 27 as Asian (0.39 percent), which is substantially unrepresentative of the current population demographics.

Considerable amounts of research have been conducted to validate these widely used measures to assess risk, but the emphasis has remained on examining their utility within majority populations. Yet, there is an abundant amount of research recognizing that suicide risk factors are not constant across all cultural groups, and that being a minority can itself be a factor related to risk (Garrison, 1992).

To appropriately assess risk in culturally diverse populations it is imperative that mental health professionals recognize unique factors that require examination to capture accurate risk levels. Culturally relevant themes have been seen to influence risk in diverse populations (Chu *et al.*, 2010; Goldston *et al.*, 2008; Joe and Kaplan, 2001; Langhinrichsen-Rohling *et al.*, 2009; Meyer, 2013). Yet, these themes are not specifically assessed for by any of the previously identified measures and there appears to be no research specifically considering the psychometric properties of these assessments for use within culturally diverse populations.

Cultural theory and model of suicide

One reason for the lack of measurements specifically considering these factors may be due to the fact that until recently these culturally relevant themes were not easily distinguishable among the plethora of research examining specific aspects regarding risk factors among cultural minority populations (Leach and Long, 2008). Without an existing comprehensive theory, assessing risk in cultural minorities, including both ethnic and sexual minorities, could not be performed in an accurate and consistent way (Lester, 2009). Yet, with the growing number of individuals identified within minority populations, and the increasing rates of risk seen in some of these groups (CDC 2009; Joe and Kaplan, 2001), the need for a guiding theory was prominent (Leach and Long, 2008; Lester, 2009).

The cultural theory and model of suicide were created through a technique utilizing the amalgamation of pre-existing data examining minority status and suicide to identify overarching commonalities influencing suicide in cultural minority populations (Chu *et al.*, 2010). Specifically, risk factors associated with African American, Asian American, Latino/a American, and sexual minority (LGBTQ) groups were examined to guide the theory's construction, with an emphasis on identifying risk factors specific to each of the aforementioned cultures. This included identifying 'categories separate from simple minority status as an ethnic or sexual minority individual; in particular, cultural factors are defined to include beliefs, values, norms, practices, or customs held by ethnic and sexual minority groups that have been shown to influence suicide' (Chu *et al.*, 2010, p. 27).

In total, 144 articles, published between 1991 and 2011, considering suicide in cultural minority populations aided in the construction of this theory (Chu *et al.*, 2010). These articles provided 240 specific risk factors related to suicidal behaviors within the four prior identified cultural groups. These specific risk factors were then gathered into themes based on common attributes. Across these four cultural minority populations (African Americans, Asian Americans, Latino/a Americans, and sexual minorities (LGBTQ)), it was found that 228 of the 240 risk factors (95 percent) could be encompassed within one of four culturally relevant themes:

Cultural sanctions

Cultural sanctions recognize specific suicide-related values, such as moral protestations, related to the acceptability of suicide. Additionally it considers attitudes, such as shame or acceptance, toward life occurrences that may precipitate risk.

Idioms of distress

Idioms of distress consider variations in the probability that risk will be communicated, how symptoms associated with risk are expressed, and how suicide attempts may be manifested.

Minority stress

Minority stress examines the experience of cultural minorities based on levels of acculturation, maltreatment, and social inequalities.

Social discord

Social discord considers how social, family, and community support influences an individual. Specifically, identifying how conflict or estrangement impact level of risk.

These themes construct a working cultural model of suicide. This two-part model initially recognizes the role of *life stressors* in one's ability or inability to cope with exterior stressors (Chu *et al.*, 2010). While both personal and social stressors contribute to one's life stressors, social stressors in particular have been found to be quite influential for individuals identifying as cultural minorities (Balsam *et al.*, 2011; Huynh *et al.*, 2012; Meyer, 2013). Social stressors encompass three of the previously identified themes: minority stress, social discord, and cultural sanctions. Additionally this model considers the role of *cultural meaning*, which influences the model in two ways. First, it influences the way in which an individual experiences life stressors based on their understanding of, or the significance attributed to the event. In this regard, 'the cultural sanctions factor is particularly salient in the mediating mechanism of cultural meaning'

(Chu *et al.*, 2010, p. 35). Second, it is seen to be a meaningful factor in one's decision to attempt or commit suicide (Chu *et al.*, 2010). With regard to the act of suicide, Cultural Meaning and Cultural Sanctions 'determine whether one's tolerance threshold for distress is surpassed and ultimately whether a person acts on suicide intention or impulse' (Chu *et al.*, 2010, p. 35). This model identified by Chu *et al.* is also guided by three larger theoretical principles, consisting of the themes and model factors previously discussed. The first principle is directly associated with Idioms of Distress, and recognizes that culture influences how suicidal thoughts and acts are expressed. This considers how culture impacts the likelihood that one would reveal information regarding suicidal ideation or intent, and the method of the suicidal action. The second principle is associated with Cultural Sanctions, Minority Stress, and Social Discord. This principle recognizes that culture influences suicidal behavior vulnerability based on the specific stressors one encounters related to the culture to which they belong. In addition to these specific cultural factors, it is imperative to recognize that other risk factors, such as past suicide attempts and hopelessness, which are experienced across majority groups, may also be present and impacting one's overall experience of suicidal ideation or intent. Finally, the third principle recognizes that cultural beliefs regarding stressors and suicidal behavior influence the overall likelihood of suicidal actions occurring (Chu *et al.*, 2010). Taken together, these themes, model, and overarching comprehensive theory provide a foundation for the standardized examination of risk within cultural minority populations.

The Cultural Assessment of Risk for Suicide (CARS)

The Cultural Assessment of Risk for Suicide (CARS) is a 39-item self-report measure for identifying culturally relevant suicide risk factors unexamined by the previously identified suicide instruments. Due to the lack of parsimony in culturally competent risk assessment, Chu *et al.* (2010) created the 'Cultural Model of Suicide' (p. 35), which attempted to address the risk and protective factors, as well as cultural disparities in suicide among four diverse groups (LGBTQ, Asian Americans, Latino/a American, and African American). Through a comprehensive literature review Chu *et al.* scrutinized the attitudes, customs, practices, and standards of these cultures in order to demonstrate how they affect suicidal behaviors. These factors were then organized into four aforementioned categories: 'Cultural Sanctions, Idioms of Distress, Minority Stress, and Social Discord' (Chu *et al.*, 2010, p. 27). These four categories of the Cultural Model of Suicide were then used to develop the CARS.

In order to test the psychometric properties of the measure, 950 participants who were diverse in ethnicity and sexual orientation were recruited from colleges and communities to complete the measure (Chu *et al.*, 2013). In addition, individuals were asked to complete the suicide item (Item 9) of the BDI, the SIS, the BHS, and provide a lifetime history of suicide attempts, assessed through Item 20 of the BSI, as a means for psychometric validation. A factor analysis was conducted in order to distinguish the underlying factor configuration of the

CARS scale. The result was an eight-factor solution including 39 items, which accounted for 57.39 percent of total variance (Chu *et al.*, 2013). Two factors, Family Discord and Social Support accounted for the most variance (28.25 percent). Convergent validity, determined by correlating the scores on the CARS with other established measures of suicidal behavior revealed significance at the $p < 0.001$ level. Furthermore, the overall CARS score demonstrated superior internal consistency ($\alpha = 0.90$; Chu *et al.*, 2013).

The CARS measure provides numerous advantages over existing suicide risk assessments. First, the CARS was constructed with cultural factors in mind (Chu *et al.*, 2013). In addition, it recognizes that a measure could not incorporate every conceivable cultural disparity in suicide behavior and risk. Furthermore, the CARS provides a method to recognize and categorize the cultural distinction within suicide. Not only does the CARS have the prospect to be used as a screening tool, it also has the capability to be utilized in the capacity of prevention and management of suicide (Chu *et al.*, 2013). It identifies critical aspects of suicide risk that can be used to generate a culturally competent safety and risk management plan.

Conclusion

Suicide rates and risk factors differ between cultural groups. An individual's cultural identity varies based on multiple facets that can impact core aspects of their inner experience. A few of the many factors impacted include risk and protective factors associated with suicide. Research has shown that varying cultures maintain beliefs regarding suicide, express symptoms related to suicide, and attempt to commit suicide in different ways from the majority population found within the United States. While these discrepancies have been identified, little emphasis has been placed on addressing and recognizing these differences in regard to risk assessment.

Most widely used measures utilized to assess for risk focus on the symptomatic presentation expressed in the majority population, which leads to uncertainties regarding the accuracy of risk assessments being conducted in populations including cultural minority group members. While research recognizes differences in risk factors present in minority populations, how to assess for these factors in a comprehensive way remained unclear until recently. The Cultural Model of Suicide addressed these concerns through the systematic examination of risk and protective factors associated with suicide among those identifying as a minority group member (African American, Asian American, Latino/a American, and LGBTQ), and constructed a measurement to accurately assess for risk.

The CARS identifies four main themes encompassing the majority of risk factors present within these groups. The themes include: Cultural Sanctions, Idioms of Distress, Minority Stress, and Social Discord. The CARS is recognized as a reliable and valid measure for identifying and categorizing risk within these minority populations, with the ability to inform potential clinical decisions such as treatment and safety planning. The full utility, both psychometrically and clinically, of the CARS will continue to expand as the quantity of individuals identifying as minority group members remains on the increase. In summary, despite having some advances over the last few years and the development of a measure such as the CARS, cultural assessment of suicide is still in its infancy and requires continued research. Future research could examine the use of the CARS with different minority populations, other countries, and languages. Additionally, further support is needed for the use of the CARS in different clinical settings or its use in standardized risk assessment procedures.

References

American Psychiatric Association. (2000). *Diagnostic and Statistical Manual of Mental Disorders* (4th edn, text revision). Washington, DC: Author.

American Psychiatric Association. (2013). *Diagnostic and Statistical Manual of Mental Disorders* (5th edn). Washington, DC: Author.

Balsam, K. F., Molina, Y., Beadnell, B., Simoni, J., and Walters, K. (2011). Measuring multiple minority stress: The LGBT People of Color Microaggressions Scale. *Cultural Diversity and Ethnic Minority Psychology*, 17(2), 163–174.

Beautrais, A. L. (2006). Suicide in Asia. *Crisis: The Journal of Crisis Intervention and Suicide Prevention*, 27(2), 55–57.

Beck, A., Brown, G., Berchick, R., Stewart, B., and Steer, R. (1990). Relationship between hopelessness and ultimate suicide: A replication with psychiatric out-patients. *The American Journal of Psychiatry*, 147(2), 190–195.

Beck, A. T., Kovacs, M., and Weissman, M. (1979). Assessment of suicidal intention: The scale for suicide ideation. *Journal of Consulting and Clinical Psychology*, 47(2), 343–352.

Beck, A. T. and Steer, R. A. (1987). *Manual for Beck Depression Inventory*. San Antonio, TX: Psychological Corporation.

Beck, A. T. and Steer, R. A. (1988). *Manual for the Beck Hopelessness Scale*. San Antonio, TX: Psychological Corporation.

Beck, A. T. and Steer, R. A. (1991). *Manual for the Beck Scale for Suicide Ideation*. San Antonio, TX: Psychological Corporation.

Braun, K. L. and Nichols, R. (1997). Death and dying in four Asian American cultures: A descriptive study. *Death Studies*, 21(4), 327–359.

Brown, G., Beck, A., Steer, R., and Grisham, J. (2000). Risk factors for suicide in psychiatric outpatients: A 20-year prospective study. *Journal of Consulting and Clinical Psychology*, 68(3), 371–377.

Chu, J., Floyd, R., Diep, H., Pardo, S., Goldblum, P., and Bongar, B. (2013). A tool for the culturally competent assessment of suicide: The cultural assessment of risk for suicide (CARS) measure. *Psychological Assessment*, 25(2), 424–434.

Chu, J. P., Goldblum, P., Floyd, R., and Bongar, B. (2010). A cultural theory and model of suicide. *Applied and Preventive Psychology*, 14(1–4), 25–10.

Centers for Disease Control and Prevention. (2009). *Web-based Injury Statistics Query and Reporting System (WISQARS): Fatal Injury Reports*. Atlanta, GA: National Center for Injury Prevention and Control. Retrieved from www.cdc.gov/ncipc/wisqars.

Centers for Disease Control and Prevention. (2010). *Web-based Injury Statistics Query and Reporting System (WISQARS): Fatal Injury Reports*. Atlanta, GA: National

Center for Injury Prevention and Control. Retrieved from www.cdc.gov/ncipc/wisqars.

De Leo, D., Milner, A., Fleischmann, A., Bertolote, J., Collings, S., Amadeo, S., *et al.* (2013). The WHO start study: Suicidal behaviors across different areas of the world. *Crisis*, 34(3), 156–163.

Dere, J., Sun, J., Zhao, Y., Persson, T. J., Zhu, X., Yao, S., *et al.* (2013). Beyond 'somatization' and 'psychologization': Symptom-level variation in depressed Han Chinese and Euro-Canadian outpatients. *Frontiers in Psychology*, 4(377), 1–13.

Garrison, C. Z. (1992). Demographic predictors of suicide. In R. W. Mails, A. L. Berman, J. T. Maltsberger, and R. I. Yufit (Eds), *Assessment and Prediction of Suicide* (pp. 484–498). New York: Guilford Press.

Gibbs, J. T. (1997). African-American suicide: A cultural paradox. *Suicide and Life-Threatening Behavior*, 27(1), 68–79.

Goldston, D., Molock, S., Whitbeck, L., Murakami, J., Zayas, L., and Hall, G. (2008). Cultural considerations in adolescent suicide prevention and psychosocial treatment. *American Psychologist*, 63(1), 14–31.

Huynh, Q., Devos, T., and Dunbar, C. M. (2012). The psychological costs of painless but recurring experiences of racial discrimination. *Cultural Diversity and Ethnic Minority Psychology*, 18(1), 26–34.

Joe, S. and Kaplan, M. S. (2001). Suicide among African American Men. *Suicide and Life-Threatening Behavior*, 31(Suppl.1), 106–121.

Kawanishi, Y. (2008). On karo-jisatsu (suicide by overwork): Why do Japanese workers work themselves to death? *International Journal of Mental Health*, 37(1), 61–74.

Kemp, J. and Bossarte, R., (2012). *Suicide Data Report*. Department of Veterans Affairs, Mental Health Services, Suicide Prevention Program.

Langhinrichsen-Rohling, J., Friend, J., and Powell, A. (2009). Adolescent suicide, gender, and culture: A rate and risk factor analysis. *Aggression and Violent Behavior*, 14(5), 402–414.

Leach, M. M., and Leong, F. T. L. (2008). Challenges for research on suicide among ethnic minorities. In F. T. L. Leong, and M. M. Leach (Eds), *Suicide Among Racial and Ethnic Minority Groups: Theory, Research, and Practice* (pp. 297–318). New York: Routledge.

Lester, D. (2009). Theories of suicide. In F. T. L. Leong and M. M. Leach (Eds), *Suicide Among Racial and Ethnic Minority Groups: Theory, Research, and Practice* (pp. 39–53). New York: Routledge.

Luxton, D. D., Rudd, M., Reger, M. A., and Gahm, G. A. (2011). A psychometric study of the suicide ideation scale. *Archives of Suicide Research*, 15(3), 250–258.

Mathy, R., Cochran, S., Olsen, J., and Mays, V. (2011). The association between relationship markers of sexual orientation and suicide: Denmark, 1990–2001. *Social Psychiatry and Psychiatric Epidemiology*, 46(2), 111–117.

Meyer, I. H. (2013). Prejudice, social stress, and mental health in lesbian, gay, and bisexual populations: Conceptual issues and research evidence. *Psychological Bulletin*, 129(5), 674–697.

Meyer, I. H., Schwartz, S., and Frost, D. M. (2008). Social patterning of stress and coping: Do disadvantaged social statuses confer more stress and fewer coping resources? *Social Science and Medicine*, 67(3), 368–379.

O'Donnell, S., Meyer, I. H., and Schwartz, S. (2011). Increased risk of suicide attempts among Black and Latino lesbians, gay men, and bisexuals. *American Journal of Public Health*, 101(6), 1055 –1059.

Organista, K. C. (2008). *Solving Latino Psychosocial and Health Problems: Theory, Practice, and Populations*. Hoboken, NJ: John Wiley and Sons.

Plöderl, M., Wagenmakers, E., Tremblay, P., Ramsay, R., Kralovec, K., Fartacek, C., and Fartacek, R. (2013). Suicide risk and sexual orientation: A critical review. *Archives of Sexual Behavior*, 42(5), 715–727.

Rowell, K. L., Green, B. L., and Eddy, J. (2008). Factors associated with suicide among African American adult men: A systematic review of the literature. *Journal of Men's Health*, 5(4), 274–281.

Rudd, M. D. (1989). The prevalence of suicidal ideation among college students. *Suicide and Life-Threatening Behavior*, 19(2), 173–183.

Seifsafari, S., Firoozabadi, A., Ghanizadeh, A., and Salehi, A. (2013). A symptom profile analysis of depression in a sample of Iranian patients. *Iranian Journal of Medical Sciences*, 38(1), 22–29.

Steer, R. A., Beck, A. T., Brown, G. K., and Beck, J. S. (1993). Classification of suicidal and nonsuicidal outpatients: A cluster-analytic approach. *Journal of Clinical Psychology*, 49(5), 603–614.

Tatum, B. D. (1997). *Why Are All the Black Kids Sitting Together in the Cafeteria? And Other Conversations About Race*. New York: Basic Books.

Tryon, W. W. (2008). Whatever happened to symptom substitution? *Clinical Psychology Review*, 28(6), 963–968.

Waza, K., Graham, A. V., Zyzanski, S. J., and Inoue, K. (1999). Comparison of symptoms in Japanese and American depressed primary care patients. *Family Practice*, 16(5), 528–533.

Wilder, H., and Wilder, J. (2012). In the wake of 'don't ask don't tell': Suicide prevention and outreach for LGB service members. *Military Psychology*, 24(6), 624–642.

Zhou, X., Dere, J., Zhu, X., Yao, S., Chentsova-Dutton, Y., and Ryder, A. G. (2011). Anxiety symptom presentations in Han Chinese and Euro-Canadian outpatients: Is distress always somatized in China? *Journal of Affective Disorders*, 135(1–3), 111–114.

16 Ethical and legal issues in dealing with suicidal behaviour

Swati Mukherjee and Updesh Kumar

The most common understanding of the term suicide is of an act leading to termination of one's own life. Suicide is the fatal outcome of an act that is deliberately initiated and performed by the deceased him- or herself, in the knowledge or expectation of its fatal outcome, the outcome being considered by the actor as instrumental in bringing about desired changes in consciousness and/or social conditions (Retterstøl, 1993). Suicide is a universal human phenomenon and a universal cause of concern across the globe. Every 40 seconds a human life is lost to suicide somewhere in the world. Every year around 5 to 12 million people die by suicide worldwide. A host of professionals across disciplines are engaged in providing support services and care to suicide survivors and suicidal individuals. Suicide is a social issue, a public health concern, or a result of mental illness when viewed from the perspective of those who are entrusted with the responsibility of preventing it. However, for the individual who takes the extreme step of ending one's own life, it marks a cry of pain, a cry for help, a desperate attempt to get away from a situation one perceives uncontrollably painful, and perhaps also a desperate attempt to achieve a desirable goal that is perceived as unattainable otherwise. Even within the fraternity of helping professionals, suicide may be defined differently depending on the purpose of the definition – medical, legal, or administrative. Despite suicide being a universal cause of human concern, it is a matter of perspective that provides a particular definition to an act of self-inflicted violence. Such discrepancies of definition often get fore-grounded in the discourses regarding perceived righteousness of a particular act by a group contrasted with the opposite group ostracizing the same act as undesirable or harmful. Simple examples might be given of the Japanese 'Kamikaze pilots' during World War II who rammed their explosive-laden airplanes into the enemy ships and of the Viet-minh 'death volunteers' post World War II who blew up enemy tanks using long stick-like explosives-thereby causing huge damage to the enemy, though losing one's own life in the act. In recent times, the suicide bombers of the Western world see themselves as martyrs for the cause of their nations or communities. Similarly, the contemporary debate about permissibility of euthanasia or 'mercy killing' highlights the difference of perspective in considering the act as an act of compassion or of cruelty. Further it highlights the moral dilemma involved in accepting the absolute right an individual has over his or her life, and death. Such a difference of perspective or philosophical stance is trans-lated in the legislation formulated by different countries regarding euthanasia.

Society's perspective on suicide is often influenced by and shaped through its specific socio-historic circumstances, its value system, its religious beliefs and per-ceptions about the meaning of human life. The self-sacrifice of wives on the death pyre of the husband (*Sati*) or the customary mass suicides embraced by wives of *Rajput* warriors when their husbands were out fighting their last battle (*Johar*) are such practices that were prescribed by religious dogma and customs in India in the Middle Ages. Alvarez (1971) mentions acts of suicide being viewed in a positive manner in the warrior society of the Vikings, which believed a violent death to be a mandatory prerequisite for attaining heaven. Ancient Greeks, on the other hand, abhorred suicide and viewed suicidal behaviour negatively in general. Though Plato allowed for some exceptional circumstances that could make sui-cide morally acceptable, the general opinion of thinkers and larger society was alike in condemning suicide by terming it as a cowardly act, and an act that deprives the state of a citizen. Alvarez (1971, p. 58) links the extreme abhorrence of the ancient Greeks to suicide to their 'more profound horror of killing one's own kin. By inference, suicide was an extreme case of this, and the language barely distinguishes between self-murder and murder of kindred.' Though the specific views and beliefs regarding suicide in these earlier ages hardly have a bearing on the current practices and theoretical stances, these serve well to highlight the need to keep the specific socio-historical milieu of a society in focus while prescribing appropriate ways of dealing with suicidal behaviours.

Any ethical guideline or a legal code that deals with the complex issues of suicide and suicide prevention needs to be cognizant and reflective of the prevalent cultural-moral value systems of the society. Leenars and colleagues (2000) provide a detailed discussion about the multiplicity and variation prevalent in ethical and legal standards prevailing in different cultures regarding issues pertaining to suicide. While recognizing that a comprehensive review of multifarious issues involved is a difficult task, they nonetheless provide a broad discussion about the ethical and legal issues involved in suicide and attempted suicide, euthanasia and assisted suicide, standards of reasonable and prudent care, responsibility for care, failure in care, liability and malpractice across a number of countries and cultures. They emphasize, 'ethical and legal standards are defined according, first, to the standards of community practices, and second, to the resources available and hence what can reasonably be expected' (p. 434). Though it is difficult to provide an inclusive code for care of suicidal individuals, a global guideline could be drawn up based upon the basic principles of ethical practice in counselling.

The profession of counselling is well regulated by professional organizations in most countries. In their attempt to ensure ethical professional practice these professional bodies enact and endorse ethical guidelines and norms, yet mere awareness of ethical standards is neither sufficient nor adequate to answer the ethical dilemmas that arise while dealing with clients (Bond, 2000). A counsellor needs to develop a deep-rooted understanding of the cultural ethos and general ethical parameters of the society, and use these in designing the specific pathways tailored to the needs of individual client.

Suicide, being the commonest psychiatric emergency, the role of a support professional or a counsellor begins with accurate estimation of suicide risk and adopting an appropriate management strategy based on the level of risk. Given the commitment of their profession to human well-being, a counsellor must have a deep and unwavering belief in the sanctity of human life that enables her to put all her efforts towards its preservation and enrichment. In a way a counsellor must be driven by the universal moral imperative of reducing suicidal risk. Yet, in practice two core considerations remain – the moral status of suicide and the morality of intervening to prevent suicide. The central question arising out of this dilemma is of reconciling the premise of sanctity of human life with the right of the individual over his or her own life.

The moral status of suicide

Through the ages philosophers have deliberated upon many dilemmas regarding the act of taking one's own life. These deliberations have involved core questions regarding morality and rationality of suicide. Kagan (2007) distinguishes between the two, first, if suicide could ever be considered as a rational act and under what circumstances (the rationality question); and, second, if suicide could be construed as a morally legitimate or a morally acceptable thing to do, and under what circumstances (the morality question). There are varied opinions and analyses of the issue, however, generally all thinkers have been opposed to grant any sanctity to suicide on moral grounds. The arguments given for this range from theologically based doctrine of all life belonging to God, to the egalitarian argument of sanctity of human life and dignity. A related argument is often raised, asking if the human life is intrinsically valuable. Is life itself worth having? Kagan (2007) talks about a range of propositions he terms as 'container theories' – neutral container, valuable container or fantastic container, which draw the simile of human life to a container. According to the neutral container theories, when evaluating the worth of somebody's life one needs to look only at the contents of life – life itself is only a container that might hold good or bad content. Valuable container theories propose that the very fact that somebody is alive is valuable. It adds positive value to the balance of good and bad happenings or contents in one's life. Going further along the continuum, the fantastic container theories propagate that the fact of being alive is so valuable as to be worthwhile in itself even when the sum total of good and bad happening in one's life end up on the negative side. Accepting life as a 'valuable container' implies acceptance of a total sanctity for life, without taking into consideration whether the actual living conditions are facilitative of living. On the other hand, conceptualizing life as a 'neutral container' entails that life is only as good as its contents, or the individual's satisfaction or dissatisfaction with the life conditions. It has been a matter of perpetual contemplation and deliberation for thinkers across the ages what it actually means to live. Is life merely constituted of biological existence or has it a deeper meaning? For example, when a person feels grateful for 'merely being alive', does she actually mean so, or does she presume the presence of certain conditions and factors that enrich her life and well-being?

The meaning of life: a psychological perspective

'What does it mean to be alive?' 'What makes life valuable and worth living?' These and many such questions pertaining to the essence of life have always intrigued the thinkers and philosophers of Eastern and Western societies alike. Explanations range from theological doctrines to modern-day biological and evolutionary explications. In modern times 'meaning in life' has been an important construct for the psychologists too, though they frame the question in a slightly different manner by asking 'When and how does one experience a sense of fulfilment and well-being in life?' or 'What does it take to ensure one's subjective well-being?'

There are variety of definitions and varied paths to achieve meaning in life. The main components that can be discerned from these definitions are: a sense of coherence in one's life (Battista and Almond, 1973; Reker and Wong, 1988); goal directedness or purposefulness (Ryff and Singer, 1998); or sense of commitment (Thompson and Janigian, 1988). Wong (1998) emphasizes that an individual derives sense of meaning in life by appraising oneself in the socio-cultural context (cognitive component), that in turn provides one with satisfaction and fulfilment (affective component), and motivates one to strive for valuable goals (motivational component). As Frankl (1965) says, since there cannot be any universal meaning of life to fit all, it is a subjective and individual pursuit for the individual to cultivate meaning in life. Frankl (1963) argues that humans are driven by an innate need to find meaning in life ('will to meaning') and a situation of existential vacuum, which could arise as a result of a sense of complete emptiness and an absence of purpose for continuing to live, leads to 'loss of meaning' (Frankl, 1967). Such experiences of loss have been found to trigger feelings of despair, chronic anxiety, depression, addictions and also suicidal behaviours (Debats *et al.*, 1993; Harlow *et al.*, 1986). On the other hand, having more meaning in life has been found to correlate with happiness and well-being (Chamberlain and Zika, 1988; Debats *et al.*, 1993).

Meaning in life has especially been an important construct in the field of humanistic psychology and in the recent years in positive psychology. Humanistic psychology began as a movement in the late 1950s and the early 1960s against the deterministic and negative view of individual life and psyche. Humanists restored the agency and dignity of individuals by emphasizing that the individual be seen and analysed holistically, and be acknowledged as a worthwhile person beyond genetic or environmental endowments. With Abraham Maslow and Carl Rogers as helm bearers, the humanists emphasized that individuals' behaviour is determined by their subjective perceptions and personal meanings they attribute to these; and that each individual is intrinsically motivated to strive and fulfil their inherent potential. Despite the early differences that positive psychology had with the humanist movement, and despite standing on different epistemological and methodological ground, the fundamental propositions made by the positive psychol-ogy movement apparently match seamlessly with its predecessor (Schneider, 2011). The positive psychology movement was initiated by Seligman and Csikszentmihalyi (2000), with a proclamation 'psychology of positive human functioning will arise that achieves a scientific understanding and effective inter-ventions to build thriving in individuals, families, and communities' (p. 5), with a focus on recognizing and building upon the inherent potentialities of the individuals in order to help them attain happiness, fulfilment and well-being. They conceptualized positive psychology initiatives resting on three conceptual foundations: positive subjective experiences, positive traits and positive environ-ment. Apparently, both humanistic and positive approaches delve into the issue of meaning of human life beyond the hedonistic conceptualizations of pleasure-pain, and endorse the eudemonic constructions that emphasize personal growth and cultivation of psychological strengths as the path to attain fulfilment and well-being.

Humanistic perspectives have made a vast impact not only on the discipline of psychology, but on the wider culture and society too. One of the seeds sown by the movement has led to the foundation of the profession of counselling and shaped the contours of client-centred approaches by recognizing the all-important role of 'self' in alleviating distress and instilling a drive towards fulfilment and actualization of potentials. In a way, the humanistic approach has influenced the research and practice of psychology by providing a unique per-spective to human life that informs and enlightens the path of psychology professionals. Both positive and humanist approaches look beyond the medical model of psychology and emphasize efficiencies over deficiencies. A therapist or counsellor hence does not merely aim at mitigating crisis, but seeks to build a supportive environment where the individual feels free to share his/her lived experiences, and through empathetic listening nurtures and strengthens the positive potentials lying dormant within the individual. Such a conceptual and theoretical grounding leads to easy enunciation of an ethical framework for professionals supporting individuals in distress.

Ethical issues in providing support services to suicidal individuals

Etymologically, the term ethic derives from the Greek 'ethos', meaning habits or customs. However, ethics have come to connote something more than mere habits or customs. Ethics are those standards of behaviour that a group or society prescribes for its members and expects them to adhere to these in a normative manner. In setting the normative standard of behaviour, the ethics prescribed by a group, organization or society set an evaluative norm that actively discriminates the desirable from undesirable and offers value-based judgements on the accept-ability of behaviour. Leong *et al.* (2008) define ethics as 'the agreed upon stand-ards of aspirational and mandatory behaviours and practices' (p. 182). Ethics set an aspirational standard of behaviour in a manner that distinguishes the *malum in se* (bad in itself) from *malum prohibitum* (wrong only because law prohibits it). This implies an ethical code subsumes any legal codes on a given issue, and demands a moral virtue of compliance even in the absence of fear of being reprimanded. The key attribute that place ethics on a higher level than the law is the freedom of choice – choice that one makes in adhering to good and refraining from bad even in the absence of a binding authority.

Being able to distinguish the good from bad on one's own volition and deciding an appropriate course of action, thus appears to be the core competence any support professional must strive to inculcate, in order to deal with the individuals facing a crisis, including suicidal behaviours. This is not an easy task to accomplish, as there cannot be a straightforward prescription of dos and don'ts. A support professional needs to actively listen to the individual in crisis, infer the hidden meanings, assess the issue at hand and design an intervention strategy to ensure optimum welfare of the person.

Fisher (2009) describes the general principles that form the basis for constituting the ethical standards in the profession of counselling. Though these are general ethical principles for the helping professionals, these set an aspirational standard that they must strive to achieve in order to fulfil the professional goals of welfare and beneficence.

The first principle, that of *Beneficence and Non-maleficence* reiterates the need to maintain a balance between the dual roles played by a psychologist or support professional while providing support services to a distressed client – providing benefits in the best interest of the client, at the same time avoiding harm to the client. Beneficence implies a duty to improve the conditions of others through the use of one's professional knowledge and wisdom. A support professional benefits a client by structuring all intervention keeping the client's welfare as primacy. The clause of 'non-maleficence' puts the onus on the support professional to avoid or minimize any harm to the client. Originating from the Hippocratic Oath, the principle of non-maleficence calls for avoiding all acts that can potentially harm the client, and directs to minimizing the effects in case any harm has been caused inadvertently or under unavoidable circumstances.

The second ethical principle concerns with *Fidelity and responsibility*. Fidelity implies faithfulness of one human being to another (Ramsey, 2002). This includes keeping one's words, discharge and acceptance of responsibilities and maintenance of relationships including scientific, professional and teaching relationships. A support professional must realize the importance of providing intervention to individuals in crisis and the responsibility it entails. In keeping with the sanctity of such a role, they need to adhere to a high standard of professional competence and ethical fidelity in their work. Gardener (2012) enumerates the ethical behaviours that mark the principle of fidelity for the professionals working for suicide prevention. These are: (a) the responsibility to keep promises and contracts; (b) to perform duties in a responsible manner and avoid actions that violate the ethical standards; (c) being trained in current methods of treating suicide ideation and behaviours; (d) not being silent when it comes to the safety of the client; (e) not using deceptive practices or encouraging deception in others; and (f) maintaining confidentiality and allowing the client to know when confidentiality is not possible and/or what the limits might be. The principle of fidelity serves the crucial function of cultivating a trusting relationship between the distressed individual and the support professional that facilitates a comprehensive exploration of suicidality.

The third ethical principle, closely related to fidelity is of maintaining absolute *Integrity*. Integrity implies honest communication, telling facts as it is to the client and also keep the commitments made to the clients.

The fourth principle concerns ensuring equitable *Justice* to all clients. This means that the counsellor is obliged to treat all individuals with care and consistency, not discriminating on the basis of socio-economic status, role or religion, and to guard against his/her own inadvertent prejudices in providing care to the clients. This also implies that the policies, procedures and norms for providing care to suicidal individuals must provide a consistent method of identification and treatment.

The fifth principle of ethical conduct put forth by Fisher is about ensuring *Respect for People's Rights and Dignity*. This implies being aware of cultural sensitivities of the client and respecting the race, ethnicity and religion of the client. The counsellor needs to be competent enough to understand the choices made by the client and the limits placed by such subjectivities. An ethical mandate for ensuring the right and dignity of the distressed individual makes it essential for the counsellor to determine what and how much of personal information is essential to be shared for the purpose of therapy (Fisher, 2009).

Beauchamp and Childress (1979) and Gardener (2012) add another important dimension to the ethical considerations – that of the autonomy of the client to make decisions regarding health options, and right of self-determination in order to preserve one's dignity.

This places an obligation on the counsellor or the support professional to provide all the relevant information to the client in order to help her make an informed decision regarding various issues, like consent for disclosing information, consent for receiving medication, consent for referral or hospitalization and any other issue concerning her welfare. Explicating the principle of autonomy of the client, Gardener (2012) emphasizes that among all other information the counsellor must include and explain to the client the 'information regarding suicide and how it is a choice resulting from a psychological breakdown of defences and increased vulnerability' (p. 28).

This gets one back to the core dilemma in the case of suicidal individuals – the dilemma between providing autonomy to the client on one hand and commitment for ensuring beneficence of the client on the other. The premise on which autonomous decision-making by the client rests is informed consent. However, the circumstances and psychological conditions leading a person towards suicidal behaviours also limit the repertoire of choices available to the person to make autonomous informed decisions. Simply put, mental illness or psychological distress often compromise informed consent. Given the ethical guideline of beneficence and non-maleficence, it might be even simpler to assume the role of a paternalistic protector of the client's life from the damage that he/she can cause to him/herself. However, as Gardener (2012) asserts, the resolution of the dilemma between autonomy and beneficence lies in structuring the support in a manner that it works to restore autonomy in a positive manner and strengthens the resources of the person in order to improve coping. It might be asserted that in many cases it is escaping from a painful situation, and not death *per se*, that pushes the suicidal individual towards taking the fatal step. It is not impossible to dissuade the suicidal person from ending one's own life, if the support professional succeeds in helping him visualize the possibility of other solutions, thereby alleviating helplessness.

Another core issue of practical concern that emerges when dealing with suicidal individuals is of the dilemma between commitment to maintain confidentiality and minimize harm to the client. Relying on the trust built in a therapeutic relationship the distressed individual might reveal a history or probability of suicidal behaviours, and the counsellor might be left with making the difficult decision of sharing the information with the family of the client or honouring the confidentiality code and keeping mum. Dilemma deepens when there is a legal obligation to share information with appropriate agencies, or when the law of the land views suicide as a culpable act or even as a punishable crime. These are difficult situations and there cannot be any straightforward answers, however, with an in-depth understanding of the case and an unshaken commitment to ethical behaviour, the counsellor needs to figure out the solution.

Resolving the legal issues

There is a wide variation across nations and cultures in the manner the act of suicide is viewed from the legal perspective. While most Western countries have decriminalized the act, many nations of the Global South continue to penalize suicide attempters. Notwithstanding the age-old cultural taboos and prohibitions that continue to impact societal views about suicide, it is quite ironic that a distressed individual who attempts to extinguish one's own life, presumably due to extreme hopelessness and despair, is viewed as a criminal by the society and its legal system, and put behind the bars, instead of being provided care and support. It is ironic too that criminalization of the act and fear of punishment fail to deter the suicidal individuals from attempting the act. There are five widely accepted purposes that criminal legislation purports to achieve through prescribing punishments, these are: retribution, deterrence, incapacitation, rehabilitation and restoration. In criminalizing suicide and prescribing a punishment for attempting the act, the law attempts (and usually fails) to coercively attain only two of these five purposes, those of deterrence and rehabilitation. Apparently, a legal code that criminalizes suicide views it as deadly violence against the self and not as a mental health issue, meriting any supportive intervention for deterrence. It has been proposed that the law of the land is reflective of the general ethos of society, and keeps evolving as a result of historical forces, scientific-medical evidence, and political change. The wider ethos is usually shaped by the ruling or dominant classes of the society that determine whether a particular act or behaviour be considered harmful and criminalized. Given the influence of historical forces and socio-cultural circumstances, the act of suicide has been proscribed or prescribed under varying circumstances and in varied contexts. In certain circumstances intentional behaviour leading to extinguishing of one's life is even termed differently and eulogized as 'self-sacrifice', 'martyrdom', or a moral duty towards one's religion, society, or nation. The issue of societal and legal prescriptions regarding suicidal behaviours also brings into focus the philosophical debates regarding individual autonomy, free will and right over one's own life. Indian law on suicide and the way it has been interpreted by the highest court of law of the nation provide an interesting case for discussing the issues of sanctity of life and right to live juxtaposed with the right to die.

Suicide legislation: the case of India

India continues to be one of the few nations that criminalize the self-harm behaviours. Though suicide is not listed as a crime, the legal provisions in India make attempted suicide an offence punishable under Indian Penal Code. The relevant section reads thus: 'Whoever attempts to commit suicide and does any act towards the commission of such offence shall be punished with simple imprisonment for a term which may extend to one year or with fine, or with both.' This legal provision has been contrasted with the overriding constitutional provision of 'Right to life' (Article 21 of the Constitution of India) that guarantees the right to life as a fundamental right to all the citizens. Article 21 of the Constitution provides for protection of life and personal liberty and reads thus: 'No person shall be deprived of his life or personal liberty except according to procedure established by law.'

The Right to life as enshrined in the Constitution has been interpreted liberally in many landmark cases by the Supreme Court of India and has led to the conceptualization of life as definitely meaning much more than mere biological existence or survival. Various rights have been held to be covered by Article 21; such as right to go abroad, right to privacy, right against solitary confinement, right to speedy trial, right to shelter, right to breathe in an unpolluted environment, right to medical aid, right to education, etc. (*Maneka Gandhi v. Union of India*, AIR 1978 SC 597). At a particular juncture it has also been interpreted by the apex court that the right to live brings in its trail the right not to live a forced life (*P. Rathinam v. Union of India*, AIR 1994 SC 1844), and accordingly the act of suicide stands decriminalized. However, further deliberations in another case (*Gian Kaur v. State of Punjab*, AIR 1996 SC 946) have led the apex court to lay down the position that the 'Right to life' cannot be construed to include within it the 'right to die'. Explaining the fundamental opposition of death with life the apex court observed that right to life includes right to live in a dignified manner, though not a right to end one's life.

As to date India remains one of the very few nations that criminalize suicide. The Law Commission of India tasked with a periodic review of the legislative laws makes a recommendation in its report (2008) of decriminalizing suicide by repealing the relevant section (Sec. 309 Indian Penal Code) of the criminal law. In their report they enumerate the difficulties that arise in preventing suicide merely because it is a criminal act. Quoting from the report:

> Emergency treatment for those who have attempted suicide is not readily accessible as they are referred by local hospitals and doctors to tertiary centers as it is termed as Medico Legal case. The time lost in the golden hour will save many lives. Those who attempt suicide are already distressed and in psychological pain and for them to face the ignominy of police interrogation causes increased distress, shame, guilt and further suicide attempt. At the time of family turmoil dealing with police procedure adds to the woes of the family. It also leads to a gross under-reporting of attempted suicide and the magnitude of the problem is not unknown. Unless one is aware of the nature of extent of the problem, effective intervention is not possible. As many attempted suicides are categorized in the guise of accidental poisoning etc. emotional and mental health support is not available to those who have attempted as they are unable to access the services.
>
> (pp. 34–35)

Concluding comments

Suicide is an individual act, yet the antecedents and consequences of the act concern the entire society. Beginning with socializing the individual in a particular manner, making one accept and internalize the social mores and values in general and the value of a human life specifically, the society structures the individual in all aspects. Going beyond viewing suicide merely as a mental health issue, the role societal values and cultural prescriptions can play in its prevention becomes evident. A culture tolerant of suicidal behaviour, a society normalizing a particular form of suicidal behaviour, or a religious dogma eulogizing specific forms of suicide provide a potent ground for suicidal behaviours. Further, a legal framework that attempts to prevent suicide through criminalizing the act, thereby squarely holding the individual responsible for the wrong done, summarily absolves the society of any responsibility for creating and providing minimum conditions that make a dignified existence possible for the individual.

A support professional working for suicide prevention has to trudge through this minefield in the course of his/her daily work. The task of alleviating distress might prove to be immensely rewarding, but at the same time immensely challenging. Despite the availability of elaborate professional guidelines and legal advisories the counsellor needs to consider each situation on its own merit, giving due credit to its specificities and an empathetic understanding of the needs of the client. A multi-dimensional perspective along with professional competence are the handy tools a counsellor must rely upon in order to enable ethical decision-making.

At the group level, a body of professionals working for suicide prevention and mitigation needs to articulate the ethical stance relied upon and work to bring in positive interventions not only for the distressed individuals, but also at the societal level, striving to make the social environment suited for a fulfilling and thriving human existence.

References

Alvarez, A. (1971). *The Savage God*. New York. Random House.

Battista, J. and Almond, R. (1973). The development of meaning in life. *Psychiatry*, 36(4), 409–427.

Beauchamp, T., and Childress, J. (1979), *Principles of Biomedical Ethics*, New York: Oxford University Press.

Bond, T. (2000). *Standards and Ethics for Counseling in Action*, 2nd edn. London: Sage.

Chamberlain, K., and Zika, S. (1988). Measuring meaning in life: An examination of three scales. *Personality and Individual Differences*, 9(3), 589–596.

Debats, D. L., van der Lubbe, P. M., and Wezeman, F. R. A. (1993). On the psychometric properties of the Life Regard Index (LRI): A measure of meaningful life. *Personality and Individual Differences*, 14(2), 337–345.

Fisher, C. B. (2009). *Decoding the Ethics Code: A Practical Guide for Psychologists*. Thousand Oaks, CA: Sage.

Frankl, V. E. (1963). *Man's Search for Meaning: An Introduction to Logotherapy*. New York: Washington Square Press.

Frankl, V. E. (1965). *The Doctor and the Soul: From Psychotherapy to Logotherapy*. New York: Vintage Books.

Frankl, V. E. (1967). *Psychotherapy and Existentialism: Selected Papers on Logotherapy*. New York: Simon and Schuster.

Gardener, G. (2012). Ethical considerations for suicide prevention. Show me you care about suicide prevention conference. Retrieved from http://media. mimhtraining.com/slides/suicideconf2012/Ethical%20Consideration%20 for%20 Suicide%20Prevention%20for%20Show%20Me%20You%20Care%20Conf% 20Truman%209-14-12.pdf.

Harlow, L. L., Newcomb, M. D., and Bentler, P. M. (1986). Depression, self-derogation, substance use, and suicide ideation: Lack of purpose in life as a mediational factor. *Journal of Clinical Psychology*, 42(1), 5–21.

Kagan, S. (2007). Death (Yale University: Open Yale Courses), Retrieved from http://oyc.yale.edu. License: Creative Commons BY-NC-SA.

Leenars, A., Cantor, C. H., Connolly, J., EchoHawk, M., Gailiene, D., He, Z. X., *et al.* (2000). Ethical and legal issues. In K. Hawton and K. van Heeringen (Eds), *The International Handbook of Suicide and Attempted Suicide* (pp. 421–435). Chichester: John Wiley and Sons Ltd.

Leong, F. T. L., Altmaier, E. M., and Johnson, B. D. (2008). *Encyclopaedia of Counseling*, Vol. 1. Thousand Oaks, CA: Sage.

Ramsey, P. (2002). *The Patient as Person: Explorations in Medical Ethics* (2nd edn). New Haven, CT: Yale University Press.

Reker, G. T. and Wong. P. T. P. (1988). Aging as an individual process: Toward a theory of personal meaning. In J. E. Birren and V. L. Bengston (Eds), *Emergent Theories of Aging* (pp. 214–246). New York: Springer.

Report of the Law Commission of India (2008). *Humanization and Decriminalization of Attempt to Suicide*. Report No. 210. Government of India. Retrieved from http://lawcommissionofindia.nic.in/reports/report210.pdf.

Retterstøl, N. (1993). *Suicide: A European Perspective*. Cambridge: Cambridge University Press.

Ryff, C. D., and Singer, B. (1998). The contours of positive human health. *Psychological Inquiry*, 9(1), 1–28.

Schneider, K. J. (2011). Toward a humanistic positive psychology: Why can't we just get along? *Existential Analysis*, 22(1), 32–38.

Seligman, M. and Csikszentmihalyi, M. (2000). Positive psychology: An introduction. *American Psychologist*, 55(1), 5–14.

Thompson, S. C. and Janigian, A. S. (1988). Life schemes: A framework for understanding the search for meaning. *Journal of Social and Clinical Psychology*, 7(2–3), 260–280.

Wong, P. T. (1998). Spirituality, meaning and successful aging. In P. T. Wong and S. F. Prem (Eds), *The Human Quest for Meaning: A Handbook of Psychological Research and Clinical Applications* (pp. 395–435). Mahwah, NJ: Lawrence Erlbaum Associates.

Index

Milton Keynes UK
Ingram Content Group UK Ltd.
UKHW031146141024
449569UK00024B/1026